Sleep and Psychosomatic Medicine

Sleep and Psychosomatic Medicine

Edited by

SR Pandi-Perumal MSc
Comprehensive Center for Sleep Medicine
Mount Sinai School of Medicine
New York, NY
USA

Rocco R Ruoti MD
Associate Director of the Psychiatric Consultation and Liaison Service
Maimonides Medical Center
Brooklyn, NY
USA

Milton Kramer MD
Director of Psychiatric Research
Maimonides Medical Center
Brooklyn, NY
USA

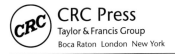

CRC Press
Taylor & Francis Group
Boca Raton London New York

CRC Press is an imprint of the
Taylor & Francis Group, an **informa** business

CRC Press
Taylor & Francis Group
6000 Broken Sound Parkway NW, Suite 300
Boca Raton, FL 33487-2742

© 2007 by Taylor & Francis Group, LLC
CRC Press is an imprint of Taylor & Francis Group, an Informa business

No claim to original U.S. Government works

ISBN-13: 978-0-415-39499-4 (hbk)

Cover

The schematic brain drawing in the *background* shows key components of the ascending arousal system originating from a series of cell groups in the brain stem (from Saper CB, Scammell TE, Lu J. Hypothalamic regulation of sleep and circadian rhythms. Nature 2005; 437: 1257–63).

The eight brain images on the *left side* of the cover show regions with significant declines in relative metabolism from waking to non-rapid eye movement (NREM) sleep in healthy people (from Nofzinger EA, Buysse DJ, Germain A, et al. Alterations in regional cerebral glucose metabolism across waking and non-rapid eye movement sleep in depression. Arch Gen Psychiatry 2005; 62: 387–96).

The six brain images on the *right side* show waking to rapid eye movement sleep activations in healthy subjects (column 1) and depressed subjects (column 2), and interactions showing regions where depressed subjects' waking to rapid eye movement activations are greater than those of healthy subjects (column 3) (from Nofzinger EA, Buysse DJ, Germain A, et al. Increased activation of anterior paralimbic and executive cortex from waking to rapid eye movement sleep in depression. Arch Gen Psychiatry 2004; 61: 695–702).

Dedication

To our wives and families,
Who are the reasons for any of our accomplishments
Who have taught and aided us
In much of what we know and do!

Contents

Contributors

David M Biondi DO
Harvard Medical School
Boston, MA
USA

Karl Heinz Brisch MD
Pediatric Psychosomatic Medicine and
  Psychotherapy
Dr von Hauner Children's Hospital
Ludwig-Maximilians University
Munich
Germany

Blynn G Bunney PhD
Brain Imaging Center
University of California
Irvine, CA
USA

Chien-Lin Chen MD
Buddhist Tzu Chi Hospital and
  Medical School
Hulien
Taiwan

C Robert Cloninger MD
Sansone Family Center for Well-Being
Washington University School of Medicine
St Louis, MO
USA

Ming Ding PhD
Department of Pharmacology
Southern Illinois University School
  of Medicine Springfield, IL
USA

Jacob L Gordon MD MS
Wayne State University School of Medicine
  and John D Dingell Veterans
  Affairs Medical Center
Detroit, MI
USA

M Goswami MPH PhD
Narcolepsy Institute
Montefiore Medical Center
  and Albert Einstein College
  of Medicine
Bronx, NY
USA

Max Hirshkowitz PhD
Michael E. DeBakey Veterans Affairs Medical
  Center Sleep Center and
  Baylor College of Medicine
Houston, TX
USA

Samuel J Huber MD
Washington University School of Medicine
St Louis, MO
USA

Sheldon Kapen MD
Chief, Neurology Section
Wayne State University School of Medicine
  and Veterans Administration Medical Center
Detroit, MI
USA

Matcheri S Keshavan MD FRCPC MRCPsych
Wayne State University School of Medicine
Detroit, MI
USA

Milton Kramer MD
Director of Psychiatric Research
Maimonides Medical Center
Brooklyn, NY
USA

Vahid Mohsenin MD
Yale Center for Sleep Medicine
Yale University School of Medicine
New Haven, CT
USA

Christoph Nissen MD
Western Psychiatric Institute and Clinic
University of Pittsburgh School of Medicine
Pittsburgh, PA
USA

Eric A Nofzinger MD
Western Psychiatric Institute and Clinic
University of Pittsburgh School
 of Medicine
Pittsburgh, PA
USA

Zvjezdan Nuhic MD
Maimonides Medical Center
Brooklyn, NY
USA

William C Orr PhD
Lynn Health Science Institute
Oklahoma University Health
  Sciences Center
Oklahoma City, OK
USA

JF Pagel MD
University of Colorado School of Medicine
Sleep Disorders Center of Colorado
Pueblo, CO and
  Sleepworks
Colorado Springs, CO
USA

SR Pandi-Perumal MSc
Comprehensive Center for Sleep Medicine
Mount Sinai School of Medicine
New York, NY
USA

Donald B Penzien PhD
University of Mississippi Medical Center
Jackson, MS
USA

J Steven Poceta MD
Scripps Clinic Sleep Center
Scripps Clinic
La Jolla, CA
USA

Steven G Potkin MD
Brain Imaging Center
School of Medicine
University of California
Irvine, CA
USA

Jeanetta C Rains PhD
Clinical Director, Center for Sleep Evaluation
  at Elliot Hospital
Manchester, NH
USA

Vadim Rotenberg MD PhD DSC
Tel-Aviv University
Bat-Yam
Israel

Neomi Shah MD
Yale Center for Sleep Medicine
Yale University School of Medicine
New Haven, CT
USA

Amir Sharafkhaneh MD PhD
Michael E DeBakey Veterans
  Affairs Medical Center and
  Baylor College of Medicine
Houston, TX
USA

Arthur J Spielman PhD
Sleep Disorders Center
The City College of the
  City University of New York
New York, NY
USA

Deborah Suchecki PhD
Department of Psychobiology
Federal University of Sao Paulo
Sao Paulo
Brazil

Paula A Tiba MSc
Department of Psychobiology
Federal University of Sao Paulo
Sao Paulo
Brazil

Linda A Toth DVM PhD
Southern Illinois University School of Medicine
Springfield, IL
USA

Rita A Trammell PhD
Department of Internal Medicine
Southern Illinois University School of Medicine
Springfield, IL
USA

Sergio Tufik MD PhD
Department of Psychobiology
Federal University of Sao Paulo
Sao Paulo
Brazil

Daniel J Wallace MD
Clinical Professor of Medicine
Cedars–Sinai Medical Center
David Geffen School of Medicine at UCLA
USA

Joseph C Wu MD
Brain Imaging Center
School of Medicine
  University of California
Irvine, CA
USA

Chien-Ming Yang PhD
National Cheng-Chi University
Taipei
Taiwan

Foreword

I would like to dedicate this foreword to Dr Leonid Kayumov who recently committed suicide. Dr Kayumov had made valuable contributions to this field but in a situation of considerable stress developed a psychosomatic illness and depression. We (his colleagues) who knew his abilities mourn his death.

A recent Australian study entitled 'Factors Predicting Sleep Disruption in Type II Diabetes'[1] opens with the statement 'a rapidly growing body of evidence suggests that sleep complaints are particularly common in patients with medical illness' and cites a study I coauthored.[2] This growing awareness of the inter-relationship between sleep, psychiatry and medical illnesses is at the core of this book. The surge in interest in the relationship between sleep and psychosomatic illness is attested to by the number of articles in three key psychosomatic journals. In the last five years there have been 77 publications in the Journal of Psychosomatic Medicine specifically referencing sleep in the title. In Psychosomatics the number is 12, in the same period in the Journal of Psychosomatic Research (perhaps because of a favorable bias by the editor) the number of sleep related papers has been 175. Of course, the publication of articles that report on the interface between sleep issues and general medicine is not restricted to these

journals and probably the vast majority of papers are either published in specialty journals or in general sleep journals. An example of this would be the subject of obesity, diabetes and the relationship of these issues to sleep and sleep disruption are predominantly in the 'diabetes literature'[3–5] rather than in the psychosomatic literature.

With the explosion of interest in sleep and the rapid broadening of the scope of the discipline of sleep, it would be almost impossible for a book entitled 'Sleep and Psychosomatic Medicine' to be comprehensive. However, this volume certainly provides a broad sweep of many of the major topics that are relevant for the clinician and theoreticians dealing with the sleep–psychosomatic interface.

The timely and taut chapter on 'Infection and Sleep' states in the conclusion 'Infectious disease and sleep appear to exert bi-directional influences on each other via effect on the immune system'. This observation by leaders in the field is notable in that the first part of that statement could be applied to many psychosomatic related issues. The issue of obesity and sleep has received much attention lately and there is clearly a bi-directional impact. The notion that cardiovascular health might influence sleep and sleep may influence cardio-vascular health is gaining momentum[6] and there are many other areas where the same might be said to apply. For example, Boethel[7] states 'it now appears that in addition to causing daytime drowsiness, cardio-vascular disease, mood and memory disturbances, impotence and car wrecks, obstructive sleep apnea also promotes insulin resistance'. This observation clearly marks a broadening of the understanding of the role of sleep in psychosomatic disorders. In a delightfully worded introduction Rains et al with a multicentered authored chapter entitled 'Sleep and Headache Disorders' point to some early observations by Wright in 1871[8] that recognized the role of sleep in 'both provoking and relieving headaches'. They go on to point out that the mechanisms are not well defined but that Paiva et al[9] has formulated the hypothetical associations that may occur between sleep and headache. The two important points that 'headache may be a cause as well as a consequence of sleep disorder or disturbance' and that 'the value of sleep regulation is a key component of head pain management for a substantial proportion of headache sufferers' are well worth noting.

The chapter on Stress and Sleep opens with three references by authors from three continents.[10–12] The personal relevance has been that I have published with each of these authors and it makes one appreciate that the theme of stress is central to much of what is published in the psychosomatic field and that it is a very international pursuit.

Hirshkowitz and Sharafkhaneh in their chapter on Sleep and Respiratory Disorders take a more medical than psychosomatic perspective. They do note the impact of nocturnal asthma in causing decreased sleep efficiency, increased awakenings during sleep, daytime tiredness and impaired cognitive functioning. The sections on asthma and chronic obstructive pulmonary disease are particularly helpful but the psychosomatic dimension is only cursorily mentioned. One of the intriguing aspects of nocturnal asthma (sleep related asthma) is that it was described in 1698 by Floyer[13] who wrote: 'I have omitted to mention this, that my fits never feize me but in the Night, and then awake me with

a heavinefs and fo grow worfe and worfe immediately. I am always moft eafy when I am Lac'd, and my fit goes frequently off on a fudden, fo as to be perfectly well in half an hours time' and was effectively rediscovered by Turner-Warwick in the mid 1970s[14] and with further advances in this field since.[15] The learning point being that physicians often deal with their patients during the day and patients with nocturnal asthma were not examined to allow their condition to be clearly identified. There is a literature on the lack of dream recall or awareness in patients with asthma [16,17] and the possible role of REM sleep in triggering nocturnal asthma attacks. The latter may lead to treatment interventions which have not been systematically explored.

The last comments are put into a context by the detailed review by Kramer and Nuhic on Dreaming in Psychiatric Patients which comes to the minimalistic conclusion that 'the mysteries of psychosis have not been revealed through the study of dreams' but that particularly in relation to depression and post traumatic stress there is a 'greater body of scientifically credible information about dreaming in a field that is fraught with lack of scientific rigor'.

In the laudable wide ranging chapter on psychosocial socio-economic and public health considerations in Narcolepsy, the authors provide some practical management approaches stating that along with medications prescribed by physicians, the psychosocial management of the impact of the clinical symptoms, diagnosis, and treatment needs to be provided by special counselors. Many psychiatrists and psychologists might view narcolepsy as a neurological disorder and at least twice in this chapter the authors make that statement. I in fact think that Narcolepsy is perhaps par excellence a psychosomatic disorder. There clearly is a genetic basis but in addition twin studies point to an environmental contribution and the role of stress as a triggering factor of narcolepsy is unfortunately omitted from this chapter. A similar claim could be made for Tourettes Syndrome which also has clear biological and psychological inputs but does not merit an independent chapter in this monograph.

The issue of alertness rather than sleepiness could have been a greater focus in the description of narcolepsy but there is perhaps still insufficient information dealing with this facet of narcolepsy in particular and in sleep related psychosomatic disorders in general.[18] The issue of driving which has implications for alertness and sleepiness is discussed and one anticipates will be an area of greater concern in the field of psychosomatic medicine in the future.[19]

The chapter on Sleep and Coronary Artery Disease takes a more purely medical perspective and no attempt at what might be viewed as the softer science of dream implications which have been documented in literature[20,21] is attempted. Unfortunately, a replication of the study by Smith[21] has not to the best of my knowledge been attempted. The authors of this chapter do however note the circadian variation in coronary deaths with differences in patients with and without sleep disorders.[22,23] The implications of sleep being a dangerous time[24] as well as a restorative time[25] needs to be grappled with both in the general medical sense and in the psychosomatic sense.

This seeming paradox is compounded by the observation in the chapter 'Sleep Deprivation as an Antidepressant' in which the phenomenon of sleep restriction has had beneficial effects in terms of change in mood whereas for most patients who are not depressed, the loss of sleep clearly leads to an increased likelihood of depression.

In focusing on the interrelationship between sleep and gastrointestinal functioning Chen et al very usefully provide the physiological changes in sleep which have clinical consequences and practical treatment interventions that arise from this knowledge. This chapter is peppered with useful insights and references, for example to the observation that sedating drugs such as benzodiazepines and alcohol prolong acid clearance during sleep[26,27] and so one could intuit that something that might be viewed as sleep promoting can in fact have an impact on the bowel and create a secondary cause

for sleep disruption. The authors delve into the more psychosomatic realm of Irritable Bowel Syndrome noting that many studies that observe sleep disruption in this population but also noting the contradictory nature of the findings. The insightful synthesis that these authors come to is that 'there are central nervous system alterations in patients with functional bowel disorders and that these alterations are perhaps uniquely identified during sleep'. Our own research has shown that patients with dyspepsia have more sleep difficulties and greater daytime fatigue.[28]

The review on sleep and neurological disorders unfortunately notes at the beginning that for reasons of space it is limited to discussing three topics, Parkinsons, stroke and traumatic brain injury but there is nary a mention of the psychosomatic aspects of these disorders. The topic is potentially too broad to be comprehensively reviewed and even in this limitation key papers of note e.g.[29–31] are omitted. This notwithstanding the chapter provides a useful introduction to these areas.

The chapter on 'Sleep and Depression: A Functional Neuroimaging Perspective' by Nissen and Nofzinger provides an exciting sweep through current developments in Neuroimaging and how the information in this area might inform our understanding of both sleep and mood and the interaction between the two. This research has built on the studies in the 1970s and 1980s on regional change in cerebral blood flow (e.g.[32]) and the neuroimaging studies especially in the 1990s (e.g.[33]). The clarity of this chapter makes it accessible to all psychiatrists, not only those interested in psychosomatics and one anticipates will be much quoted. The breadth of the implications of the research these authors describe is emphasized in their final sentence, 'Eventually this approach may help to characterize brain processes and the clinical symptomatology in depression on an individual level, and may guide the development and individual application of therapy including medications, psychotherapy and other therapies'.

It is useful in a monograph such as this that there are a couple of chapters specifically devoted to treatments. The chapter on medication effects on sleep provides some useful tables although not everyone would agree with all the specifics cited in the tables and they are not referenced. It does however, give an overview. The content of the chapter has some notable omissions. For example, most would think that a small section on cataplexy should not only mention a single less used agent.

By contrast the review on Behavioral Interventions for Sleep Disorders by Yang is a tour-de-force which will act as a ready primer for most clinicians needing to get an overview of this area. The clear documentation of the five categories of dysfunctional cognitions about sleep into (a) misconceptions regarding the causes, (b) misattributions or amplifications of the consequences, (c) unrealistic sleep expectations, (d) diminished perception of control, and (e) predictability of sleep is helpful and pivotal in the therapy.[34]

The potential for group therapy as a treatment modality is underemphasized[35] and the perseveration of referring to 'sleep restriction therapy' when reference to it being more accurately described as 'bed restriction' has been made in the literature[36] is somewhat frustrating. The recognition of the role of behavioral interventions to facilitate compliance with treatment is an important issue in many psychosomatic disorders and this chapter gives due emphasis to this facet.

The chapter by Keshavan concerning sleep alterations in schizophrenia provides a balanced view of current knowledge and the potential of studies in this area. It does not have a heavy psychosomatic slant but is a useful complement to the chapter on neuroimaging in depression mentioned above.

This slightly lengthy foreword has attempted to give an overview of the unevenness of the information contained in this book on psychosomatic aspects of sleep. Clearly a field in its infancy and one can anticipate that it will develop rapidly. Ten years ago when a fellow of mine initiated a study on sleep patterns in cancer there was only a single small study in the literature. Currently there is an explosion of interest for both clinical and fundamental research reasons in this subject. The absence of a chapter

dealing with Nephrology or Obesity or Diabetes is notable but perhaps an indication that as the field develops and matures there will be a better synthesis and understanding of what the psychosomatic aspects of sleep disorders might reveal and the treatments that might be useful specifically at this interface between psychiatry, sleep and medicine. The editors are to be complimented for producing this first in the field.

Colin M Shapiro BSC(HON) MBBCH PHD MRCPSYCH FRCP(C)
Professor of Psychiatry and Ophthalmology

1. Lamond N, Tiggemann M, Dawson D. Factors predicting sleep disruption in type II diabetes. Sleep 2000; 23(3): 1–2.
2. Shapiro CM, Devins GM, Hussain MRG. Sleep problems in patients with medical illness. Br Med J 1993; 306: 1532–5.
3. Bjorkelund C, Bondyr-Carlsson D, Lapidus L, et al. Sleep disturbances in midlife unrelated to 32-year diabetes incidence: the prospective population study of women in Gothenburg. Diabetes Care 2005; 28(11): 2739–44.
4. Meyers L. Sleep apnea and diabetes. Diabetes Forecast 2005; 58(7): 32.
5. Bixler EO, Vgontzas AN, Lin HM, et al. Excessive daytime sleepiness in a general population sample: the role of sleep apnea, age, obesity, diabetes and depression. J Clin Endocrinol Metab 2005; 90(8): 4510–15.
6. Dhillon S, Chung SA, Fargher T, Huterer N, Shapiro CM. Sleep apnea, hypertension and the effects of CPAP. Am J Hypertens 2005; 18: 594–600.
7. Boethel CD. Sleep and the endocrine system: new associations to old diseases. Curr Opin Pulmonary Med 2002; 8: 502–5.
8. Wright H. Headaches: Their causes and their cures. Philadelphia, PA: Lindsay & Blakiston, 1871.
9. Paiva T, Batista A, Martins P, Martins A. The relationship between headaches and sleep disturbances. Headache 1995; 35(10): 590–6.
10. Holdstock TL, Verschoor GJ. Student sleep patterns before, during and after an examination period. South African J Psychol 1974; 4: 16–24.
11. Knowless J, Beaumaster E, MacLean A. The sleep of skydivers: a study of stress. In: Second International Sleep Research Congress, Edinburgh, 1975; 119.
12. Goncharenko AM, Schakhnarovich VM, Rotenberg VS. Changes of sleep at various types of reactions to an

emotional stress. Journal Visshey Nervnoy Deyatelnosti 1977; 27: 837 (in Russian).

13. Floyer J. A Treatise of the Asthma. London: Witkin & Innys, 1698.

14. Turner-Warwick M. On observing patterns of airflow obstruction in chronic asthma. Br J Dis Chest 1977; 71: 73–86.

15. Turner-Warwick M. Epidemiology of nocturnal asthma. Am J Med 1988; 85(1B): 6–8.

16. Catterall JR, Douglas NJ, Calverley PM, et al. Irregular breathing and hypoxaemia during sleep in chronic stable asthma. Lancet 1982; 1(8267): 301–4.

17. Montplaisir J, Malmo JL, Walsh J, Monday J. Nocturnal asthma: sleep and dream analysis. In: WP Koella, ed. Sleep 1980 Karger Basle, 1981: 397–9.

18. Shapiro CM, Catterall JR, Montgomery I, Raab G, Douglas NJ. Do asthmatics suffer bronchoconstriction during rapid eye movement sleep? B M J l986; 292: 116–5.

19. Shapiro CM, Auch C, Reimer M, et al. A new approach to the construct of alertness. J Psychosom Res 2006; 60: 595–603.

20. Bulmash EL, Moller HJ, Kayumov L, et al. Psychomotor disturbance in depression: Assessment using a driving simulator paradigm. J Affec Disord (2006); 93: 213–18.

21. Smith RD. A possible biologic role for dreaming. Psychother Psychosom 1984; 41: 167–76.

22. Katz M, Shapiro CM. Dreams and medical illness. B M J 1993; 306: 993–5.

23. Muller JE, Stone PH, Turi ZG, et al. Circadian variation in the frequency of onset of acute myocardial infarction. N Engl J Med 1985; 313: 1315–22.

24. Gami AS, Howard DE, Olson EJ, et al. Day-night pattern of sudden death in obstructive sleep apnea. N Engl J Med 2005; 352: 1206–14.

25. Flanigan MJ, Shapiro CM. Sleep solutions: Dangers of sleep. Solutions Sommeil: Dangers du sommeil. St. Laurent, Kommunicom Publications, 1992; 3: 1–20.

26. Shapiro CM. Energy expenditure and restorative sleep. Biol Psychol 1982; 15: 229–39.

27. Shoenut JP, Kerr P, Micfikier AB, Yamashiro Y, Kryger M. The effect of nasal CPAP on nocturnal reflux in patients with aperistaltic esophagus. Chest 1994; 106: 738–41

28. Vitale GC, Cheadle WG, Patel B, et al. The effect of alcohol on nocturnal gastroesophageal reflux. JAMA 1987; 258: 2077–9.

29. Dhillona S, Chunga SA, Chatooa K, Ladhaa N, Shapiro CM. Sleepiness and Fatigue in Dyspepsia Patients (draft manuscript being submitted for publication)

30. Postuma RB, Lang AE, Massicotte-Marquez J, Montplaisir J. Potential early markers of Parkinson disease in idiopathic REM sleep behavior disorder. Neurology 2006; 28, 66(6): 846–51.

31. Razmy A, Shapiro CM. Interactions of sleep and Parkinson's disease. Semin Clin Neuropsychiatry 2000; 5: 20–32.

32. Razmy A, Lang AE, Shapiro CM. Predictors of impaired daytime sleep and wakefulness in patients with Parkinsons disease treated with older (ergot) vs newer (nonergot) dopamine agonists. Arch Neurol 2004; 61: 97–102

33. Shapiro CM, Rosendorff C. Local hypothalamic blood flow during sleep. Electroenceph. Clin Neurophysiol 1975; 39: 365–9.

34. Maquet P, Dequeldre C, Delfiore G, et al. Functional neuroimaging of slow wave sleep. J Neurosci 1997; 17(8): 2807–12.

35. Morin CM. Insomnia: Psychological Assessment and Management. New York: Guilford 1993.

36. Kupych-Woloshyn N, Macfarlane J, Shapiro CM. A group approach for the management of insomnia. J Psychosom Res 1993; 37(Suppl 1): 39–44.

37. Sloan EP, Hauri P, Bootzin R, et al. The nuts and bolts of behavioral therapy for insomnia. J Psychosom Res 1993; 37(Suppl 1): 19–38.

Preface

The topic of sleep medicine has emerged during the last few decades as an area of intense medical and scientific interest. It also reflects the philosophy of the editors that the aspects of psychosomatics should be well understood so as to produce skilled sleep practitioners. Sleep and psychosomatic medicine is an intensely personal, inherently interesting, and fascinating field of medical science. Its subject matter touches all facets of our health and well-being, particularly in the sleep field; it overlaps with neuropharmacology, pharmacology, psychiatry, basic and clinical medical disciplines. We have striven to present valuable chapters in order to make the reading enjoyable as well as meaningful.

The chapters have been written by experts in the field in order to provide physicians of widely ranging interests and abilities with a highly readable exposition of the principal results, which include numerous well-articulated examples and a rich discussion of applications. In particular, we have tried to indicate how psychosomatics can be applied to sleep medicine, and vice versa.

This book is intended primarily for sleep researchers, general and neuropharmacologists, psychiatrists, and physicians who evaluate and treat sleep disorders. In addition, the volume will be extremely useful for pharmacologists, pharmacists, medical students, and clinicians of various disciplines who want to get an overall grasp of both sleep and psychosomatic medicine. Nineteen chapters have been written for this purpose by authors who are experts in their fields. The chapters have been written in a readable and easily understood manner. The book presents topics of current interest, ranging from attachment disorders to personality disorders and stress and psychosomatic factors implicated in various medical illnesses.

This book explores many of these new and exciting developments in the field of sleep and psychosomatics. Unfortunately, it is impossible in a volume such as this to include all recent advances – but that is what makes this field unique and such an exciting field to study and read and write about.

New concepts are discussed in this book. The reader may feel confident that the information presented is based on the most recent literature on sleep and psychosomatic medicine. Furthermore, the importance of neuroimaging of sleep is stressed. It is our hope that we have succeeded in accomplishing this goal.

As usual, we welcome communications from our readers concerning this book, especially any errors or deficiencies that may remain.

Acknowledgments

Many individuals played instrumental roles in the development of this volume. It is our pleasure to acknowledge some of these here.

This volume provides an introduction to the interphase between sleep and psychosomatic medicine. An enterprise of this sort is bound to be contentious and challenging, and editors who attempt such things need all the help they can get. Several people were instrumental in the production of *Sleep and Psychosomatic Medicine*.

We were delighted to experience warm, professional, and highly enthusiastic support from Ms Rupal Malde, Development Editor, Medical Books. Her commitment to excellence was a strong guiding force throughout the development of this volume. The wonderfully talented people of Informa Healthcare, Oxford, UK made this project an especially pleasurable one. In particular, we wish to acknowledge the invaluable help of Nick Dunton, Head of Medical Book Publishing, and Lindsay Campbell, Editorial Assistant, who gave support from start to finish.

A very special debt of gratitude and appreciation is owed to the several reviewers who made numerous helpful suggestions. Their candid comments and insights were invaluable.

To all the people who contributed to this project, we want to say 'thank you'. They make our work possible and enjoyable.

Our greatest gratitude goes to our families for their wisdom, creativity, patience, and support. Last, but certainly not least, we owe everything to our wonderful wives and families. Without the love and support of our families and friends, we could not have completed this project. They saw the work through from conception to completion with unwavering optimism and encouragement. You are the source of joy and inspiration for us – Thank you!

Color Plates

(a) Healthy control

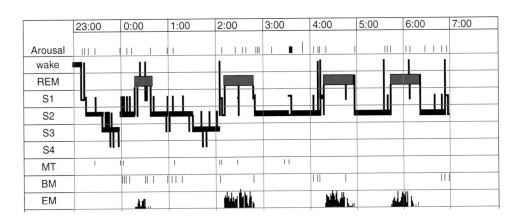

(3) Sleep continuity disturbances

(b) Depressed patient

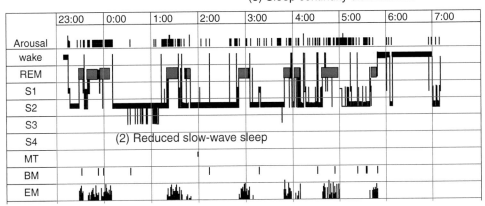

(1) Shortened REM sleep latency

Figure 5.1 Polysomnograms showing the characteristics of healthy sleep (a) in comparison with sleep in a depressed patient (b). (1) In depression, the period between sleep onset and the first occurrence of rapid eye movement (REM) sleep, shown in red, is markedly reduced (reduced REM latency). (2) The depressed patient spends less time in sleep stages 3 and 4 (reduced slow-wave sleep). (3) In depression, the number of awakenings and arousals is increased and the patient awakens early in the morning (disturbed sleep continuity). The sleep stages (REM and sleep stages 1–4 (S1–S4)) are given across the time. BM, body movement; EM, eye movement

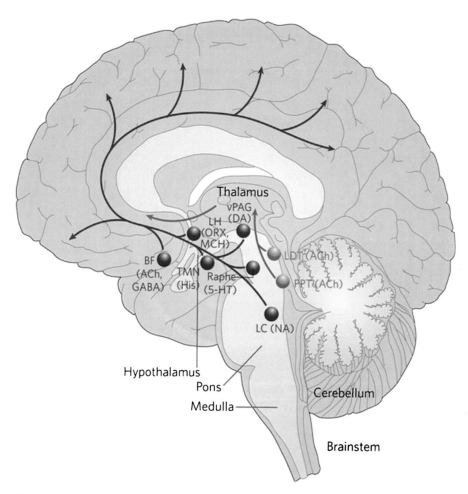

Figure 5.2 Key components of the ascending arousal system (assending reticular activating system, ARAS). A major input to the thalamus (yellow pathway) originates from cholinergic (ACh) cell groups in the pons: the pedunculopontine (PPT) and laterodorsal tegmental (LDT) nuclei. These inputs facilitate thalamocortical transmission. A second, non-thalamic, pathway (red) activates the cerebral cortex to facilitate the processing of inputs from the thalamus. This pathway comprises neurons in monoaminergic cell groups, including the locus ceruleus (LC) containing norepinephrine (noradrenaline, NA), the raphe nucleus containing serotonin (5-hydroxytryptamine, 5-HT), the tuberomammillary nucleus (TMN) containing histamine (His), and neurons in the ventral periaqueductal gray matter (vPAG) containing dopamine (DA). This pathway also receives contributions from neurons in the lateral hypothalamus (LHA) containing orexin (ORX) or melanin-concentrating hormone (MCH), and from basal forebrain (BF) neurons containing γ-aminobutyric acid (GABA) or ACh (reprinted, by permission from Macmillan Publishers Ltd: Saper CB, Scammell TE, Lu J. Hypothalamic regulations of sleep and circadian rhythms. Nature 437:1257–63, Copyright 2005)[20]

(a)

Prefrontal cortex

Parietal cortex

Temporal cortex

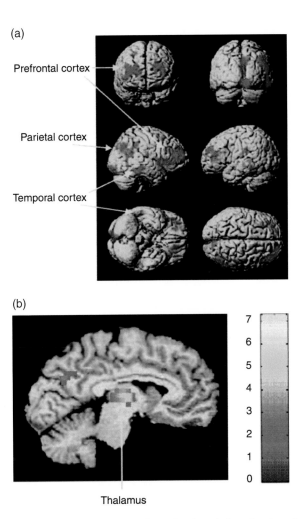

(b)

Thalamus

Figures 5.3   NREM sleep in healthy subjects. (a) Three-dimensional rendering of regions demonstrating significantly less relative metabolism during NREM sleep in relation to waking in healthy subjects. (b) Sagittal section showing regions of the thalamus demonstrating less relative metabolism during NREM sleep in relation to during waking (reproduced from Nofzinger EA et al. Brain 2002; 125:1105–15 by permission of Oxford University Press)[13]

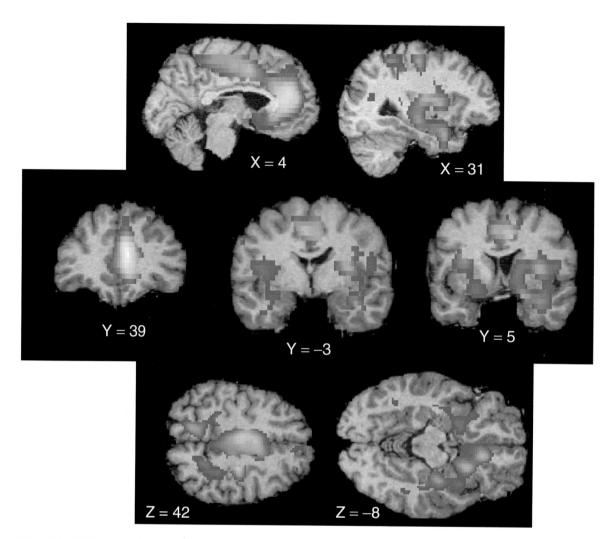

Figure 5.4   REM sleep in healthy subjects: brain structures where relative metabolism is greater in REM sleep than in waking in healthy subjects. This general pattern includes limbic and paralimbic structures, hippocampus, amygdala, ventral striatum, basal ganglia, supplementary motor area, anterior cingulate cortex, and medial prefrontal cortex (reprinted from Sleep Medicine Reviews, Vol 9, Nofzinger EA, Newimaging and sleep medicine, pp 157–72, Copyright 2005, with permission from Elsevier)[7]

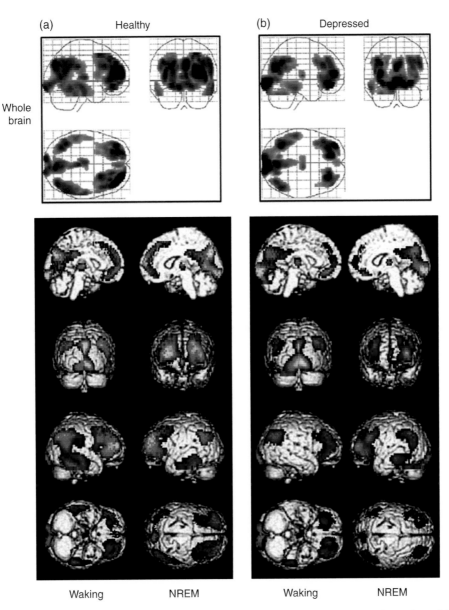

Figure 5.5   NREM sleep in depression, 'Glass brain' and 3-dimensional brain-rendering images showing regions with significant declines in relative metabolism from waking to NREM sleep, including the prefrontal cortex, cuneus, precuneus, and the temporoparietal cortex: (a) healthy subjects. (b) depressed subjects. Note that, despite a generally similar pattern of metabolism, depressed patients showed less frontal activity during waking ('hypofrontality') in comparison with healthy subjects and a relative lack of deactivation from waking to NREM sleep (reproduced from Nofzinger EA et al. Arch Ger Psychiatry 2005; 62:387–96. Copyright © 2005, American Medical Association. All rights reserved.)[25]

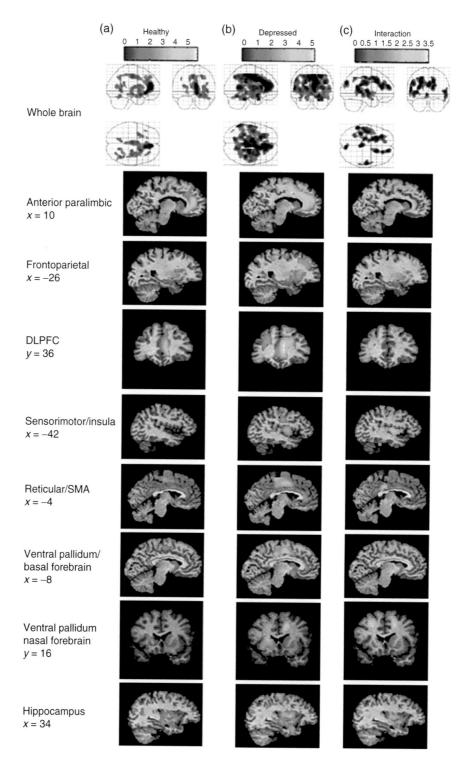

Figure 5.6 REM sleep in depression. Waking-to-REM sleep activations in healthy subjects (column a), depressed subjects (column b), and interactions showing regions where the depressed subjects' waking-to-REM activations are greater than those

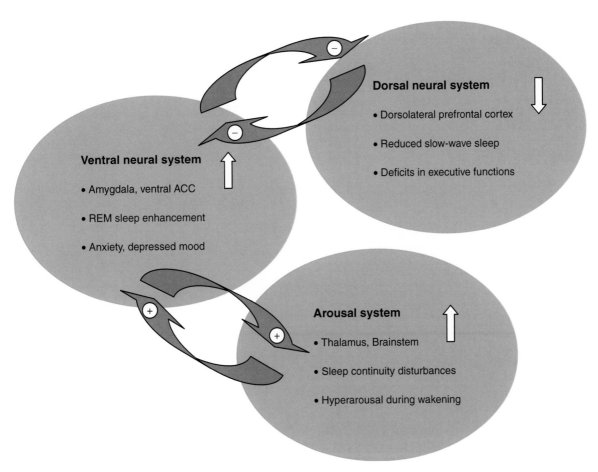

Figure 5.7   Sleep-neuroscience model of depression. The model aims to integrate findings from brain imaging studies, polysomnographic studies, and cognitive/affective neuroscience studies in depression. It proposes that three neural systems (arousal system, ventral emotional system, and dorsal executive system) are critically implicated in the pathophysiology of depression. The white arrows indicate the level of activity in each system in depressed patients in comparison with healthy controls. This level of activity is linked to polysomnographic characteristics and cognitive or affective symptoms in depression. The curved arrows reflect that the neural systems and their correlates on the polysomnographic and clinical levels are anatomically and functionally closely connected ('+' indicates functional enhancement. '−' indicates functional inhibition). REM, rapid eye movement; ACC, anterior cingulate cortex

of healthy subjects (column c). Brain regions of greater activation from waking to REM sleep in depressed patients in comparison with healthy subjects include the brainstem reticular formation, the limbic and anterior paralimbic cortex, and parts of the executive cortex. DLPFC, dorsolateral prefrontal cortex; SMA, supplementary motor area; x and y are the Talairach x- and y-coordinates (reproduced from Nofzinger EA et al. Arch Ger Psychiatry 2004; 61:695–702 by permission of …)[31]

1

Sleep and gastrointestinal functioning

Chien-Lin Chen, William C Orr

INTRODUCTION

Interest in sleep and gastrointestinal (GI) functioning has increased substantially over the past several years. These discoveries have led to a remarkable broadening of the focus and importance of the applications of basic sleep physiology to numerous areas of clinical medicine. In this chapter, the manifestation and/or pathogenesis of GI functioning and the relationship to GI disorders during sleep will be reviewed.

NOCTURNAL SYMPTOMS

The manifestation of GI symptoms during sleep is quite familiar to the practicing gastroenterologist. Perhaps the most obvious and common example is the occurrence of epigastric pain characteristically awakening the patient from sleep in the early morning hours. This pattern of awakening from sleep is quite predictable by the patient and can help significantly in establishing a diagnosis of duodenal ulcer disease. Patients may also have awakenings from sleep with symptoms that ostensibly are not related to GI disorders. For example, individuals may complain of sleep disruption secondary to awakening from sleep with chest pain, heartburn, or regurgitation into the throat. Asthmatics may be awoken from sleep by exacerbation of bronchial asthma that can be secondary to gastroesophageal reflux (GER). Numerous studies are accumulating

to suggest that respiratory complications secondary to GER are common, and these symptoms are noted primarily secondary to sleep-related GER.[1]

Other symptoms encountered by the practicing gastroenterologist that may occur during the day but whose occurrence during sleep adds a disconcerting dimension to the symptom include nocturnal diarrhea, fecal incontinence, chest pain, and the respiratory disorders noted above. Although a denial of symptoms thought to be related to GI problems such as GER does not necessarily preclude the occurrence of the sleep-related abnormalities, a positive symptom history would enhance the probability of the existence of a nocturnal GI disorder, as may be the case in patients with functional bowel disorders such as irritable bowel syndrome (IBS) and functional dyspepsia.

Nocturnal acid secretion

Patients with duodenal ulcer disease maintain a circadian pattern of gastric acid secretion, and studies have shown that the levels of secretion are enhanced.[2] The study by Feldman and Richardson[2] showed that the peak of basal acid secretion occurs at approximately midnight, with minimal acid secretion occurring during the day in the absence of food ingestion. In addition, there does not appear to be any relation between the stages of sleep and gastric acid secretion. However, the study by Orr et al[3] demonstrated a failure to inhibit acid during the first 2 hours of sleep in patients with duodenal ulcer disease. Multicenter trials with bedtime administration of histamine H_2 receptor antagonists have documented the efficacy of healing duodenal ulcers through nocturnal acid suppression.[4, 5] These studies uniformly documented that duodenal ulcer-healing rates were at least as good with a once-a-day, bedtime dose of these potent acid-suppressing compounds as with the more conventional multiple daily dosing regimens. Howden et al[6] reviewed the published data on nocturnal dosing of H_2 receptor antagonists in more than 12 000 patients with duodenal ulcer disease. They concluded that nocturnal dosing showed a clear advantage over multiple daily doses. These data strongly support the notion that nocturnal acid suppression alone is sufficient to heal a duodenal ulcer.

Other studies in patients with refractory duodenal ulcer suggest that nocturnal acid suppression is not only sufficient but also necessary for duodenal ulcer healing. In a study by Gledhill et al,[7] it was demonstrated that a reduction in nocturnal acid secretion through parietal cell vagotomy produced an enhanced healing rate in patients who were unresponsive to conventional cimetidine treatment. In a similar study by Galmiche et al,[8] 20 patients with duodenal ulcers who were resistant to conventional cimetidine treatment received 150 mg ranitidine twice daily for 6 weeks. They demonstrated that the ulcer was healed in 8 patients, whereas it remained unhealed in 12 patients. Patients whose ulcer healed had a substantial suppression of nocturnal acid secretion, whereas patients whose ulcer again failed to heal maintained a nocturnal peak in gastric acid secretion. A subsequent study found that in persons who had had a parietal cell vagotomy, nocturnal acid secretion was significantly greater in those who experienced ulcer recurrence than in those who did not.[9] Further support for the important role of nocturnal acid secretion in the pathogenesis of duodenal ulcer disease comes from data showing that the maintenance of a modest degree of nocturnal acid suppression will effectively prevent the recurrence of duodenal ulcer disease.[10,11] These studies compared the use of 150 mg ranitidine at bedtime with 400 mg

cimetidine at bedtime, and found ranitidine to be superior in the prevention of ulcer recurrence. This finding is most likely due to the increased potency of ranitidine and its enhanced effectiveness in producing nocturnal acid suppression. A study actually documenting effective nocturnal acid suppression by 150 mg ranitidine at bedtime was reported by Santana et al,[12] who concluded that it might be relevant to the pathogenesis of duodenal ulceration that the short-lived decrease in nocturnal acidity observed in their study was sufficient to prevent relapse of ulceration in most patients.

Gastroesophageal reflux during sleep

GER, particularly with its familiar symptom of heartburn, is recognized as a common phenomenon. Most normal people will experience occasional bouts of heartburn. About 7% of the normal population experiences heartburn nearly every day.[13] Furthermore, the majority of patients with frequent heartburn complain of night-time GER symptoms, and a substantial proportion (>50%) of these patients report that their symptoms disrupt their sleep and affect their daytime functioning.[14,15] Many patients who present to a physician with a complaint of heartburn can be readily treated with simple alterations in lifestyle, such as the avoidance of certain provocative foods and the use of antacid therapy, although there are no data specifically on the utility of these measures in treating sleep-related symptoms.[16] The familiarity of this symptom and its rapid response in most instances to relatively simple therapeutic measures belie the severity and potential complications of the disease process. As will be reviewed here, the complications of GER appear to be the result of recurrent episodes of sleep-related GER.

GER events do occur during sleep, but appear to occur most commonly during brief arousals from sleep. Two studies have been published that were remarkably similar in their results in that reflux events occurred much more frequently in patients with diagnosed GER disease, and relatively infrequently in normal volunteers.[17,18]

The majority of reflux events in both studies did occur in association with polygraphically determined brief arousal responses.

Attention has been focused on the importance of different patterns of GER associated with waking and sleeping.[19] These patterns were documented in studies involving 24-hour monitoring of the distal esophageal pH. GER is identified when the pH falls below 4 for a period of more than 30 seconds, and the reflux episode is arbitrarily terminated when the pH reaches 4 or 5. In this landmark study, Johnson and DeMeester[19] described two different patterns of reflux. Reflux in the upright position occurs most often postprandially and usually consists of two or three reflux episodes that are rapidly cleared (2–3 minutes). Reflux in the supine position is usually associated with sleep and with more prolonged clearance time.

These studies documented highly significant increases in acid–mucosa contact time in patients with esophagitis, and these differences were most impressive when the supine position or sleep interval was considered; that is, there was a greater difference between patients and control subjects in the supine position compared with the upright position. The same group of investigators have also asserted that, even though acid–mucosa contact time may be equivalent in the upright and supine positions, the prolonged acid clearance times associated with sleep appeared to result in greater damage to the esophageal mucosa.[20] In another study, they attempted to correlate the relation between the patterns of GER, as determined by 24-hour esophageal pH monitoring, and the endoscopic evaluation of the esophageal mucosa.[21] They identified patients as primarily *upright* (waking) *refluxers*, *supine* (sleep) *refluxers*, and those whose reflux was evident throughout the 24-hour day, whom they termed *combined refluxers*. The severity of endoscopic change according to three grades of esophagitis was determined. Grade 1 esophagitis was defined simply as distal erythema and friability; grade 2 was defined when mucosal erosions were noted; and grade 3 involved more severe ulcerations and strictures. Their data indicated that an increasing

incidence of nocturnal acid exposure was associated with more severe esophageal mucosal damage. An additional study compared the results of 24-hour esophageal pH monitoring in patients who had either normal findings on endoscopy or erosive esophagitis.[22] The results of this study showed that total acid exposure time and the number of reflux episodes requiring longer than 5 minutes to clear were found to most reliably discriminate these two groups of patients. Furthermore, these authors found that 50% of the patients with reflux symptoms had normal 24-hour pH monitoring and that 29% of the patients with erosive esophagitis also had normal pH studies. It is of interest that the most effective variable in distinguishing the two groups of patients was the number of episodes requiring longer than 5 minutes to clear (to pH 4). An extension of these findings comes from a study by Orr et al[23] in which 24-hour pH monitoring was accomplished in a group of symptomatic patients with heartburn and normal endoscopic results and a group of patients with severe complications of GER, including erosive esophagitis, stricture, and Barrett's esophagus. The results showed that the best discriminator among the two groups was the number of episodes of prolonged acid clearance (longer than 5 minutes) in the supine position. These episodes appear to be more likely to occur during sleep, and this finding certainly confirms the notion that prolonged acid clearance is an important determinant in the development of esophagitis. Other investigators have not been as enthusiastic in their support of nocturnal GER as an important factor in the pathogenesis of reflux esophagitis. De Caestecker et al[24] found that postprandial acid exposure was the best predictor of the severity of esophagitis, and their results led them to conclude that nocturnal reflux was substantially less important in the production of esophagitis.

As previously noted, acid clearance during sleep seems to be an important contributing factor in the development of reflux esophagitis. The process of acid clearance has been well studied by Helm et al,[25] who described a two-factor theory of acid clearance.

They proposed that acid clearance takes place in two phases: an initial phase, termed *volume clearance*, and a second phase, termed *acid neutralization*. Their data indicate that the vast majority of the volume of refluxed material is cleared from the esophagus quite rapidly by the first two or three swallows. There remains a coating of acid on the esophageal mucosa, which keeps the esophageal pH well below 4. Subsequent swallows serve to deliver saliva to the distal esophagus, and, with its potent buffering capacity, the distal esophageal pH is returned to its normal level (5.5–6.5). A subsequent study confirmed these findings in that acid clearance was found to be independent of the swallowing rate but significantly altered by an anticholinergic drug that inhibits salivation.[26]

Both swallowing frequency and salivation have been shown to be markedly depressed during sleep; as a result, one would hypothesize a prolongation of acid clearance during sleep.[27,28] Lichter and Muir[27] have shown that swallowing occurs sporadically during sleep, and there are long periods (longer than 30 minutes) without swallowing. Overall, the rate of swallowing during sleep is approximately six swallows per hour, and the swallows usually occur in association with a movement arousal. The highest frequency of these events is in stages 1 and 2 and rapid eye movement (REM) sleep.[27] Similarly, a study by Orr et al[29] showed a marked reduction in swallows associated with esophageal acid infusion during sleep. Studies have focused specifically on the issue of the parameters of esophageal acid clearance during sleep. A model that incorporates the clearance of infused acid (15.0 ml 0.1 M HCl) during sleep was used in these studies. As opposed to simply analyzing spontaneous GER, this allowed the infusion of acid into the distal esophagus during specific periods of documented sleep (REM versus non-REM (NREM) sleep), and it allowed the precise timing of infusions such that the amount of sleep before each infusion could be relatively well controlled. This model also permitted a precise comparison of acid clearance during waking and during sleep under well-controlled conditions.

The initial study in this series involved a comparison of acid clearance during sleep in normal volunteers and patients with mild to moderate esophagitis.[29] The results revealed that sleep infusions in both groups were associated with a statistically significant prolongation of acid clearance time. The absolute clearance time was nearly doubled in both groups. However, there was no significant difference between the clearance times in the patients and in the control subjects. The latter finding is believed to be a somewhat academic point, because, as noted previously, normal persons rarely have reflux during sleep, whereas it is somewhat more common in patients with esophagitis. In addition, it was clear from the polysomnographic observations that clearance was invariably associated with an arousal from sleep, and if this did not occur, there was a marked prolongation in acid clearance time. To evaluate this notion more precisely, clearance intervals that were associated with greater or less than 50% of waking during the clearance interval were compared. The clearance trials that involved more than 50% of waking had significantly faster clearance times. These data led to the conclusion that both arousal responses and waking are important elements in the response to an acidic distal esophagus.

To evaluate the motor function of the esophagus during sleep and the associated arousals, a subsequent study was performed using a specially designed esophageal probe to monitor not only distal esophageal pH but also esophageal peristalsis.[30] This study also confirmed the importance of arousal responses in the efficient clearance of acid from the distal esophagus. The test was performed on normal volunteers who had a negative acid perfusion test; that is, they did not show any sensitivity to acid dripped in the distal esophagus and could not distinguish acid from water in the esophagus. However, the determination of arousal responses to these two different substances infused during sleep revealed that the acid infusions produced a significantly greater number of arousal responses. In addition, an exponential relation was described between the percentage of waking during the acid clearance interval and the acid clearance time; that is, the greater the amount of waking during the acid clearance interval, the faster the clearance time. Again, this finding substantiates those from the previous study of patients with esophagitis. This study did not document any difference between peristaltic parameters during sleep and during waking.

To more definitively test the hypothesis that complications of GER are associated with prolonged acid clearance, a group of 13 patients with Barrett's esophagus was studied.[31] Barrett's esophagus is a condition believed to be related to chronic, severe GER, which results in the replacement of normal esophageal squamous epithelium with gastric columnar epithelium. The results of this study proved to be quite surprising in that the patients with Barrett's esophagus were shown to have significantly faster acid clearance during sleep and waking compared with the control subjects. These data were, however, quite compatible with previous results in documenting the importance of arousal responses in the clearance process. The patients with Barrett's esophagus showed both a higher frequency of arousal responses and a shorter latency to the first swallow than did the control subjects.

Further illustrating the importance of these parameters in differentiating the patients with Barrett's esophagus from the control subjects is the fact that they could not be distinguished on the basis of any parameters associated with esophageal motor function, such as the amplitude of the peristaltic contraction or the esophageal transit time. It is especially notable in this study that there were a remarkable number of episodes of spontaneous GER in the group with Barrett's esophagus compared with the control subjects. These data led to the conclusion that the severe esophagitis in the patients with Barrett's esophagus is acquired through repeated episodes of spontaneous GER during sleep, which are associated with prolongation of the acid clearance time (even though this was demonstrated to be faster than in normal control subjects, the acid clearance still is substantially longer than that occurring during waking).

Therapeutic considerations

GER appears to be affected by sleeping position. In a study by Khoury et al,[32] it was determined that sleeping in the left lateral position significantly reduced the incidence of GER. The results of previously cited studies suggest that the pattern of GER during waking and sleep is important in that sleep-related reflux produces a prolongation of acid clearance.[22,23] Additional documentation of the importance of this pattern of the prolongation of acid clearance comes from studies that have shown that the back-diffusion of hydrogen ions in the esophagus is directly related to the duration of acid–mucosa contact time.[33] Further evidence for the importance of nocturnal GER comes from a clinical study that documented individuals with symptoms of nocturnal heartburn, as well as dysphagia and chest pain, were much more likely to have demonstrable esophageal disease.[34]

These results, as well as those described in the cited studies, tend to substantiate the time-honored clinical approach to persistent reflux, which is the suggestion that the patient sleep with the head of the bed elevated. This clinical axiom has survived for decades with little in the way of objective documentation that it actually is an efficacious approach to GER. Johnson and DeMeester[35] specifically tested this clinical axiom. Using intraesophageal pH monitoring during sleep, they demonstrated that sleeping with the head of the bed elevated produced a 67% improvement in acid clearance time; however, the frequency of reflux episodes remained unchanged. The use of a cholinergic drug (bethanechol) that produces an elevation in lower-esophageal sphincter pressure and increases esophageal peristaltic efficiency resulted in a decrease in both reflux frequency (30%) and acid clearance time (53%). The authors concluded that nocturnal reflux was most responsive to these therapeutic modalities. Another clinical axiom – avoidance of late evening meals – has also been directly tested in a study by Orr and Harnish.[36] They noted that reflux events during monitored sleep were not increased by a late-evening provocative meal in patients with symptomatic GER disease. However, they did note that an over-the-counter (OTC) dose (75 mg) of ranitidine at bedtime was effective in significantly reducing reflux events during sleep.

The use of H_2 receptor antagonists to suppress gastric acid secretion has been shown to be effective in the relief of heartburn.[37,38] One study using 24-hour ambulatory esophageal pH assessments in patients with symptomatic heartburn and documented GER demonstrated that increasing doses (40 mg at bedtime, 20 mg twice daily, and 40 mg twice daily) of an H_2 receptor antagonist (famotidine) produced increasing reductions in daytime and total acid–mucosa contact.[39] The three dosing regimens were equally effective in reducing nocturnal acid contact time. Thus, in contrast to duodenal ulcer disease, it does not appear that only bedtime dosing is adequate to treat GER. However, these data suggest that GER can be adequately controlled through effective gastric acid suppression. A study by Cohen et al[40] reported on the effect of a Nissen fundoplication on sleep-related GER and heartburn symptoms, as well as objective and subjective sleep measures. They noted a significant decrease in both sleep-related reflux events and symptoms after surgery. Subjective and objective sleep measures were improved after surgery. More specifically, there was a very small, but significant, increase (approximately 5%) in non-REM sleep, while there were more robust improvements in difficulty falling asleep, sleep quality, and daytime sleepiness. An interesting finding was reported by Kerr et al,[41] who showed that the administration of nasal continuous positive airway pressure (CPAP) to patients who are being treated for obstructive sleep apnea (OSA) had the additional therapeutic benefit of reducing GER during sleep and consequent esophageal acid contact time. Similar improvement was reported in patients with GER without apnea.[42] Since these studies examined only a single night of CPAP, it is important to note that this effect was replicated in a protocol that utilized 1 week of continuous CPAP treatment in patients with documented moderate/severe OSA, and abnormal acid contact

time documented by 24-hour esophageal pH monitoring.[43] In this study, patients studied at the end of 1 week of CPAP treatment were shown to have a significant decrease in sleep-related acid contact time. Also of interest with regard to OSA is a study by Graf et al[44] that determined that patients with OSA have a high incidence of GER. The authors further determined that there is no relation between severity of OSA and GER, nor is there any relation between OSA events and reflux events. A similar conclusion was reached from a study reported by Tardif et al.[45] Similar results have been reported by Ing et al,[46] but they also reported an overall increase in reflux events and acid clearance time, in spite of the fact that there was no clear relationship between OSA events and reflux events. The question remains as to what is the pathogenesis of increased sleep-related GER in patients with OSA. They clearly share some risk factors, such as obesity, alcohol consumption, and perhaps hiatal hernia, but, based on some clinical and physiologic data, obesity alone would not appear to be an adequate explanation for this relationship. Suganuma et al[47] described an association between obesity and symptoms of OSA, but they found no relationship between obesity and reflux symptoms. On the other hand, in another questionnaire study, Green et al[48] showed a significant reduction in night-time heartburn symptoms after CPAP treatment, and those with higher CPAP levels had a greater reduction in symptoms of night-time heartburn. In another study that evaluated reflux symptoms (i.e., heartburn and acid regurgitation) in patients with a diagnosis of OSA, Valipour et al[49] found that there was no difference in reflux symptoms between those with the diagnosis of OSA and those designated as 'simple snorers'. Furthermore, they found no relationship between the severity of OSA and reflux symptoms. It should be noted that, in contrast to the study by Green et al,[48] this investigation did not specifically address night-time GER symptoms. In addition, Valipour et al[49] noted in their discussion that the incidence of reflux symptoms did not appear to be greater than that noted in some general population surveys. An interesting physiologic study addressed the issue of the relationship between GER and OSA by identifying individuals with significant OSA and GER, and treating them with acid suppression with a proton pump inhibitor (PPI). In this study, Senior et al[50] noted that after treatment with the PPI for 1 month, there was a significant reduction in complete obstructive events, although the overall respiratory disturbance index (RDI) only showed a strong trend towards a reduction after treatment ($p < 0.06$). On the basis of these data, it would appear that the incidence of night-time heartburn is elevated in patients with OSA. In the study by Green et al,[48] it was noted to be 62%, which is similar to the rate noted above in patients with frequent heartburn complaints.[14] Furthermore, the frequency shows a very significant decline with CPAP treatment. This coincides nicely with other physiologic studies, which have clearly shown a significant decline in esophageal acid contact time with CPAP treatment.[41,42] The mechanism by which CPAP reduces esophageal acid contact time remains controversial, but an interesting study from this same group has suggested that some residual lower esophageal sphincter (LES) pressure (>10 mmHg) may be necessary for nasal CPAP to affect nocturnal reflux.[51]

Of considerable interest is the fact that studies have documented that commonly consumed sedating drugs such as benzodiazepines and alcohol have been shown to prolong acid clearance during sleep. A study by Vitale et al[52] showed that alcohol consumption approximately 3 hours before sleep resulted in marked prolongation of the clearance of spontaneous episodes of GER. In another investigation of the effect of the administration of commonly used hypnotic drugs, a decrease was shown in the arousal latency and a prolongation was shown in the acid clearance time with triazolam.[53]

INTESTINAL MOTILITY AND IRRITABLE BOWEL SYNDROME

Due to the technological and practical difficulties in monitoring intestinal activity, particularly in patients, relatively little has been done in terms of acquiring data on intestinal motility during sleeping and waking in patient populations of interest. However, some data have been gradually appearing in the medical literature. One study that used 24-hour ambulatory monitoring of small intestinal motility in patients with IBS was carried out by Kellow et al.[54] Although nocturnal motor patterns did not differentiate the patient group from the control subjects, the notable lack of motility activity during sleep led these investigators to suggest that the changes in motor function noted were primarily the result of reactions to various 'stressful' events occurring in the waking state. However, in a subsequent study, Kumar et al[55] noted a marked increase in REM sleep in patients with IBS. These data were interpreted as lending additional support to their speculation that this syndrome has a central nervous system (CNS) pathogenesis.

The observation by Kumar et al[55] that REM sleep was enhanced in patients with IBS has prompted a number of investigations into sleep and functional bowel disorders, including IBS and functional dyspepsia. Using subjective reports of sleep quality, Goldsmith and Levin[56] showed a strong correlation between the exacerbation of IBS symptoms and poor sleep. The obvious problems of a subjective study without physiologic measurement of sleep were noted by Wingate,[57] one of the authors of the original study on IBS and sleep. Wingate pointed out that the occurrence of waking symptomatology may unduly influence the perception of the previous night's sleep, and, without polysomnographic documentation of sleep, this influence cannot be discounted. In a study in patients with non-ulcer dyspepsia (characterized by epigastric postprandial bloating, nausea, or early satiety), two-thirds of 65 patients with non-ulcer dyspepsia complained of general sleep disturbances suggestive of non-restorative sleep (i.e., numerous wakenings after sleep onset and morning awakenings without feeling rested).[58] These were significantly more common than noted in control subjects, and 65% of those complaining of sleep disturbance attributed their sleep problem to their abdominal symptoms. Ten patients were also studied for a

24-hour period with intestinal manometric monitoring, and a change in the rhythmicity and frequency of intestinal contractions was found in the functional dyspeptics during the nocturnal recording interval. In a subsequent study, Fass et al[59] documented a marked increase in sleep complaints in patients with functional bowel disorders (i.e., IBS and functional dyspepsia) compared with normal controls. In addition, the dyspeptic patients had more complaints of sleep disturbance, perhaps due to more intense abdominal pain. Increased sleep complaints have also been documented by studies by Heitkemper et al,[60] Elsenbruch et al,[61] and Rotem et al.[62] In these studies, full polysomnography (PSG) was conducted. In the study by Elsenbruch et al,[61] no difference was found in any of the sleep measures reported between IBS subjects and normals. However, the study by Heitkemper et al[60] did show a significant prolongation of REM sleep. The study by Rotem et al[62] revealed sharply contrasting PSG data: they noted a number of significant PSG differences in the IBS subjects compared with control groups, including decreased slow-wave sleep, increased arousal responses, and increased waking after sleep onset. Further research with larger sample sizes and stratification by IBS diagnostic subtypes may help elucidate and resolve these discrepancies. The original study by Kumar et al[55] documenting the enhancement of REM sleep in patients with IBS reported on only six individuals who had a single night of sleep subsequent to small-bowel intubation for monitoring of intestinal motility. With a small number of subjects and no attempt to adapt individuals to the laboratory setting (even though a control group was used), there is a high probability that these results were spurious. Orr et al[63] attempted to replicate this study while at the same time non-invasively monitoring a gastrointestinal measure so that more natural sleep could be obtained. Nine patients with IBS and nine control subjects were studied with full PSG monitoring and gastric electrical activity monitored by the surface electrogastrogram. In this study, a statistically significant

increase in REM sleep was documented in the patients with IBS, but the absolute level of REM sleep was not nearly in the range reported by Kumar et al.[55] In addition, specific electrogastrographic changes were found to be associated with sleep in normal subjects that were not noted in patients with IBS. Normal volunteers showed a significant decrease in the spectral amplitude of the 3 cycle/min electrogastrogram rhythm during NREM sleep compared with the waking state. Of interest is the fact that during REM sleep, the amplitude was significantly increased to levels approaching those in the waking state. The patients with IBS failed to significantly modulate the amplitude of the dominant frequency of the gastric electrical rhythm during any of these states of consciousness. The lack of modulation of the dominant frequency of the electrogastrographic amplitude during sleep in patients with IBS raises the possibility that other autonomic abnormalities may be unmasked by further study of physiologic functioning during sleep.

In a subsequent study by Thompson et al,[64] it was noted that IBS patients who had dyspeptic symptoms in addition to classic symptoms of abdominal pain and cramping did not exhibit the increase in sympathetic dominance in REM sleep that was noted only in the patients with abdominal cramping alone as part of their IBS symptomatology. In a series of subsequent studies by Orr and colleagues,[62,64,65] none has replicated the finding of an increase in REM sleep in IBS patients.

Collectively, these results from various sleep investigations in patients with functional bowel disorders suggest not only that there are sleep disturbances noted in this patient population but also that the sleep disturbances may contribute to altered GI functioning. Certainly, these studies confirm the notion that there are CNS alterations in patients with functional bowel disorders and that these alterations are perhaps uniquely identified during sleep. Future studies on sleep in patients with functional bowel disorders will undoubtedly provide additional understanding of

COLONIC MOTILITY

Bassotti et al[66] monitored colonic motility for 24 hours in normal volunteers and in patients with chronic constipation. Although they documented a decrease in the number and duration of mass movements in the patients with chronic constipation, as well as a circadian pattern of decrease in mass movements during the night, no significant difference was noted between patients and control subjects with regard to the circadian pattern itself. In a similar study, Ferrara et al[67] monitored the motor activity of the distal colon, rectum, and anal canal over a 24-hour interval in patients with slow-transit constipation. These patients were compared with 10 healthy control subjects. The patients with slow-transit constipation were noted to have impaired responses to feeding on awakening from sleep in the morning.

Another interesting observation concerning alterations in anorectal functioning during sleep concerns a study by Orkin et al[68] in which the authors monitored rectal motor activity during sleep in patients who had undergone ileal–anal anastomosis. They noted that decreases in anal resting pressure coupled with marked minute-to-minute variations in pressure during sleep occurred in control subjects and in patients, and, when particularly profound, led to nocturnal fecal incontinence in some patients.

CONCLUSIONS

There appears to be an important relation between sleep and the development of various acid peptic diseases, such as duodenal ulcer disease and GER disease. The pathogenesis and treatment of these disorders rely on the control of acid secretion during sleep. The suppression of nocturnal acid secretion appears to be an essential element in the healing of duodenal ulcers, and the occurrence of nocturnal GER is an unquestionably important aspect of the development of serious complications of this disorder. Continuous monitoring of the distal esophageal pH to document nocturnal GER is becoming an important and useful diagnostic tool. In addition, prolonged monitoring of small- and large-bowel motility appears to be a promising tool in further understanding the pathogenesis of various gastrointestinal diseases and how these diseases may be altered by sleep. These sleep-related phenomena are becoming important factors in the practice of state-of-the-art gastroenterology, and future research will undoubtedly further substantiate the important role of sleep in the pathogenesis of gastrointestinal disease.

REFERENCES

1. Cuttitta G, Cibella F, Visconti A, et al. Spontaneous gastroesophageal reflux and airway patency during the night in adult asthmatics. Am J Respir Crit Care Med 2000; 161: 177–81.
2. Feldman M, Richardson CT. Total 24-hour gastric acid secretion in patients with duodenal ulcer: comparison with normal subjects and effects of cimetidine and parietal cell vagotomy. Gastroenterology 1986; 90: 540–4.
3. Orr WC, Hall WH, Stahl ML, et al. Sleep patterns and gastric acid secretion in duodenal ulcer disease. Arch Intern Med 1976; 136: 655–60.
4. Kildebo S, Aronsen O, Bernersen B, et al. Cimetidine, 800 mg at night, in the treatment of duodenal ulcers. Scand J Gastroenterol 1985; 20: 1147–50.
5. Colin-Jones DG, Ireland A, Gear P, et al. Reducing overnight secretion of acid to heal duodenal ulcers: comparison of standard divided dose of ranitidine with a single dose administered at night. Am J Med 1984; 77: 116–22.
6. Howden CW, Jones DB, Hunt RH. Nocturnal doses of H_2 receptor antagonists for duodenal ulcer. Lancet 1985; i: 647–8.
7. Gledhill T, Buck M, Paul A, et al. Comparison of the effects of proximal gastric vagotomy, cimetidine, and placebo on nocturnal intragastric acidity and acid secretion in patients with cimetidine resistant duodenal ulcer. Br J Surg 1983; 70: 704–6.
8. Galmiche JP, Tranvouez JL, Denis P, et al. L'enregistrement nocturne du pH gastrique permet-il de

prévoir la response thérapeutique des ulcères duodenaux sévères traites par la ranitidine? Gastroenterol Clin Biol 1985; 9: 583–9.

9. Gotthard R, Strom M, Sjodahl R, et al. 24-h study of gastric acidity and bile acid concentration after parietal cell vagotomy. Scand J Gastroenterol 1986; 21: 503–8.

10. Gough KR, Bardhan KD, Crowe JP, et al. Ranitidine and cimetidine in prevention of duodenal ulcer relapse. Lancet 1984; ii: 659–62.

11. Silvis SE. Final report on the United States multicenter trial comparing ranitidine to cimetidine as maintenance therapy following healing of duodenal ulcer. J Clin Gastroenterol 1985; 7: 482–7.

12. Santana IA, Sharma BK, Pounder RE, et al. 24-hour intragastric acidity during maintenance treatment with ranitidine. BMJ 1984; 289: 1420.

13. Nebel OT, Fornes MF, Castell DO. Symptomatic gastroesophageal reflux: incidence and precipitating factors. Am J Dig Dis 1976; 21: 953–6.

14. Shaker R, Castell DO, Schoenfeld PS, Spechler SJ. Nighttime heartburn is an under-appreciated clinical problem that impacts sleep and daytime function: the results of a Gallup survery conducted on behalf of the American Gastroenterological Association. Am J Gastroenterol 2003; 98: 1487–93.

15. Farup C, Kleinman L, Sloan S, et al. The impact of nocturnal symptoms associated with gastroesophageal reflux disease on health-related quality of life. Arch Intern Med 2001; 151: 45–52.

16. Orr WC. Lifestyle measures for the treatment of gastroesophageal reflux disease. In: Bayless TM, Diehl AM, eds. Advanced Therapy in Gastroenterology and Liver Disease. Hamilton: BC Decker, 2005: 59–62.

17. Freidin N, Fisher MJ, Taylor W, et al. Sleep and nocturnal acid reflux in normal subjects and patients with reflux oesophagitis. Gut 1991; 32: 1275–9.

18. Penzel T, Becker HR, Brandenburg U, et al. Arousal in patients with gastro-esophageal reflux and sleep apnea. Eur Respir J 1999; 14: 1266–70.

19. Johnson LF, DeMeester TR. Twenty-four hour pH monitoring of the distal esophagus. Am J Gastroenterol 1974; 62: 325–32.

20. DeMeester TR, Johnson LF, Guy JJ, et al. Patterns of gastroesophageal reflux in health and disease. Ann Surg 1976; 184: 459–70.

21. Johnson LF, DeMeester TR, Haggitt RC. Esophageal epithelial response to gastroesophageal reflux, a quantitative study. Am J Dig Dis 1978; 23: 498–509.

22. Schlesinger PK, Honahue PE, Schmid B, et al. Limitations of 24-hour intraesophageal pH monitoring in the hospital setting. Gastroenterology 1985; 89: 797–804.

23. Orr WC, Allen ML, Robinson M. The pattern of nocturnal and diurnal esophageal acid exposure in the pathogenesis of erosive mucosal damage. Am J Gastroenterol 1994; 89: 509–12.

24. De Caestecker, Blackwell JH, Brown J, et al. When is acid reflux most damaging to the esophagus? Gastroenterology 1985; 88: 1360 (abst).

25. Helm JF, Dodds WJ, Hogan WJ, et al. Acid neutralizing capacity of human saliva. Gastroenterology 1982; 83: 69–74.

26. Allen ML, Orr WC, Woodruff DM, et al. The effects of swallowing frequency and transdermal scopolamine on esophageal acid clearance. Am J Gastroenterol 1985; 80: 669–72.

27. Lichter J, Muir RC. The pattern of swallowing during sleep. Electroencephalogr Clin Neurophysiol 1975; 38: 427–32.

28. Schneyer LH, Pigman W, Hanahan L, et al. Rate of flow of human parotid, sublingual, and submaxillary secretions during sleep. J Dent Res 1956; 35: 109–14.

29. Orr WC, Johnson LF, Robinson MG. The effect of sleep on swallowing, esophageal peristalsis, and acid clearance. Gastroenterology 1984; 86: 814–19.

30. Orr WC, Robinson MG, Johnson LF. Acid clearing during sleep in the pathogenesis of reflux esophagitis. Dig Dis Sci 1981; 26: 423.

31. Orr WC, Lackey C, Robinson MG, et al. Acid clearance and reflux during sleep in Barrett's esophagus. Gastroenterology 1983; 84: 1265.

32. Khoury R, Camacho-Lobato L, Katz P, Mohiuddin M, Castell D. Influence of spontaneous sleep positions on nighttime recumbent reflux in patients with gastroesophageal reflux disease. Am J Gastroenterol 1999; 94: 2069–73.

33. Johnson LF, Harmon JW. Experimental esophagitis in a rabbit model: clinical relevance. J Clin Gastroenterol 1986; 8(Suppl 1): 26–44.

34. Anderson LIB, Madsen PV, Dalgaard P, et al. Validity of clinical symptoms in benign esophageal disease, assessed by questionnaire. Acta Med Scand 1987; 221: 171–7.

35. Johnson LF, DeMeester TR. Evaluation of the head of the bed, bethanechol, and antacid foam tablets on gastroesophageal reflux. Dig Dis Sci 1981; 26: 673–80.

36. Orr WC, Harnish MJ. Sleep-related gastrooesophageal reflux: provocation with a late evening meal and treatment with acid suppression. Aliment Pharmacol Ther 1998; 12: 1033–8.

37. Behar J, Brand DL, Brown FC, et al. Cimetidine in the treatment of symptomatic gastroesophageal reflux: a double-blind controlled trial. Gastroenterology 1978; 74: 441–8.

38. Sontag S, Glaxo, GERD Research Group. Ranitidine therapy for gastroesophageal reflux disease. Results of a large double-blind trial. Arch Intern Med 1987; 147: 1485–91.

39. Orr WC, Robinson MG, Humphries T. Dose response effect of famotidine on patterns of gastroesophageal reflux. Aliment Pharmacol Ther 1988; 2: 229–35.

40. Cohen JA, Arain A, Harris PA, et al. Surgical Trial Investigating Nocturnal Gastroesophageal Reflux and Sleep (STINGERS). Surg Endosc 2003; 17: 394–400.

41. Kerr P, Shoenut P, Millar T, et al. Nasal CPAP reduces gastroesophageal reflux in obstructive sleep apnea syndrome. Chest 1992; 101: 1539–44.

42. Kerr P, Shoenut JP, Steens RD, et al. Nasal CPAP: a new treatment for nocturnal gastroesophageal reflux. J Clin Gastroenterol 1993; 17: 276–80.

43. Insert Tawk manuscript Chest 2006; 130: 1003–8.

44. Graf KI, Karaus M, Heinemann S, et al. Gastroesophageal reflux in patients with sleep apnea syndrome. Z Gastroenterol 1995; 33: 689–93.

45. Tardif C, Denis P, Verdure-Poussin A, et al. Reflux gastro-oesophagien pendant le sommeil chez l'obese. Neurophysiol Clin 1988; 18: 323–32.

46. Ing AJ, Ngu MC, Breslin AB. Obstructive sleep apnea and gastroesophageal reflux. Am J Med 2000; 108(Suppl 4a):120S–5S.

47. Suganuma N, Shigedo Y, Adachi H, et al. Association of gastroesophageal reflux disease with weight gain and apnea, and their disturbance on sleep. Psychiatry Clin Neurosci 2001; 55: 255–6.

48. Green BT, Broughton WA, O'Connor JB. Marked improvement in nocturnal gastroesophageal reflux in a large cohort of patients with obstructive sleep apnea treated with continuous positive airway pressure. Arch Inter Med 2003; 163: 41–5.

49. Valipour A, Makker H, Hardy R, et al. Symptomatic gastroesophageal reflux in subjects with a breathing sleep disorder. Chest 2002; 121: 1748–53.

50. Senior BA, Khan M, Schwimmer C, Rosenthan L, Benninger M. Gastroesophageal reflux and obstructive sleep apnea. Laryngoscope 2001; 111: 2144–6.

51. Shoenut JP, Kerr P, Micfikier AB, Yamashiro Y, Kryger M. The effect of nasal CPAP on nocturnal reflux in patients with aperistaltic esophagus. Chest 1994; 106: 738–41.

52. Vitale GC, Cheadle WG, Patel B, et al. The effect of alcohol on nocturnal gastroesophageal reflux. JAMA 1987; 258: 2077–9.

53. Orr WC, Robinson MG, Rundell OH. The effect of hypnotic drugs on acid clearance during sleep. Gastroenterology 1985; 88: 1526.

54. Kellow JE, Gill RG, Wingate DL. Prolonged ambulant recordings of small bowel motility demonstrate abnormalities in the irritable bowel syndrome. Gastroenterology 1990; 98: 1208–18.

55. Kumar D, Thompson PD, Wingate DL, et al. Abnormal REM sleep in the irritable bowel syndrome. Gastroenterology 1992; 103: 12–17.

56. Goldsmith G, Levin JS. Effect of sleep quality on symptoms of irritable bowel syndrome. Dig Dis Sci 1993; 38: 1809–14.

57. Wingate D. An association between poor sleep quality and the severity of IBS symptoms. Dig Dis Sci 1994; 39: 2350–1.

58. David D, Mertz H, Fefer L, et al. Sleep and duodenal motor activity in patients with severe non-ulcer dyspepsia. Gut 1994; 35: 916–25.

59. Fass R, Fullerton S, Tung S, et al. Sleep disturbances in clinic patients with functional bowel disorders. Am J Gastroenterol 2000; 95: 1195–2000.

60. Heitkemper M, Charman AB, Shaver J, et al. Self-report and polysomnographic measures of sleep in women with irritable bowel syndrome. Nurs Res 1998; 47: 270–7.

61. Elsenbruch S, Harnish MJ, Orr WC. Subjective and objective sleep quality in irritable bowel syndrome. Am J Gastroenterol 1999; 94: 2447–52.

62. Rotem AY, Sperber AD, Krugliak P, et al. Polysomnographic and actigraphic evidence of sleep fragmentation in patients with irritable bowel syndrome. Sleep 2003; 26: 747–52.

63. Orr WC, Crowell MD, Lin B, et al. Sleep and gastric function in irritable bowel syndrome: derailing the brain–gut axis. Gut 1997; 41: 390–3.

64. Thompson JJ, Elsenbruch S, Harnish MJ, et al. Autonomic functioning during REM sleep differentiates IBS symptom subgroups. Am J Gastroenterol 2002; 97: 3147–53.

65. Elsenbruch S, Thompson JJ, Harnish MJ, et al. Behavioral and physiological sleep characteristics in women with irritable bowel syndrome. Am J Gastroenterol 2002; 97: 2306–14.

66. Bassotti G, Gaburri M, Imbimbo BP, et al. Alimentary tract and pancreas: colonic mass movements in idiopathic chronic constipation. Gut 1988; 29: 1173–9.

67. Ferrara A, Pemberton JH, Hanson RB. Motor responses of the sigmoid, rectum and anal canal in health and in patients with slow transit constipation (STC). Gastroenterology 1991; 100: A441.

68. Orkin BA, Soper NJ, Kelly KA, et al. Influence of sleep on anal sphincter pressure in health and after ileal pouch-anal anastomosis. Dis Colon Rectum 1992; 35: 137–44.

2

Sleep and respiratory disorders

Max Hirshkowitz, Amir Sharafkhaneh

INTRODUCTION

The respiratory system is designed to provide adequate oxygen (O_2) to and remove carbon dioxide (CO_2) from the circulation. In this manner, it helps maintain a chemical milieu that remains constant within a specified range. The system has two basic control systems. One is under voluntary control, while the other is involuntary and is regulated automatically. Autonomic regulation depends on chemical control systems and occurs during both sleep and wake. Although one does not have to remember to breathe when awake, an individual can override the automatic regulation and take a breath at will. On occasion, a person might overcompensate and hyperventilate, as can happen during a panic attack. By contrast, ventilation is solely under chemical control during sleep. Thus, respiratory function may be compromised during sleep when a primary respiratory disorder is present. In this chapter, we will briefly review the physiology of the respiratory system during transition from wake to sleep and during various stages of sleep. Then, we will review sleep disorders in various primary respiratory diseases.

Disorders of respiratory systems can be divided into disorders that primarily involve the airways and disorders that impose restriction on the lungs. The former include asthma, chronic obstructive pulmonary disease (COPD), cystic fibrosis, and bronchiectasis. The latter include fibrotic processes of the lung parenchyma, pleural and chest wall diseases, and respiratory pump disorders. Primary disorders of the respiratory system result in impaired ventilation and oxygenation.

RESPIRATION DURING THE TRANSITION FROM WAKEFULNESS TO SLEEP AND DURING SLEEP

Control of respiratory function

The major functions of the respiratory system are to provide the body with the required oxygen and remove carbon dioxide produced during metabolism. Additionally, the respiratory system is involved in acid–base regulation. Regulation of respiratory systems function operates through a negative feedback loop. For example, an elevated carbon dioxide level (hypercapnia) increases ventilation, while a low level (hypocapnia) decreases ventilation. Chemoreceptors and non-chemoreceptor sensory elements are involved in this regulation. The chemoreceptor component consists of peripheral and central chemoreceptors. The peripheral chemoreceptors in humans are located in the carotid body, and these receptors respond to changes in the oxygen and carbon dioxide levels in the blood. An estimated 30% of carbon dioxide chemosensitivity and 90–95% of hypoxic chemosensitivity are provided by the peripheral chemoreceptors.[1]

The carbon dioxide level is mainly regulated by central chemoreceptors that are located in the superficial layers of the ventral medulla.[2] Information from sensory receptors is relayed to the respiratory control center located in the medulla. Finally, the efferent arm of the feedback loop consists of motor output to the upper airways (especially the pharyngeal area), diaphragm, intercostals, and abdominal muscles through phrenic and intercostal nerves. In summary, the respiratory system under the control of the central respiratory control in the medulla oblongata sustains ventilation and maintains oxygen and carbon dioxide within a normal range in the blood and tissue environment. Automatic control of ventilation is maintained both during sleep and wake. However, the respiratory controller activity can be affected by behavioral and voluntary input from higher areas of the brain, including the cortex during the wakeful state and possibly during rapid eye movement (REM) sleep. With transition from wake to non-REM (NREM) and REM sleep, alveolar ventilation and consequently both carbon dioxide and oxygen concentrations change.

Control of ventilation

Ventilation is under automatic control during sleep. With initiation of sleep, minute ventilation falls about 0.5–1.5 liters per minute.[3,4] The minute ventilation change with sleep is due to reduced carbon dioxide production and oxygen uptake, absence of a wake stimulus, reduced chemosensitivity, and increased upper-airway resistance. Ventilatory response to hypercapnea diminishes as sleep deepens during NREM sleep. Similar reduction in minute ventilation is reported in REM sleep. Reduction of minute ventilation results in a 2–8 mmHg elevation of partial pressure of carbon dioxide ($PaCO_2$) elevation, an up to 10 mmHg reduction in the partial pressure of oxygen (PaO_2), and a less than 2% reduction in oxygen saturation (SaO_2).[4,5]

Upper-airway function

During the transition from wake to NREM and from NREM to REM sleep, upper-airway resistance increases. This increase is mainly in the palatal or hypopharyngeal areas,[6,7] is greater in snorers and obese subjects,[8,9] is highest during REM sleep,[10] and is induced by diminished upper-airway muscle phasic activity and loss of upper-airway protective reflexes.[8,11] With transition to REM sleep, the tonic activity of the upper-airway muscles diminishes further. Consequently, upper-airway occlusion is usually more prominent in REM sleep.

Lower-airway function

Lower-airway resistance increases in a circadian pattern, with the highest value in early morning hours in normal individuals.[12] Airways resistance follows a similar pattern in asthmatics, but with a higher amplitude.[13] The major mechanism of this change in airway caliber and increased resistance at night is a sleep-synchronized circadian rhythm largely due to changes in autonomic activity to the airways with increased cholinergic bronchoconstrictor tone and decreased non-adrenergic non-cholinergic bronchodilator function in the early-morning hours.[14]

Cough due to stimulation of airways is suppressed with sleep, and cough only occurs with arousals.[15] Thus, sleep may reduce mucociliary clearance.

Respiratory pump

Input to respiratory muscles is controlled by the respiratory center in the brainstem through phrenic and intercostal nerves. The phasic activity of the respiratory pump is state-dependent, and therefore diminishes with initiation of sleep. However, phasic activity of the diaphragm is maintained. With progression of sleep into REM, the tonic component of the respiratory muscle pump decreases. The changes in muscle activity result in increased upper-airway resistance and decreased minute ventilation.

Chemoreceptors

Hypoxic ventilatory response diminishes during sleep.[16] In NREM sleep, men show more reduction from wakefulness than women.[17] This difference is mainly due to higher ventilatory drive during wakefulness in men. With progression to REM sleep, the hypoxic ventilatory drive falls further in both men and women.[14]

Hypercapnic ventilatory response diminishes about 50% with transition from wakefulness to NREM sleep.[5,14] In REM sleep, the ventilatory response falls even further; therefore, the lowest ventilatory response to hypercapnia occurs during REM sleep.[5]

Overall, with transition from wakefulness to NREM sleep, the wake stimulus and voluntary control of ventilation are lost, leaving automatic control to prevail. In addition, carbon dioxide production and oxygen uptake diminish, upper-airway resistance increases, chemoreceptor response to hypercapnia and hypoxia falls, and operating lung volume decreases. Subsequently, $PaCO_2$ rises and PaO_2 falls. Combinations of these changes can produce respiratory instability and predispose to periodic breathing and obstruction of the upper airway during sleep. Loss of muscle tone with REM sleep makes the upper airway more prone to obstruction.

OBSTRUCTIVE AIRWAYS DISORDERS

Obstructive airways disorders may involve the upper or lower airways. Obstructive sleep apnea (OSA) is an example of upper-airway obstruction. Lower-airway obstructive disorders include asthma, COPD, cystic fibrosis, and bronchiectasis. Physiologically, obstructive disorders present with expiratory or inspiratory flow limitation that results in compromised ventilation and, in more severe cases, compromised oxygenation. Clinically, lower-airway obstructive disorders present as chronic dyspnea, cough, and sputum production. Further, episodes of rather acute worsening of symptoms or 'exacerbations' are frequently seen. Patients with obstructive airways disorders are predisposed to worsening in transition from wakefulness to sleep due to the effect of sleep on the control of breathing. Further, obstructive airways disorders are chronic diseases, and the disease itself or its treatment may result in disturbed sleep. In addition, exacerbations of the disease can further compromise the sleep.

Obstructive sleep apnea

OSA is characterized by collapse of the upper airways during sleep. The resultant cessations of breathing are called apneas if their duration is 10 seconds or longer in an adult. Increased inspiratory resistance can also produce episodes of hypopnea in which the airway narrows but does not fully collapse. These hypopnea episodes are associated with decreased tidal volume and increasing respiratory effort; however, what makes them pathophysiologic is their association with oxyhemoglobin desaturations and/or a respiratory effort-related arousal. Repeated hypoxemia or continual brief arousals fragmenting sleep produce a host of other problems by interfering with the sleep process and thereby undermining its functions.

Table 2.1 lists some of the major risk factors for and some of the common symptoms of OSA.

Table 2.1 Risk factors and symptoms of OSA	
Risk factors	*Common symptoms*
Obesity	Sleepiness, tiredness, or exhaustion
Micrognathia or retrognathia	Loud snoring with frequent awakenings
Large neck circumference	Awakening with gasping and/or choking
Nasal allergies and stuffiness	Awakening unrefreshed
Middle-age or older	Nocturia
Being male	Morning headache
Bed-partner or other witnessed sleep apnea	Falls asleep while driving or at stop lights

Most of these features are more sensitive than specific; however, pretest probability for sleep apnea is high when an excessively sleepy patient snores loudly, awakens gasping or choking, has witnessed cessation of breathing, and falls asleep when driving or at stop lights.

Table 2.2 shows some of the consequences of OSA. It is interesting to note that many consequences of OSA are also common psychosomatic symptoms. In this case, however, the etiology is well documented and the problem diminishes or disappears when the sleep-disordered breathing is treated.

Table 2.3 shows the odds ratio for cardiovascular and cerebrovascular disease based on our comparison

of the 98 735 patients diagnosed with sleep apnea with the remaining 3 548 593 cases in the US Department of Veteran Affairs Beneficiaries Database.[18]

Positive airway pressure therapy is the first-line treatment for most patients with OSA. Positive airway pressure devices come in four varieties; the most common is called continuous positive airway pressure (CPAP). CPAP provides a constant airflow that is used to 'pneumatically splint' the vulnerable portions of the nasopharyngeal airway by having air blown into the patient's nose and/or mouth using a nasal or full-face mask, nasal pillows, or nasal prongs. A second type called bilevel positive airway pressure (BPAP) provides two pressure levels – one during inhalation and a lower one during exhalation. The pressure drop during exhalation increases comfort for patients with difficulty exhaling against the incoming airflow. The third type of device is called automatic self-adjusting positive airway pressure (APAP). As the name suggests, APAP uses computer-controlled flow variations to determine and supply optimal pressure. Finally, non-invasive positive-pressure ventilation (NIPPV) devices represent a fourth type of positive pressure device. These machines are much like BPAP; however, the rate of oscillation between the two pressures is specified. Thus, NIPPV is designed to provide ventilatory assist.

CPAP for treating patients with OSA was initially described by Sullivan et al.[19] In their report, five patients with severe OSA were treated

---

Table 2.2   Clinical features associated with and consequences of OSA

- Difficulty staying awake in non-stimulating situations
- Attention deficit
- Cognitive deterioration
- Irritability and impaired coping mechanisms
- Depressed mood
- Anxiety
- Aches and pains
- Impaired eye–hand coordination
- Erectile dysfunction
- Diminished quality of life

Table 2.3   Cardiovascular and cerebrovascular comorbidities in obstructive sleep apnea[18]

Comorbidity	Odds ratio	95% confidence interval
Hypertension	2.34	2.31–2.37
Diabetes	2.52	2.48–2.55
Heart failure	3.40	3.34–3.46
Cardiovascular disease	1.84	1.82–1.87
Cerebrovascular accident	1.57	1.52–1.61

with CPAP applied through the nares. Low pressure levels (ranging from 4.5–10 cmH$_2$O) completely prevented upper-airway occlusion, allowing uninterrupted sleep.

Overall, CPAP is extremely safe and very effective in patients with OSA. Furthermore, the beneficial effects of CPAP are well sustained over time. Patients receiving CPAP and conservative therapy (sleep hygiene and weight loss) compared with those receiving only conservative therapy[20] had decreased sleepiness and improved quality-of-life measures. Similarly, sleepiness and quality of life improved in the active treatment group of a randomized, double-blind, placebo-controlled study of CPAP versus subtherapeutic CPAP.[21] However, negative study results have also been reported.[22]

A cause-and-effect relationship has been suggested between OSA and systemic hypertension. In a pioneering study, Lavie et al[23] observed a linear increase in blood pressure and the number of patients with hypertension as a function of severity of sleep apnea (indexed by the apnea + hypopnea index). Other studies also link CPAP therapy with a reduction in blood pressure.[24-26] However, not all investigators have reported similar findings, and some have argued that hypertension in OSA is more closely linked to weight loss than to CPAP therapy. Evidence for this contention can be derived from a study of 60 hypertensive patients with OSA, in which hypertension severity decreased in 40% of patients in the combined nasal CPAP and weight-loss group, in 58% of patients in the weight-loss-only group, in 29% of patients in the nasal-CPAP-only group, and in 6% of the patients in the no-treatment group.[27]

Mortality studies are difficult to design, perform, control, and validate. Nonetheless, in their landmark study, He et al[28] found greater mortality in patients with an apnea index of 20 or more compared with those with an apnea index less than 20 in a sample of 385 cases in a longitudinal database. The apnea-related mortality increase was reversed by treatment with CPAP. These data underscore the serious, potentially life-threatening nature of OSA and the benefit of effective management with positive airway pressure therapy.

Asthma

Asthma, an inflammatory disease of the airways, affects at least 5% of the population.[29] Clinically, asthma presents with shortness of breath and wheezing. Asthmatic patients may have worsening symptoms and airflow limitations during sleep due to circadian variations in airway caliber. The airflow may fall as much as 50% in some asthmatics, who are called 'morning dippers'.[30] This morning dipping may predict a subgroup of asthmatics with higher mortality.[31] Nocturnal asthma is associated with poor quality of life and increased mortality.[32] Up to 75% of asthmatics awaken weekly with symptoms of their disease, and about half of these awaken nightly.[33] In fact, asthma symptoms at night are used to rate the severity of asthma and to guide management decisions.

Nocturnal worsening of airflow results in sleep interruption and daytime tiredness, decreased sleep efficiency and total sleep time, increased awakening during sleep, and impaired cognitive function. Hypoxemia associated with the nocturnal bronchoconstrictions in stable asthmatics is not severe and is in the range of 85–90.[34]

Effective treatment of asthma with anti-inflammatory agents and bronchodilators relieves night-time symptoms and improves sleep efficiency.[35] Inhaled corticosteroids are one of the main agents used in treatment of asthma. They reduce awakening from sleep.[36] Long-acting bronchodilators such as salmeterol and formoterol also improve sleep in patients with asthma.[37]

Chronic obstructive pulmonary disease (COPD)

COPD is a major public health problem and is a leading cause of morbidity and mortality all over the world. It is currently the fourth leading cause of death and among the top 10 leading causes of disability in the USA. Recent statistics from the Third National Health and Nutrition Examination Survey reveal that COPD leads annually to 8 million physician office and hospital outpatient visits,

1.5 million emergency department visits, and 726 000 hospitalizations. It is often underdiagnosed and undertreated. As with many other chronic diseases, a multimodal approach to the management of COPD has been advocated by recently published evidence-based guidelines, including the position paper on standards for the diagnosis and treatment of patients with COPD from the American Thoracic Society and European Respiratory Society[38] and the GOLD international guidelines.[39]

Clinically, COPD patients suffer from dyspnea, cough, and sputum production. In the more advanced form of the disease, patients suffer from daytime, nocturnal, or exercise-induced hypoxia. This hypoxia may result in right-side heart failure. Pathologically, COPD is characterized by destruction of airspaces, fibrosis of small-airway walls, and occlusion of small airways with inflammatory mucus. Physiologically, COPD is characterized by expiratory flow limitation that is not fully reversible.

Sleep disorders such as insomnia, sleep apnea with a greater severity of arterial oxygen desaturation, restless leg syndrome, nightmares, and daytime sleepiness are more common in patients with COPD, with close to 50% reporting such problems.[40,41] Polysomnography shows sleep fragmentation with frequent arousals and diminished sleep-wave and REM sleep.[42]

Insomnia

More than 50% of COPD patients complain of insomnia and more than 25% report daytime sleepiness.[43] Sleep in COPD patients is characterized by longer sleep-onset latency, frequent arousals and awakenings, frequent sleep-stage shifts, and lower sleep efficiency.[44] Disturbed sleep in COPD patients is associated with the severity of airflow obstruction and decreased quality of life. Sleep disturbances also relate to poor control of disease-related symptoms and side-effects of some of the medications used for the management of COPD.

Treatment options for the treatment of insomnia in COPD patients need careful consideration. Hypnotics may have adverse effects for patients with

moderate to severe COPD. Triazolam has no obvious effect on respiration when used in single doses for patients with an awake supine $SaO_2 \geq 90\%$ and no carbon dioxide retention ($PaCO_2 \leq 45\,mmHg$). In contrast, zolpidem was tested in COPD patients with more severe lung function abnormality.[45] Thus, if the patient has supine $SaO_2 \leq 90\%$, zolpidem is clearly the first choice; and triazolam and other benzodiazepines must be used with extreme caution. Further, cognitive–behavioral therapy may be as effective as sedatives, and should be tried as first-line therapy in patients with compromised respiratory function.[46]

Nocturnal desaturations

The prevalence of sleep apnea in COPD patients does not differ from that in the non-COPD population.[47] However, COPD patients with sleep apnea have more profound oxygen desaturation compared with patients with sleep apnea and no COPD. Further, arterial oxygen desaturations during sleep are reported in COPD patients without sleep apnea. The nocturnal desaturation is mainly due to the effect of sleep-related hypoventilation. However, in many COPD patients, PaO_2 is already in the steep portion of the oxyhemoglobin dissociation curve, and sleep-induced hypoventilation results in marked reduction of arterial saturation.[48,49] In addition, decreased functional residual capacity with transition to sleep may aggravate ventilation/perfusion mismatch and result in greater oxygen desaturation. Nocturnal hypoxia is associated with increased daytime and nocturnal pulmonary artery pressure.[50] Further, nocturnal hypoxemia may increase mortality, especially during acute exacerbations of COPD.[51,52]

In COPD patients with isolated nocturnal oxygen desaturations, nocturnal oxygen therapy is recommended when complications of hypoxemia such as polycythemia and cor pulmonale are present.[53] However, optimization of medical treatment with theophylline and anticholinergic agents such as ipratropium and tiotropium can improve oxygenation.[54–56]

SUMMARY

Sleep is clearly a stimulus for changes in the respiratory system. Acting through autonomic, homeostatic, and circadian mechanisms, dysfunctions of sleep, as well as abnormalities within the respiratory system, can lead to or exacerbate sleep disturbance. Manifestations of respiratory-related sleep disturbances share many symptoms with a wide variety of psychosomatic illnesses. While OSA is the most common sleep disorder within this grouping, nocturnal asthma and COPD are important and widespread. More research is needed to better elucidate the mechanisms involved and how sleep contributes to and is altered by respiratory disorders.

REFERENCES

1. Honda Y, Tani H. Chemical control of breathing. In: Altose MD, Kawakami Y, eds. Control of Breathing in Health and Disease. New York: Marcel Dekker, 1999: 41–87.
2. Mitchell RA. Respiratory chemosensitivity in the medulla oblongata. J Physiol 1969; 202: 3P–4P.
3. Hudgel DW, Martin RJ, Johnson B, Hill P. Mechanics of the respiratory system and breathing pattern during sleep in normal humans. J Appl Physiol 1984; 56: 133–7.
4. Chokroverty S. Physiologic changes in sleep. In: Chokroverty S, ed. Sleep Disorders Medicine, Basic Science, Technical Considerations, and Clinical Aspects, 2nd edn. Boston, MA: Butterworth Heinemann, 1999: 95–126.
5. Douglas NJ, White DP, Pickett CK, Weil JV, Zwillich CW. Respiration during sleep in normal man. Thorax 1982; 37: 840–4.
6. Lopes JM, Tabachnik E, Muller NL, Levison H, Bryan AC. Total airway resistance and respiratory muscle activity during sleep. J Appl Physiol 1983; 54: 773–7.
7. Hudgel DW, Hendricks C. Palate and hypopharynx – sites of inspiratory narrowing of the upper airway during sleep. Am Rev Respir Dis 1988; 138: 1542–7.
8. Dempsey JA, Smith CA, Harms CA, Chow C, Saupe KW. Sleep-induced breathing instability. Sleep 1996; 19: 236–47.
9. Skatrud JB, Dempsey JA. Airway resistance and respiratory muscle function in snorers during NREM sleep. J Appl Physiol 1985; 59: 328–35.
10. Orem J, Lydic R. Upper airway function during sleep and wakefulness: experimental studies on normal and anesthetized cats. Sleep 1978; 1: 49–68.
11. Krieger J. Respiratory physiology: breathing in normal subjects. In: Kryger MH, Roth T, Dement WC, eds. Principles and Practice of Sleep Medicine, 3rd edn. Philadelphia, PA: WB Saunders, 2000: 229–41.
12. Lewinsohn HC, Capel LH, Smart J. Changes in forced expiratory volumes throughout the day. BMJ 1960; vol I(5171): 462–4.
13. Hetzel MR, Clark TJ. Comparison of normal and asthmatic circadian rhythms in peak expiratory flow rate. Thorax 1980; 35: 732–8.
14. Douglas NJ. Asthma. In: Kryger MH, Roth T, Dement WC, eds. Principles and Practice of Sleep Medicine, 3rd edn. Philadelphia, PA: WB Saunders, 2000: 955–64.
15. Douglas NJ. Respiratory physiology: control of ventilation. In: Kryger MH, Roth T, Dement WC, eds. Principles and Practice of Sleep Medicine, 3rd edn. Philadelphia, PA: WB Saunders, 2000: 221–8.
16. Hedemark LL, Kronenberg RS. Ventilatory and heart rate responses to hypoxia and hypercapnia during sleep in adults. J Appl Physiol 1982; 53: 307–12.
17. White DP, Douglas NJ, Pickett CK, Weil JV, Zwillich CW. Hypoxic ventilatory response during sleep in normal premenopausal women. Am Rev Respir Dis 1982; 126: 530–3.
18. Sharafkhaneh A, Richardson P, Hirshkowitz M. Sleep apnea in a high risk population: a study of Veterans Health Administration beneficiaries. Sleep Med 2004; 5: 345–50.
19. Sullivan CE, Issa FG, Berthon-Jones M, Eves L. Reversal of obstructive sleep apnoea by continuous positive airway pressure applied through the nares. Lancet 1981; i: 862–5.
20. Ballester E, Badia JR, Hernandez L, et al. Evidence of the effectiveness of continuous positive airway pressure in the treatment of sleep apnea/hypopnea syndrome. Am J Respir Crit Care Med 1999; 159: 495–501.
21. Jenkinson C, Davies RJ, Mullins R, Stradling JR. Comparison of therapeutic and subtherapeutic nasal continuous positive airway pressure for obstructive sleep apnoea: a randomised prospective parallel trial. Lancet 1999; 353: 2100–5.
22. Barnes M, Houston D, Worsnop CJ, et al. A randomized controlled trial of continuous positive airway pressure in mild obstructive sleep apnea. Am J Respir Crit Care Med 2002; 165: 773–80.

23. Lavie P, Herer P, Hoffstein V. Obstructive sleep apnoea syndrome as a risk factor for hypertension: population study. BMJ 2000; 320: 479–82.

24. Faccenda JF, Mackay TW, Boon NA, Douglas NJ. Randomized placebo-controlled trial of continuous positive airway pressure on blood pressure in the sleep apnea-hypopnea syndrome. Am J Respir Crit Care Med 2001; 163: 344–8.

25. Mayer J, Becker H, Brandenburg U, et al. Blood pressure and sleep apnea: results of long-term nasal continuous positive airway pressure therapy. Cardiology 1991; 79: 84–92.

26. Akashiba T, Minemura H, Yamamoto H, et al. Nasal continuous positive airway pressure changes blood pressure "non-dippers" to 'dippers' in patients with obstructive sleep apnea. Sleep 1999; 22: 849–53.

27. Rauscher H, Formanek D, Popp W, Zwick H. Nasal CPAP and weight loss in hypertensive patients with obstructive sleep apnoea. Thorax 1993; 48: 529–33.

28. He J, Kryger MH, Zorick FJ, Conway W, Roth T. Mortality and apnea index in obstructive sleep apnea. Experience in 385 male patients. Chest 1988; 94: 9–14.

29. Anon. Improving care and quality of life for all asthma patients. Qual Lett Health Lead 2001; 13: 2–13.

30. Douglas NJ. Asthma at night. Clin Chest Med 1985; 6: 663–74.

31. Bateman JR, Clarke SW. Sudden death in asthma. Thorax 1979; 34: 40–4.

32. Holimon TD, Chafin CC, Self TH. Nocturnal asthma uncontrolled by inhaled corticosteroids: theophylline or long-acting β_2 agonists? Drugs 2001; 61: 391–418.

33. Turner-Warwick M. Epidemiology of nocturnal asthma. Am J Med 1988; 85: 6–8.

34. Catterall JR, Douglas NJ, Calverley PM, et al. Irregular breathing and hypoxaemia during sleep in chronic stable asthma. Lancet 1982; i: 301–4.

35. D'Alonzo GE, Ciccolella DE. Nocturnal asthma: physiologic determinants and current therapeutic approaches. Curr Opin Pulm Med 1996; 2: 48–59.

36. Meltzer EO, Lockey RF, Friedman BF, et al. Efficacy and safety of low-dose fluticasone propionate compared with montelukast for maintenance treatment of persistent asthma. Mayo Clin Proc 2002; 77: 437–45.

37. Campbell LM, Anderson TJ, Parashchak MR, et al. A comparison of the efficacy of long-acting β_2-agonists: eformoterol via Turbohaler and salmeterol via pressurized metered dose inhaler or Accuhaler, in mild to moderate asthmatics. Force Research Group. Respir Med 1999; 93: 236–44.

38. Celli BR, MacNee W; ATS/ERS Task Force. Standards for the diagnosis and treatment of patients with COPD: a summary of the ATS/ERS position paper. Eur Respir J 2004; 23: 932–46.

39. Pauwels RA, Buist AS, Ma P, et al. Global strategy for the diagnosis, management, and prevention of chronic obstructive pulmonary disease: National Heart, Lung, and Blood Institute and World Health Organization Global Initiative for Chronic Obstructive Lung Disease (GOLD): Executive summary. Am J Respir Crit Care Med 2001; 46: 798–825.

40. George CF, Bayliff CD. Management of insomnia in patients with chronic obstructive pulmonary disease. Drugs 2003; 63: 379–87.

41. Kutty K. Sleep and chronic obstructive pulmonary disease. Curr Opin Pulm Med 2004; 10: 104–12.

42. Cormick W, Olson LG, Hensley MJ, Saunders NA. Nocturnal hypoxaemia and quality of sleep in patients with chronic obstructive lung disease. Thorax 1986; 41: 846–54.

43. Klink M, Quan SF. Prevalence of reported sleep disturbances in a general adult population and their relationship to obstructive airways diseases. Chest 1987; 91: 540–6.

44. George CF, Bayliff CD. Management of insomnia in patients with chronic obstructive pulmonary disease. Drugs 2003; 63: 379–87.

45. Girault C, Muir JF, Mihaltan F, et al. Effects of repeated administration of zolpidem on sleep, diurnal and nocturnal respiratory function, vigilance, and physical performance in patients with COPD. Chest 1996; 110: 1203–11.

46. Jacobs GD, Pace-Schott EF, Stickgold R, Otto MW. Cognitive behavior therapy and pharmacotherapy for insomnia: a randomized controlled trial and direct comparison. Arch Intern Med 2004; 164: 1888–96.

47. Sanders MH, Newman AB, Haggerty CL, et al. Sleep and sleep-disordered breathing in adults with predominantly mild obstructive airway disease. Am J Respir Crit Care Med 2003; 167: 7–14.

48. Hudgel DW, Martin RJ, Capehart M, Johnson B, Hill P. Contribution of hypoventilation to sleep oxygen desaturation in chronic obstructive pulmonary disease. J Appl Physiol 1983; 55: 669–77.

49. Phillips B, Cooper K, Burke T. The effect of sleep loss of breathing in chronic obstructive pulmonary disease. Chest 1987; 91: 29–32.

50. Levi-Valensi P, Weitzenblum E, Rida A, et al. Sleep-related oxygen desaturation and daytime pulmonary hemodynamics in COPD patients. Eur Respir J 1992; 5: 301–7.

51. Fletcher E, Miller J, Divine G, Fletcher J, Miller T. Nocturnal oxyhemoglobin desaturations in COPD patients with arterial oxygen tensions above 60 mmHg. Chest 1987; 92: 604–8.

52. Connaughton JJ, Caterall JR, Elton RA, Stradling JR, Douglas NJ. Do sleep studies contribute to the management of patients with severe chronic obstructive pulmonary disease? Am Rev Respir Dis 1988; 138: 341–4.

53. Celli BR, MacNee W. ATS/ERS Task Force. Standards for the diagnosis and treatment of patients with COPD: a summary of the ATS/ERS position paper. Eur Respir J 2004; 23: 932–46.

54. Mulloy E, McNicholas WT. Theophylline improves gas exchange during rest, exercise and sleep in severe chronic obstructive pulmonary disease. Am Rev Respir Dis 1993; 148: 1030–6.

55. Martin RJ, Bucher BL, Smith P, et al. Effect of ipratropium bromide treatment on oxygen saturation and sleep quality in COPD. Chest 1999; 115: 1338–45.

56. McNicholas WT, Calverley PMA, Edwards C, Lee A. Effects of anticholinergic therapy (Tiotropium) on REM-related desaturation and sleep quality in patients with COPD. Am J Respir Crit Care Med 2001; 163(Suppl): A281.

3

Sleep and coronary artery disease

Neomi Shah, Vahid Mohsenin

INTRODUCTION

Coronary artery disease is highly prevalent and claims many lives. Sleep is a part of everybody's life, and – contrary to what is often thought – it is actually an active, organized process. Sleep-related breathing disorders have been linked to coronary artery disease (CAD). In this chapter, we will see how normal sleep affects the heart, specifically the coronary circulation. We will also discuss the effects of normal sleep and sleep-related breathing disorders, specifically obstructive sleep apnea (OSA), on the coronary circulation and cardiovascular system. We will describe several mechanisms by which sleep-related breathing disorders can cause atherosclerosis and contribute to CAD. Finally, the treatment of sleep-related breathing disorders and its impact on CAD-related morbidity and mortality will be addressed.

CORONARY CIRCULATION

The energy requirements of the human heart are greater than those of any other organ in the body. The myocardium normally extracts approximately 75% of the delivered arterial oxygen, in contrast to the 25% removed by most other organs, and is largely flow-dependent for its oxygen supply.[1] Unlike blood flow in other organs, arterial flow is exclusively diastolic and venous outflow is systolic.

Coronary microvessels are surrounded by myocytes, which contract and relax and exert periodic mechanical influences on coronary vessels and flows. Direct observation of deeper intramyocardial microvessels in beating porcine or canine left ventricles revealed compression of arterioles and venules by 10–20% during systole, while the subepicardial arteriolar diameter changed little.[2,3] Coronary blood flow is a direct function of blood pressure and is inversely related to small-vessel resistance. Under physiologic conditions, decreases in coronary vascular resistance and increases in coronary flow and oxygen consumption are regulated precisely to meet the metabolic demands of the myocardium.[4] In general, the amount of work that the myocardium does determines the amount of blood flow through it. The exact nature of the link between work and flow is not known. It seems to be a local mechanism, since it is still seen after the heart is completely denervated. Mechanisms of coronary flow regulation are based on the integration of many metabolic and neurohumoral factors: adenosine triphosphate (ATP)-sensitive potassium channels (K_{ATP}), endothelium-derived hyperpolarizing factor (EDHF), nitric oxide (NO), carbon dioxide, hydrogen ions, oxygen, norepinephrine (noradrenaline), and acetylcholine.[5] Local tissue hypoxia is the most important stimulus to increase the coronary blood flow.[6] It has also been suggested that the release of adenosine (a potent coronary vasodilator) from the breakdown of adenine nucleotides may represent the final pathway through which coronary blood flow is regulated.[5] When the oxygen content of the coronary arterial blood is reduced, an acceleration in coronary blood flow occurs. In animals, when the oxygen content decreased from 18 to 4 vol%, coronary blood flow increased fivefold without any great change in cardiac work. In fact, Eckenhoff[7] showed that there is an excellent correlation between myocardial oxygen consumption and coronary blood flow, and based on his animal studies, he concluded that the metabolic demands of the heart, of which, that for oxygen is the most important, is the regulating determinant of coronary flow.

The coronary arterial system is densely innervated with sympathetic and parasympathetic nervous systems and non-adrenergic/non-cholinergic nerves. Neurotransmitters released from nervous tissues and wide variety of humoral substances significantly affect microvascular tone.[5] If the

sympathetic nerves to the heart are stimulated, the heart rate, strength of ventricular contractility, and coronary blood flow increase. Similarly, the direct effects of vagal stimulation and exogenous acetylcholine increase the coronary flow conductance.[8] The imposition of these neurohumoral factors on coronary microvascular tone, in addition to myogenic, flow-induced, and local metabolic controls, participate in integrating the coronary vascular resistance to determine the supply of oxygen and nutrition to the myocardium (Figure 3.1).[5]

Cardiovascular responses differ significantly between the state of wakefulness and that of sleep. There are numerous studies that focus on the effects of sleep on the overall cardiovascular system; however, there are very limited data on the consequences of sleep on the coronary circulation. Kirby et al[9] observed sizable episodic surges in heart rate and coronary blood flow with corresponding decreases in coronary vascular resistance during

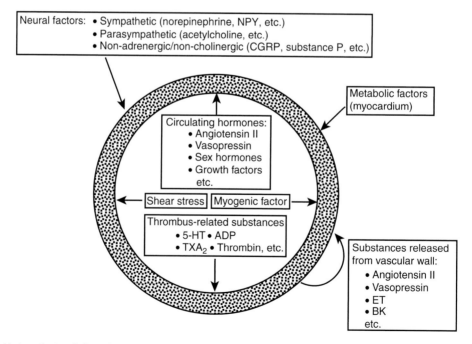

Figure 3.1 Various factors influencing coronary microvascular tone. NPY, neuropeptide Y; CGRP, calcitonin gene-related peptide; 5-HT, 5-hydroxytryptamine (serotonin); ADP, adenosine diphosphate; TXA₂, thromboxane A₂; ET, endothelin; BK, bradykinin (reprinted from Pharmacological Therapy, Vol 86, Komara T, Kanatsuka H, Shirato K, Coronary microcirculation: physiology and pharmacology, pp 217–61, Copyright 2000, with permission from Elsevier)[5]

rapid eye movement (REM) sleep in dogs. There were no appreciable changes in mean arterial blood pressure. In contrast, during slow-wave sleep, there were moderate but significant reductions in heart rate, 9% decreases in left coronary blood flow, and increases in coronary vascular resistance. These surges were eliminated by stellectomy, indicating that they were mediated by the sympathetic nervous system. Similarly, decreases in mean arterial pressure, total peripheral resistance, and coronary vascular resistance in REM sleep were observed in a chronically instrumented pig. The decreases were eliminated by α-adrenergic blockade.[10] The phasic portion of REM sleep is associated with periods of sinus tachycardia. During the transition from non-REM (NREM) to REM sleep, increases in vagal tone can lead to respiratory sinus arrhythmias and observed sinus pauses in cardiac rhythm that are subsequently followed by increases in coronary blood flow.[11]

EFFECT OF SLEEP ON THE CARDIOVASCULAR SYSTEM

Reliable data on blood pressure levels during sleep have so far been documented in seven species, including humans. A small reduction in blood pressure is often described during synchronized (slow-wave) sleep. During desynchronized (REM) sleep, the blood pressure undergoes frequent marked oscillations, sometimes falling below the levels measured during synchronized sleep and at other times rising to levels above waking values. During REM sleep, blood pressure can reach the lowest levels of the circadian cycle, in adults and infants. The difference in the blood pressure responses, particularly during REM sleep, is probably a consequence of the relative amounts of tonic and phasic periods that occur.[12]

It has been shown that the slow-wave stages of NREM sleep are accompanied by hypotension, bradycardia, and a reduction in cardiac output and systemic vascular resistance. It has also been shown that the bradycardia is due mainly to an increase in vagal activation, whereas the hypotension is due to a reduction in sympathetic vasomotor tone, since surgical sympathectomy markedly attenuates the drop in blood pressure.[13] In addition, there is evidence suggesting that the cardiovascular influence of sleep is more complex than a generalized inhibition of the sympathetic nervous system. The most striking example is REM sleep, during which sympathetic drive decreases in the splanchnic and renal circulation but increases in skeletal muscle blood vessels. Furthermore, an initial pronounced decrease in blood pressure is interrupted by large transient increases in blood pressure and heart rate, during which sympathetic vasoconstriction in muscle further increases.[14]

Somers et al[15] confirmed that in humans slow-wave sleep causes hypotension and bradycardia and that both changes become more pronounced as sleep progresses from its minimal to its maximal slow-wave pattern (from stage 1 to stage 4 NREM). They also confirmed that during REM sleep, large transient increases in blood pressure reverse the hypotension that characterizes the preceding slow-wave stages and raise the mean blood pressure to levels observed during wakefulness. Further, by direct recording of sympathetic nerve traffic for several hours, these investigators provided solid evidence that sympathetic activity is reduced by more than half from wakefulness to stage 4 NREM sleep, but increases to levels above waking values during REM sleep. These data strongly suggest a primary role for the sympathetic nervous system in the generation of both the inhibitory and the excitatory cardiovascular phenomena of sleep.[6]

Measurements of cardiac output during wakefulness and sleep have been performed in cats[16] and humans,[17] and both studies have shown a reduction in cardiac output during sleep, although the results have not been consistent.[18] In humans, the cardiac output decreased by approximately 10%, with a decrease of 745 ml/min in NREM sleep from a mean cardiac output of 7639 ml/min.

PREVALENCE OF CAD IN SLEEP-DISORDERED BREATHING

There is a high prevalence of sleep-related breathing disorders in patients with CAD. This association is supported by several case–control and cross-sectional epidemiologic studies. Mooe et al[19,20] have shown that the prevalence of sleep-related breathing disorders is high in both men and women with known CAD. They examined 142 men with angina and angiographically verified CAD for the occurrence of sleep apnea, and found that men with CAD had a high occurrence of sleep-related breathing disorders. Thirty seven percent of the men in their study had an apnea–hypopnea index (AHI, events/hour slept) ≥ 10. Similarly, in a case–control study of women with CAD, they found that 54% had AHI ≥ 5 or more, and 30% had AHI ≥ 10. They also reported that sleep apnea was a significant predictor of CAD after adjustment for age, body mass index, hypertension, smoking habits, and diabetes. Schafer et al[21] also reported a high prevalence (31%) of OSA in patients with angiographically proven CAD. However, limited data have been published on the rate of CAD as a complication in patients with OSA. Maekawa et al[22] investigated the prevalence of CAD (documented by cardiac stress test, radionuclide myocardial scintigraphy, and/or coronary angiography) in 386 subjects suspected of OSA with heavy snoring. They defined OSA as an AHI ≥ 10, and found the prevalence of CAD among these patients with untreated OSA to be 23.8%. In a prospective cohort study conducted in Sweden, 408 patients aged 70 years or younger with verified CAD were followed for a median period of 5.1 years. Those with AHI ≥ 10 had a risk ratio of 1.62 (95% confidence interval (CI) 1.09–2.41; $p = 0.017$) for composite endpoint of death, cerebrovascular events, and myocardial infarction compared with the comparison group with AHI < 10.[23] The results of these studies show that sleep-related breathing disorders in patients with CAD are associated with worse long-term outcome. Interestingly, there appears to be a circadian effect on CAD-related mortality. Reports in the world literature going back as far as 1960 have described a circadian periodicity in the onset of myocardial infarction, and have documented a peak incidence in the hours between 6 AM and noon[24] and a nadir from midnight to 6 AM. The risk of sudden death from cardiac causes in the general population is significantly greater during the morning hours after waking (i.e., from 6 AM to noon) than during the other 6-hour intervals of the day.[25] However, patients with OSA have a significant alteration in this well-established day–night pattern of sudden death from cardiac causes evident in the general population. In a study by Gami et al,[26] a marked nocturnal peak in sudden death from cardiac causes was observed in OSA patients. In more than half of OSA patients, sudden death from cardiac causes occurred between 10 PM and 6 AM. In contrast, the persons without OSA had a day–night pattern of sudden death from cardiac causes very similar to that in the general population, with a peak in sudden death from cardiac causes from 6 AM to noon. The presumed mechanism is that the process begins with the development of a vulnerable atherosclerotic plaque, which may become disrupted during sleep and after rising, due to alterations in blood pressure, as described previously, creating shearing forces within the coronary blood vessels and promoting a thrombogenic focus.[27]

EFFECT OF SLEEP APNEA ON CORONARY BLOOD FLOW AND CARDIOVASCULAR SYSTEM

The impact of sleep on the cardiovascular system is significantly altered during OSA. Patients with OSA are exposed to repetitive episodes of obstructed breathing during sleep. While the pathophysiology of the obstruction is not well delineated, the consequences have been studied extensively. As a result of obstructed breathing, patients with sleep apnea experience repeated and prolonged episodes of arterial oxygen desaturation and carbon dioxide retention. During recurrent apneas, hypoxemia and retained carbon dioxide can stimulate chemoreceptors, leading to an increase in sympathetic tone. The duration of apnea and the level of oxygen desaturation are key determinants in sympathetic activation. The sympathetic tone increases progressively during the obstructive event, reaching its peak after arousal. On release of the airway obstruction and resumption of breathing, increased cardiac output, together with the vasoconstricted peripheral vasculature, result in marked increases in blood pressure. In a subject who is normotensive during wakefulness, the blood pressure surge at the end of the apneic event can reach levels as high as 250/110 mmHg. Other factors, such as increased muscle tone and arousal, may also contribute to the increased blood pressure at the end of apnea.[28,29] Oxyhemoglobin saturation decreases during apnea and recovers only slowly after apnea termination. Therefore, the sudden increase in cardiac output at arousal with increased myocardial oxygen demand is met with low oxygen delivery to the myocardium and increased risk of cardiac ischemia. Thus, we see that there are nocturnal variations in the sympathetic activity during hypoxic states seen during obstructive apneas. In addition to this nocturnal sympathetic drive in OSA, there is also evidence of persistence of this heightened sympathetic drive during awake normoxic conditions in patients with OSA.[30]

Norepinephrine (noradrenaline) is the primary neurotransmitter for the postganglionic sympathetic nervous system. Baylor et al[31] analyzed plasma samples from patients who were highly suspected of sleep apnea by history, over a 5.5-hour sleeping period, and found that as the oxygen desaturation fell cyclically, the variability in plasma norepinephrine increased and that patients with the most severe degree of cyclic desaturation had the greatest variability in plasma norepinephrine levels. The surges in norepinephrine concentrations were greatest in those with the greatest desaturations. It should also be noted that changes in norepinephrine levels across the night are related to the degree of cyclic oxygen desaturation and not to the AHI. It has also been suggested that plasma epinephrine (adrenaline) levels

play a minor role, if any, in this disease. It is possible that the increased cardiovascular morbidity and mortality associated with sleep apnea are, in part, related to these hormonal changes.[32]

In addition to blood gas changes and sympathetic nervous system activation, swings in the intrathoracic pressure as low as $-80 \, cmH_2O$ as a result of inspiratory efforts during apneic events (similar to the Müller maneuver) can impose significant strain and stress on the cardiovascular system.[33,34] Virolainen et al[35] showed that during a sustained Müller maneuver, most of the intrathoracic pressure drop is transmitted into the pericardial cavity, increasing the left ventricular (LV) transmural pressure gradient and LV afterload. They also demonstrated that the LV relaxation rate becomes impaired during this maneuver, which further impedes LV filling and preload. Increased afterload and reduced preload together lead to a reduction in stroke volume and cardiac output during the apnea. With arousal and resumption of breathing, venous return increases, potentially distending the right ventricle and causing the interventricular septum to shift to the left, resulting in impaired LV compliance and LV diastolic filling.[14]

Myocardial hypertrophy may be associated with compression of endocardial capillaries, impaired myocardial perfusion, and ischemia.[21] In a study by Cloward et al,[36] 83% of the patients who were normotensive and had underlying OSA were found to have LV hypertrophy. Similarly, Hedner et al[37] compared 61 men with OSA with 61 control subjects, and reported that LV mass and LV mass index (obtained by dividing the LV mass by the body surface area) were significantly higher among the OSA patients. The LV mass index was approximately 15% higher in the normotensive OSA patients compared with normotensive control subjects.

ACCELERATED ATHEROSCLEROSIS IN SLEEP APNEA

Recent years have witnessed progress in the understanding of the natural evolution of cardio- and cerebrovascular diseases. Atherosclerosis, the pathogenetic mechanism underlying cardiovascular and cerebrovascular events, is viewed as a dynamic and progressive disease arising from the subclinical condition of endothelial dysfunction.[38] Likewise, oxidative stress and inflammation are gaining widespread attention as fundamental mechanisms that participate in the initiation and progression of atherosclerate – both have been shown to be exaggerated in patients who have OSA.[39–41] Oxygenation–reoxygenation with production of reactive oxygen species due to intermittent obstructive apneas initiates an inflammatory cascade with

production of cytokines and adhesion molecules promoting endothelial dysfunction and atherosclerosis (Figure 3.2).[42] It is, therefore, reasonable to assume that alterations in these fundamental mechanisms in the setting of OSA may promote cardio- and cerebrovascular events.[43]

Endothelial NO is a key regulator of vascular homeostasis; it induces vasorelaxation by generating cyclic guanosine monophosphate (cGMP) in the underlying smooth muscle cells, and prevents monocyte adhesion to the endothelium, platelet activation, and smooth muscle cell proliferation. Hence, impaired NO release from the injured

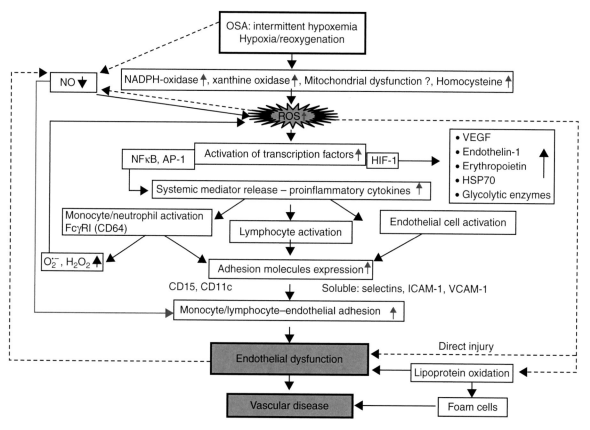

Figure 3.2 Intermittent hypoxia due to OSA results in hypoxia–reoxygenation with generation of reactive oxygen species (ROS), activation of proinflammatory cytokines, release of adhesion molecules, and inactivation of nitric oxide (NO), with subsequent endothelial dysfunction and initiation of atherosclerotic process. NADPH, reduced form of nicotinamide adenine dinucleotide phosphate; NFκB, nuclear factor κB; AP-1, activator protein 1; HIF-1, hypoxia inducible factor 1; VEGF, vascular endothelial growth factor; HSP70, heat-shock protein 70; O_2^-, superoxide radical anion; H_2O_2, hydrogen peroxide; ICAM-1, intercellular adhesion molecule 1; VCAM-1, vascular cell adhesion molecule 1 (reprinted from Sleep Medical Reviews, Vol 7, Lavie L, Obstructive sleep apnoea syndrome – an oxidative stress disorder, pp 35–51, Copyright 2003, with permission from Elsevier)[42]

endothelial cells is regarded as an initiator and promoter of arteriosclerosis. Endothelial nitric oxide synthase (eNOS) is responsible for the production of endothelial NO. eNOS is inhibited by endogenous inhibitors such as asymmetric dimethylarginine (ADMA). Increased concentrations of ADMA are associated with coronary risk factors, i.e., hypertension, hyperlipidemia, diabetes, etc. This suggests that ADMA may be responsible for endothelial dysfunction. Endothelium-dependent vasodilatation is impaired in patients with OSA,[44] which improves after treatment with continuous positive airway pressure (CPAP: see below), with a rise in the plasma concentrations of NO and a reduction in the level of ADMA, suggesting that patients with OSA have enhanced endothelial dysfunction via lack of NO-mediated vascular homeostasis.[45]

Studies have demonstrated that increased serum levels of C-reactive protein (CRP), interleukin (IL)-6, and tumor necrosis factor (TNF)-α are important risk factors for atherosclerosis, stroke, and cardiovascular diseases.[46–48] It has been shown that levels of CRP and IL-6 and spontaneous production of IL-6 by monocytes are elevated in patients with OSA.[49] Spontaneous production of TNF-α by monocytes and serum levels of TNF-α are also elevated in patients with moderate to severe OSA, as shown by Minoguchi et al.[50] One of the initial events in the development of atherosclerosis is the adhesion of monocytes to endothelial cells, with subsequent transmigration into the vascular intima.[51] Leukocyte and vascular cell adhesion molecules, such as selectins, integrins, vascular cell adhesion molecule 1 (VCAM-1), and intercellular adhesion molecule 1 (ICAM-1), affect this process. Although the origins, metabolism, and functional importance of soluble cell adhesion molecules are not fully understood, levels of these molecules may serve as surrogate markers of the cellular expression of cell adhesion molecules.[52] For example, the risk of myocardial infarction has been associated with increased concentrations of soluble ICAM-1.[53] Chin et al[54] found that patients with OSA have elevated levels of serum soluble ICAM-1. Fibrinogen, which is an independent risk factor for coronary

heart disease and is elevated in OSA, mediates leukocyte adhesion to the vascular endothelium through an ICAM-1-dependent pathway, thereby enhancing the atherosclerotic process.[55,56] Hypoxia is the major stimulus of vascular endothelial growth factor (VEGF), which is a potent angiogenic cytokine. Lavie et al[57] described the results of their experiments in which plasma concentrations of VEGF were measured in patients with sleep apnea. They found that AHI was found to be a significant independent predictor of morning VEGF concentrations in 85 male subjects investigated in their sleep laboratory, of whom 47 had AHI > 20. VEGF concentrations measured hourly during the sleep period were found to be significantly higher in a group of five sleep apnea patients compared with six age-similar snorers and six normal young adults (129.1 ± 43.4 pg/ml vs 74.6 ± 11.5 pg/ml and 32.5 ± 12.8 pg/ml, respectively; $p < 0.007$). Others have also shown similar results indicating that plasma levels of VEGF are increased in patients with OSA.[58]

Non-invasive imaging techniques can be used to directly identify and monitor preclinical atherosclerosis in human arteries. B-mode ultrasound imaging can directly quantitate the atherosclerotic burden. Measurement of carotid arterial wall intima–media thickness (IMT) made with high-resolution B-mode ultrasound imaging was first presented as a means of assessing atherosclerotic changes in the aorta in 1986. Studies of excised aorta showed close correlation between ultrasonically measured IMT and the same thickness measured by light microscopy. Carotid IMT has been recognized as a surrogate measure of atherosclerosis and a useful index of subclinical cardiovascular disease. Epidemiologic studies have shown that carotid IMT is a strong independent risk factor for predicting future CAD and stroke, even after adjusting for traditional risk factors.[59–62] Silvestrini et al[63] found that the IMT of the common carotid arteries of patients with OSA was significantly greater than that of control subjects (1.429 ± 0.34 vs 0.976 ± 0.17 mm; $p < 0.0001$). Similarly, since atherosclerosis (atheroma formation) of the extracranial carotid artery can be recognized on panoramic radiographs, Friedlander et al[64] conducted a study comparing the prevalence of atheromas in subjects with OSA and normal controls, and found that 22% of the patients with OSA showed atheromas on their radiographs, as opposed to only 3.7% of the patients in the control group. It has been demonstrated that the severity of OSA is independently related to atherosclerosis and that the severity of OSA-related hypoxemia is more important than the frequency of obstructive events.[65] Based on the above studies, it is evident that OSA is independently associated with the progression of atherosclerosis.

This concept of accelerated atherosclerosis and adverse cardiovascular outcomes in patients with OSA has been investigated in a large observational cohort study by Marin et al,[66] where they compared the incidence of fatal (death from myocardial infarction or stroke) and non-fatal (non-fatal myocardial infarction, non-fatal stroke, coronary artery bypass surgery, and percutaneous transluminal coronary angiography) cardiovascular events in simple snorers, patients with untreated OSA, patients with treated OSA (with CPAP), and healthy men from the general population. They showed that untreated severe OSA significantly increased the risk of fatal (odds ratio (OR) 2.87, 95% CI 1.17–7.51) and non-fatal (OR 3.17, 95% CI 1.12–7.51) cardiovascular events compared with healthy participants. In a large prospective study in males and females with no prior history of stroke and cardiovascular events, the presence of OSA increased the risk of stroke and death by 1.97-fold (95% CI 1.12–3.48), independently of other cardiovascular risk factors, including hypertension.[67]

EFFECT OF THERAPY OF OSA ON CAD OUTCOME

Positive airway pressure therapy is the treatment of choice for most patients with OSA. The most common type of positive airway pressure therapy provides a constant pressure throughout the respiratory cycle and is called continuous positive airway pressure (CPAP). Other treatment options for OSA include oral appliances such as mandibular advancement splints, surgical treatment options such as uvulopalatopharyngoplasty, genioglossus advancement, maxillomandibular advancement, and tracheostomy. Of these, CPAP therapy is effective and is the most widely used modality in patients with moderate to severe disease.[68]

Hanly et al[69] found that 30% of consecutively enrolled patients with OSA and no history of CAD had ST-segment depression during sleep indicating myocardial ischemia. The CPAP treatment resulted in a reduction in AHI, arousal index, and time spent with oxygen saturation less than 90%, with a shortening of the duration of ST-segment depression. Similarly, it has been shown that nocturnal angina diminishes and the number of nocturnal myocardial ischemic events also reduces during treatment of sleep apnea by CPAP.[70]

CPAP therapy has been shown to decrease the incidence of cardiovascular outcomes in patients with concomitant OSA and CAD. Milleron et al[71] conducted a long-term prospective study to evaluate the effect of treating OSA on the rate of cardiovascular events in CAD. They followed 54 patients with both CAD and OSA over a period of 86.5 ± 39 months. OSA patients were treated with CPAP (85%) and/or upper-airway surgery (15%). Cardiovascular events as defined by cardiovascular death, acute coronary syndrome, hospitalization for heart failure, or need for coronary revascularization occurred in 58% of untreated patients with OSA, compared with 24% of the patients who were treated. CPAP therapy has also been shown to decrease the incidence of cardiovascular outcomes in patients with OSA without concomitant CAD or other cardiovascular disease. In a prospective observational study of 182 Swedish men with no prior history of cardiovascular disease or hypertension, the diagnosis of OSA increased the risk of incident cardiovascular event by 4.9-fold (95% CI 1.8–13.6). Cardiovascular events occurred in 56.7% of incompletely treated OSA patients, compared with 6.7% of the optimally treated group ($p < 0.001$).[72] Doherty et al[73] compared the cardiovascular outcomes of OSA patients who were intolerant of CPAP (untreated group) with those continuing CPAP therapy. They noted that there was a significant excess of cardiovascular deaths in the untreated group (nine deaths, 14.8%), compared with two deaths (1.9%) in the treated group ($p = 0.009$). Furthermore, the total number of cardiovascular events (death and new cardiovascular disease combined) was significantly greater in the untreated group compared with that in the CPAP group (31% vs 18%; $p < 0.05$). In another large prospective observational study conducted in Spain, patients with severe untreated OSA had a significantly higher risk of fatal and non-fatal cardiovascular events than the CPAP-treated group.[66] These data show that patients with sleep apnea are at risk of cardiovascular events and death, and that the treatment of this condition improves survival and cardiovascular outcome.

In summary, sleep-disordered breathing, especially if associated with hypoxemia, causes endothelial dysfunction and vasculopathy through oxygenation–reoxygenation mechanisms inducing systemic inflammation and atherosclerosis with high cardiovascular and cerebrovascular morbidity and mortality. Effective treatment of sleep-disordered breathing reverses the pathogenetic mechanisms and improves survival. Patients with established cardiovascular disease or those with risk factors for vascular disease should be screened for underlying sleep-related breathing disorders.

REFERENCES

1. Messer JV, Neill WA. The oxygen supply of the human heart. Am J Cardiol 1962; 9: 384–94.
2. Hiramatsu O, Goto M, Yada T, et al. In vivo observations of the intramural arterioles and venules in beating canine hearts. J Physiol 1998; 509: 619–28.
3. Yada T, Hiramatsu O, Kimura A, et al. In vivo observation of subendocardial microvessels of the beating porcine heart using a needle-probe videomicroscope with a CCD camera. Circ Res 1993; 72: 939–46.
4. Alella A, Williams FL, Bolene-Williams C, et al. Interrelation between cardiac oxygen consumption and coronary blood flow. Am J Physiol 1955; 183: 570–82.
5. Komaru T, Kanatsuka H, Shirato K. Coronary microcirculation: physiology and pharmacology. Pharmacol Ther 2000; 86: 217–61.
6. Berne RM. Regulation of coronary blood flow. Physiol Rev 1964; 44: 1–29.
7. Eckenhoff JE. The physiology of the coronary circulation. Anesthesiology 1950; 11: 168–77.
8. Roddie IC. Modern views on physiology. XXIV. Autonomic nervous system. Practitioner 1970; 205: 828–34.
9. Kirby DA, Verrier RL. Differential effects of sleep stage on coronary hemodynamic function during stenosis. Physiol Behav 1989; 45: 1017–20.
10. Zinkovska S, Rodriguez EK, Kirby DA. Coronary band total peripheral resistance changes during sleep in a porcine model. Am J Physiol 1996; 270: H723–9.
11. Shaheen F, Bowman TJ, Sisson JH. Sleep Physiology. In: Bowman TJ, ed. Review of Sleep Medicine. Burlington, MA: Butterworth Heinemann, 2003: 43.
12. Coote JH. Respiratory and circulatory control during sleep. J Exp Biol 1982; 100: 223–44.
13. Baccelli G, Guazzi M, Mancia G, et al. Neural and non-neural mechanisms influencing circulation during sleep. Nature 1969; 223: 184–5.
14. Mancia G. Autonomic modulation of the cardiovascular system during sleep. N Engl J Med 1993; 328: 347–9.
15. Somers VK, Dyken ME, Mark AL, et al. Sympathetic-nerve activity during sleep in normal subjects. N Engl J Med 1993; 328: 303–7.
16. Mancia G, Baccelli G, Adams DB, et al. Vasomotor regulation during sleep in the cat. Am J Physiol 1971; 220: 1086–93.
17. Khatri IM, Freis ED. Hemodynamic changes during sleep. J Appl Physiol 1967; 22: 867–73.
18. Bristow JD, Honour AJ, Pickering TG, et al. Cardiovascular and respiratory changes during sleep in normal and hypertensive subjects. Cardiovasc Res 1969; 3: 476–85.
19. Mooe T, Rabben T, Wiklund U, et al. Sleep-disordered breathing in men with coronary artery disease. Chest 1996; 109: 659–63.
20. Mooe T, Rabben T, Wiklund U, et al. Sleep-disordered breathing in women: occurrence and association with coronary artery disease. Am J Med 1996; 101: 251–6.

21. Schafer H, Koehler U, Ewig S, et al. Obstructive sleep apnea as a risk marker in coronary artery disease. Cardiology 1999; 92: 79–84.

22. Maekawa M, Shiomi T, Usui K, et al. Prevalence of ischemic heart disease among patients with sleep apnea syndrome. Psychiatry Clin Neurosci 1998; 52: 219–20.

23. Mooe T, Franklin KA, Holmstrom K, et al. Sleep-disordered breathing and coronary artery disease: long-term prognosis. Am J Respir Crit Care Med 2001; 164: 1910–13.

24. Muller JE, Stone PH, Turi ZG, et al. Circadian variation in the frequency of onset of acute myocardial infarction. N Engl J Med 1985; 313: 1315–22.

25. Cohen MC, Rohtla KM, Lavery CE, et al. Meta-analysis of the morning excess of acute myocardial infarction and sudden cardiac death. Am J Cardiol 1997; 79: 1512–16.

26. Gami AS, Howard DE, Olson EJ, et al. Day–night pattern of sudden death in obstructive sleep apnea. N Engl J Med 2005; 352: 1206–14.

27. Muller JE. Circadian variation and triggering of acute coronary events. Am Heart J 1999; 137: S1–8.

28. Narkiewicz K, Somers VK. Cardiovascular variability characteristics in obstructive sleep apnea. Auton Neurosci 2001; 90: 89–94.

29. Hahn PY, Olson LJ, Somers VK. Cardiovascular complications of obstructive sleep apnea. In: Lee-Chiong TL, ed. Sleep: A Comprehensive Handbook. New York: Wiley, 2005: 267–73.

30. Somers VK, Dyken ME, Clary MP, et al. Sympathetic neural mechanisms in obstructive sleep apnea. J Clin Invest 1995; 96: 1897–904.

31. Baylor P, Mouton A, Shamoon HH, et al. Increased norepinephrine variability in patients with sleep apnea syndrome. Am J Med 1995; 99: 611–15.

32. Marrone O, Riccobono L, Salvaggio A, et al. Catecholamines and blood pressure in obstructive sleep apnea syndrome. Chest 1993; 103: 722–7.

33. Shamsuzzaman AS, Gersh BJ, Somers VK. Obstructive sleep apnea: Implications for cardiac and vascular disease. JAMA 2003; 290: 1906–14.

34. Shiomi T, Guilleminault C, Stoohs R, et al. Leftward shift of the interventricular septum and pulsus paradoxus in obstructive sleep apnea syndrome. Chest 1991; 100: 894–902.

35. Virolainen J, Ventila M, Turto H, et al. Effect of negative intrathoracic pressure on left ventricular pressure dynamics and relaxation. J Appl Physiol 1995; 79: 455–60.

36. Cloward TV, Walker JM, Farney RJ, et al. Left ventricular hypertrophy is a common echocardiographic abnormality in severe obstructive sleep apnea and reverses with nasal continuous positive airway pressure. Chest 2003; 124: 594–601.

37. Hedner J, Ejnell H, Caidahl K. Left ventricular hypertrophy independent of hypertension in patients with obstructive sleep apnoea. J Hypertens 1990; 8: 941–6.

38. Davignon J, Ganz P. Role of endothelial dysfunction in atherosclerosis. Circulation 2004; 109(23 Suppl 1): III27–32.

39. Libby P. Inflammation in atherosclerosis. Nature 2002; 420: 868–74.

40. Lefer DJ, Granger DN. Oxidative stress and cardiac disease. Am J Med 2000; 109: 315–23.

41. Babior BM. Phagocytes and oxidative stress. Am J Med 2000; 109: 33–44.

42. Lavie L. Obstructive sleep apnoea syndrome – an oxidative stress disorder. Sleep Med Rev 2003; 7: 35–51.

43. Lavie L. Sleep-disordered breathing and cerebrovascular disease. A mechanistic approach. Neurol Clin 2005; 23: 1059–75.

44. Carlson JT, Rangemark C, Hedner JA. Attenuated endothelium-dependent vascular relaxation in patients with sleep apnea. J Hypertens 1996; 14: 577–84.

45. Ohike Y, Kozaki K, Iijima K, et al. Amelioration of vascular endothelial dysfunction in obstructive sleep apnea syndrome by nasal continuous positive airway pressure – possible involvement of nitric oxide and asymmetric *NG, NG*-dimethylarginine. Circ J 2005; 69: 221–6.

46. Burke AP, Tracy RP, Kolodgie F, et al. Elevated C-reactive protein values and atherosclerosis in sudden coronary death: association with different pathologies. Circulation 2002; 105: 2019–23.

47. Ridker PM, Rifai N, Stampfer MJ, et al. Plasma concentration of interleukin-6 and the risk of future myocardial infarction among apparently healthy men. Circulation 2000; 101: 1767–72.

48. Ridker PM, Rifai N, Pfeffer M, et al. Elevation of tumor necrosis factor-α and increased risk of recurrent coronary events after myocardial infarction. Circulation 2000; 101: 2149–53.

49. Yokoe T, Minoguchi K, Matsuo H, et al. Elevated levels of C-reactive protein and interleukin-6 in patients with obstructive sleep apnea syndrome are decreased by nasal continuous positive airway pressure. Circulation 2003; 108: 1129–34.

50. Minoguchi K, Tazaki T, Yokoe T, et al. Elevated production of tumor necrosis factor-alpha by monocytes

in patients with obstructive sleep apnea syndrome. Chest 2004; 126: 1473–9.

51. Ross R. Atherosclerosis – an inflammatory disease. N Engl J Med 1999; 340: 115–26.

52. Abe Y, El-Masri B, Kimball KT, et al. Soluble cell adhesion molecules in hypertriglyceridemia and potential significance on monocyte adhesion. Arterioscler Thromb Vasc Biol 1998; 18: 723–31.

53. Ridker PM, Hennekens CH, Roitman JB, et al. Plasma concentration of soluble intercellular adhesion molecule-1 and risks of future myocardial infarction in apparently healthy men. Lancet 1998; 351: 88–92.

54. Chin K, Nakamura T, Shimizu K, et al. Effects of nasal continuous positive airway pressure on soluble cell adhesion molecules in patients with obstructive sleep apnea syndrome. Am J Med 2000; 109: 562–7.

55. Languino LR, Plescia J, Duperray A, et al. Fibrinogen mediates leukocyte adhesion to vascular endothelium through an ICAM-1 dependent pathway. Cell 1993; 73: 1423–34.

56. Chin K, Ohi M, Kita H, et al. Effects of NCPAP therapy on fibrinogen levels in obstructive sleep apnea syndrome. Am J Respir Crit Care Med 1996; 153: 1972–6.

57. Lavie L, Kraiczi H, Hefetz A, et al. Plasma vascular endothelial growth factor in sleep apnea syndrome: effects of nasal continuous positive air pressure treatment. Am J Respir Crit Care Med 2002; 165: 1624–8.

58. Schulz R, Hummel C, Heinemann S, et al. Serum levels of vascular endothelial growth factor are elevated in patients with obstructive sleep apnea and severe nighttime hypoxia. Am J Respir Crit Care Med 2002; 165: 67–70.

59. Kuller LH, Shemanski L, Psaty BM, et al. Subclinical disease as an independent risk factor for cardiovascular disease. Circulation 1995; 92: 720–6.

60. Bots ML, Hoes AW, Koudstaal PJ, et al. Common carotid artery intima–media thickness and risk of stroke and myocardial infarction: the Rotterdam Study. Circulation 1997; 96: 1432–7.

61. O'Leary DH, Polak JF, Kronmal RA, et al. Carotid-artery intima and media thickness as a risk factor for myocardial infarction and stroke in older adults. Cardiovascular Health Study. N Engl J Med 1999; 340: 14–22.

62. O'Leary DH, Polak JF. Intima–media thickness: a tool for atherosclerosis imaging and event prediction. Am J Cardiol 2002; 90: 18–21.

63. Silvestrini M, Rizzato B, Placidi F, et al. Carotid artery wall thickness in patients with obstructive sleep apnea syndrome. Stroke 2002; 33: 1782–5.

64. Friedlander AH, Yueb R, Littner MR. The prevalence of calcified carotid artery atheromas in patients with obstructive sleep apnea syndrome. J Oral Maxillofac Surg 1998; 56: 950–4.

65. Suzuki T, Nakano H, Maekawa J, et al. Obstructive sleep apnea and carotid-artery intima–media thickness. Sleep 2004; 27: 129–33.

66. Marin JM, Carrizo SJ, Vincente E, et al. Long-term cardiovascular outcomes in men with obstructive sleep apnoea-hypopnoea with or without treatment with continuous positive airway pressure: an observational study. Lancet 2005; 365: 1046–53.

67. Yaggi HK, Concato J, Kernan WN, et al. Obstructive sleep apnea as a risk factor for stroke and death. N Engl J Med 2005; 353: 2034–41.

68. Sullivan CE, Issa FG, Berthon-Jones M, et al. Reversal of obstructive sleep apnoea by continuous positive airway pressure applied through the nares. Lancet 1981; i: 862–5.

69. Hanly P, Sasson Z, Zuberi N, et al. ST-segment depression during sleep in obstructive sleep apnea. Am J Cardiol 1993; 71: 1341–5.

70. Franklin KA, Nilsson JB, Sahlin C, et al. Sleep apnoea and nocturnal angina. Lancet 1995; 345: 1085–7.

71. Milleron RS, Pilliere R, Foucher A, et al. Benefits of obstructive sleep apnoea treatment in coronary artery disease: a long-term follow-up study. Eur Heart J 2004; 25: 728–34.

72. Peker Y, Hedner J, Norum J, et al. Increased incidence of cardiovascular disease in middle-aged men with obstructive sleep apnea: a 7-year follow-up. Am J Respir Crit Care Med 2002; 166: 159–65.

73. Doherty LS, Kiely JL, Swan V, McNicholas WT. Long-term effects of nasal continuous positive airway pressure therapy on cardiovascular outcomes in sleep apnea syndrome. Chest 2005; 127: 2076–84.

4

Sleep and genitourinary systems

Max Hirshkowitz, Amir Sharafkhaneh

INTRODUCTION

Genitourinary symptoms and disorders intersect sleep physiology in five important areas: the symptoms nocturia and enuresis, the conditions erectile dysfunction (impotence) and sleep-related painful erections, and sleep alterations associated with the menstrual cycle. In this chapter, we will describe these problems from a clinical sleep perspective, review their etiology, describe the relevant pathophysiology, and review current therapeutics, where appropriate.

NOCTURIA

Definition and description

Nocturia is the need to void during sleep. It can occur without disease, commonly resulting from excessive evening fluid intake. However, nocturia is often a non-specific symptom, and when it occurs more than twice nightly, it can significantly disturb sleep. Underlying causes range from prostatism (due to bladder neck obstruction) to renal, liver, or heart failure.

Treatment

In the primary care setting, four-step management has been proposed: (1) clinical evaluation, (2) simple investigations, (3) provisional diagnosis, and (4) diagnosis-driven management.[1] Bladder retraining, anticholinergic drug therapy, or both are recommended in cases where the cause is an overactive bladder. The use of sedative hypnotics is discouraged in older adults, for whom loop diuretics in the afternoon should be considered. For younger patients desmopressin is suggested, but this should be used cautiously in older patients because of the risk of hyponatremia. Finally, a recent study found that the adrenoreceptor antagonist terazosin objectively and subjectively reduced nocturia episode frequency in some men with prostate-related lower urinary tract symptoms.[2]

Special association with sleep

In sleep clinical settings, we frequently note nocturia as a symptom of sleep-related breathing disorders (SRBDs). Furthermore, treatment with continuous positive airway pressure (CPAP) significantly reduces nocturia episodes.[3] In one study, 97 patients (75 men and 22 women), mean age 55 years, with a mean respiratory disturbance index of 34 were tested. The mean number of awakenings to urinate went from 2.5 times nightly at baseline to 0.7 after 1–3 months following CPAP therapy ($p < 0.001$). In a retrospective analysis, Fitzgerald et al[4] found that age, diabetes, and SRBD severity correlated with nocturia frequency. Moreover, CPAP significantly reduced the frequency of nocturia episodes.

NOCTURNAL ENURESIS

Definition and description

Commonly called bedwetting, enuresis is normal in children up to age 3 years. If it persists, it becomes increasingly problematic. Sleep enuresis is a disorder in which the individual urinates during sleep while in bed long after the usual developmental milestones have been passed or begins again after the occurrence of some medical or psychologic event. Bedwetting frequency ranges from nightly to monthly. Psychologic consequences range from mild embarrassment to severe shame and guilt.[5,6] Moreover, enuresis has two very different forms: primary and secondary.

In children, primary sleep enuresis is the persistence of bedwetting from infancy until after age 2 or 3 years. Usually, after toilet training, bedwetting spontaneously resolves before age 6 years. Prevalence progressively declines from 30% at age 4, to 10% at age 6, to 5% at age 10, and to 3% at age 12. If a parent had primary enuresis, this increases the likelihood that the children will be enuretic. A single recessive gene is suspected. It may be associated with delayed lower urinary tract neuromuscular maturation or disease. Diseases include urethral infection, stenosis, posterior urethral valve problems, and neurogenic bladder.

Secondary enuresis refers to relapse after toilet training has been completed and there has been a period during which the child remained dry. Secondary enuresis in children may occur with the birth of a sibling and represent a 'cry for attention'. Secondary enuresis can also be associated with nocturnal seizures, sleep deprivation, and urologic anomalies. In adults, sleep enuresis is occasionally seen in patients with sleep-disordered breathing. In most cases, embarrassment is the most serious consequence. Nonetheless, if sleep enuresis is not addressed, it may leave psychosocial scars.

Treatment

A variety of medications have also been used to treat sleep enuresis, including imipramine, oxybutynin chloride, and synthetic vasopressin. Behavioral treatments – including bladder training, use of conditioning devices (bell and pad), and fluid restriction – reportedly have good success when properly administered. Other treatments include psychotherapy, motivational strategies, and hypnotherapy. Glazener et al[7] conducted an evidence-based medicine review of 15 randomized and quasi-randomized trials examining enuresis treatment in children. They concluded that 'there was weak evidence to support the use of hypnosis, psychotherapy, acupuncture and chiropractic but it was provided in each case by single small trials, some of dubious methodological rigour.' In an earlier review, Glazener et al[8] examined six Cochrane Reviews evaluating simple behavioral interventions, complex behavioral or educational interventions, alarms, and drugs (desmopressin, tricyclic antidepressants, and other drugs). They found that most evidence was of poor quality and that there were few head-to-head comparisons between interventions. Nonetheless, alarms were ranked as the most effective treatment for nocturnal enuresis in children, with desmopressin as a good choice for temporary relief. After reviewing all papers published between 1980 and 2002 that sampled 10 or more children (38 papers in total), Butler and Gasson[9] also concluded that the enuresis alarm reduced or eliminated nocturnal enuresis. Effectiveness varied, with there being important individual factors related to its appropriateness for any particular child. Finally, another review of randomized controlled trials found that enuresis alarms produced durable (3 months post-treatment) treatment effect.[10] Less durable, but acutely effective, outcome was produced by desmopressin and tricyclic antidepressants (but the effect was not sustained after cessation of dosing).

Special association with sleep

Like nocturia, enuresis has a special relationship with sleep-disordered breathing. A chart review of 326 cases of child (age 2–18 years) tonsillectomy or adenotonsillectomy found that 107 (33%)

were enuretic.[11] All of these 107 were having the surgery to treat SRBDs, and 53% agreed to participate in the follow-up study. Postoperatively, 61% had complete cessation of enuresis, 23% had a partial reduction, and the remainder did not change. Thus, enuresis is common in children with SRBDs, and the vast majority improve after treatment of the sleep-disordered breathing. Similarly, enuresis can be a symptom of sleep apnea in adults.[12] The mechanism posited involves a negative intrathoracic pressure-evoked release of atrial natriuretic peptide resulting from cardiac distension. This peptide increases sodium and water excretion while inhibiting fluid volume regulation. As expected, enuresis ceases or dramatically declines after treatment of the sleep-related breathing problem.

ERECTILE DYSFUNCTION (IMPOTENCE)

Definition and description

Erectile dysfunction is the inability to attain or sustain an erection satisfactory for coitus. In the USA, erectile dysfunction afflicts 10–20 million men (males aged 18 years or greater). Prevalence increases with age. Erectile failure may be due to psychologic factors, organic factors, or both. Psychologic factors include sexual guilt, fear of intimacy, depression, and severe anxiety. Organic factors include hormonal imbalances, vascular disease, neurologic disorders, and iatrogenic side-effects of medication. Hormonal problems include diminished testosterone, elevated prolactin, hypothyroidism and hyperthyroidism, and Cushing syndrome. Relevant vascular disorders include penile arterial atherosclerotic disease and venous leaks. Diseases that accelerate atherosclerosis (e.g., diabetes, smoking, and hypertension) adversely affect erectile function. Complementarily, vascular tone regulation (e.g., nitric oxide, NO) provides a potential treatment avenue. Neurologic disorders include stroke, temporal lobe seizures, multiple sclerosis, sensory and autonomic dysfunction, and spinal cord injuries. Of men undergoing

transurethral resection of the prostate (TURP), 40% experience problems with erections. Drugs are estimated as causing about 25% of erectile dysfunction.

Treatment

A wide range of treatments are available to treat erectile dysfunction. These include psychotherapy, sexual counseling, vacuum devices, 'cock-rings' to prevent venous leakage, androgen replacement therapy, revascularization surgery, surgical implantation of a penile prosthesis, vasodilator injection, transurethral prostaglandin E_1 (PGE$_1$) administration, and the use of phosphodiesterase inhibitors or other drugs that potentiate the vascular smooth muscle effects of NO. Many of the treatments are specific to the etiology. In other words, some treatments for psychogenic problems would not be helpful for treating organic erectile dysfunction. Furthermore, very invasive treatments for severe organic impairment (e.g., implantation of a penile prosthesis) should not be used when the main and nearly exclusive problem is largely psychologic. Endocrine panels can reveal specific hormonal problems that can be treated with hormone replacement therapies. Thus, currently there is an array of treatments in our armamentarium; consequently, reassurance that treatment is possible is crucial. Finally, individuals have many misconceptions concerning sexuality, and misinformation must be dispelled as part of the treatment regimen.

Special association with sleep

Traditionally, there were no objective tests to differentiate organic and psychogenic influences. When Brantley Scott developed the inflatable prosthesis, he wanted, as a prerequisite for implantation, to be reasonably certain that the patient did not have psychogenic impotence. Part of the reason was that the surgical procedure destroys any existing mechanisms. Given the invasive nature of the treatment intervention the availability of an objective method would be highly desirable.

As fate would have it, Ismet Karacan was conducting research concerning sleep-related erections and their diagnostic utility literally across the street at Baylor College of Medicine. This was the beginning of a long and fruitful collaboration.[13]

What are sleep-related erections (SREs)?

Sleep-related erections (SREs – also known as nocturnal penile tumescence, NPT) refer to the cycle of penile erections that occur episodically in all healthy, sexually potent men. These involuntary erections can be objectively assessed and can be used to differentiate psychogenic from organic erectile dysfunction. A normal pattern of sleep erections occurs in patients with psychogenic impotence, in contrast to the diminished erectile response characteristic of men with neurologic, endocrine, or vascular erectile dysfunction. Over the past four decades, we have learned much about SREs. Perhaps the pivotal finding is the great consistency with which they occur. This consistency, coupled with non-invasive recording techniques, has provided researchers an unparalleled approach for physiologically investigating erectile function.

Thus, SREs are naturally occurring and involuntary. They are closely associated with rapid eye movement (REM) sleep. The discovery that dreaming and REM sleep are concurrent posed the question of whether sleep erections were related to dream content. A case series by Fisher and co-workers[14,15] suggested that they were; however, more systematic work by Karacan[16] failed to find such a relationship. Subsequent research[17,18] revealed that dream reports infrequently contain overt sexual content, notwithstanding the expected four to six REM sleep episodes occurring nightly.

Presleep sexual arousal evoked by presenting videotapes depicting sexually explicit activity does not alter the SRE profile.[19] Twelve sexually potent young adult males were presented erotic, dysphoric, and neutral videotape segments on different nights before laboratory SRE testing. No differences were found for frequency, magnitude, duration, architecture, or coordination between REM sleep and SREs between experimental nights. Using a similar protocol, SRE patterns were not altered by sexual abstinence or presleep sexual activity in young adult potent volunteers.[20,21]

Age-related changes in SREs have been well researched.[22–25] SRE recordings in potent young boys, young adults, middle-aged men, and the elderly who were free from significant physical disease revealed modest but statistically reliable declines in SRE frequency, SRE duration, and the frequency of REM sleep-related erections.[22] Other researchers confirmed small age-related decreases in SRE frequency, and also found a lower percentage of REM sleep associated with tumescence in older subjects.[23] However, no significant differences between age groups were found for penile rigidity. In another study, greater age-related declines were reported among subjects aged 65–74 years when samples included men with intermittent erectile failure.[24] Thus, SREs appear to persist throughout the lifespan in healthy, sexually potent men.

By contrast, SRE alterations have been shown in men complaining of erectile failure associated with a variety of medical conditions, including diabetes,[26,27] chronic obstructive pulmonary disease (COPD),[28] alcoholism,[29] spinal lesions,[30] end-stage renal disease,[31] and hypertension.[32,33] Decreased SREs are also reported in men suffering from major depressive disorder.[34] Men with longstanding androgen deficiency have markedly diminished SREs.[35] Furthermore, hypogonadal men treated with androgen replacement therapy who recover potency have normalized SRE activity.[36] Similar SRE androgen dependence has been reported by Carani et al;[37] however, response to visual erotic stimuli appeared to be androgen-independent. Bancroft[38] further posited the involvement of a central noradrenergic mechanism in erectile activity, citing that α_2-adrenoceptor antagonists restore sexual behavior in castrated rats. He also noted that SREs during REM sleep occur at a time when there is virtual cessation of peripheral sympathetic activity. This provides the framework for a model of psychogenic erectile dysfunction that involves high-level central α_2 tone diminishing central nervous system (CNS) arousal capability.

Noradrenergic mechanisms likely play a role in androgen-induced SRE changes; however, the relationship is likely complex.

How are SREs measured?

The most common approach to measuring SREs is to continuously record penile circumference throughout the night. This is usually accomplished by placing strain gauges around the penis. As an erection occurs and penile girth increases, the gauge stretches. Stretching elongates and narrows the gauge's tubing, producing an increased electrical resistance that can be transformed to direct-current voltage by a bridge amplifier. This voltage can be calibrated to accurately reflect penile expansion. Laboratory sleep studies are expensive; therefore, non-laboratory approaches have emerged.[39–41] Non-laboratory tests are more prone to artifact and erroneous outcome than laboratory testing.[42–45]

Standard laboratory technique

The traditional laboratory-based polysomnographic approach for evaluating SREs grew out of early research projects attempting to link erectile activity, REM sleep, and dreaming. Penile circumference increase was recorded concurrently with electroencephalography (EEG), electro-oculography (EOG), and electromyography (EMG) during the night while subjects slept in the sleep laboratory. Modern practice includes EEG (central), EOG (left and right eyes), EMG (submentalis and anterior tibialis), electrocardiography (ECG), nasal and oral airflow, respiratory effort (using abdominal and thoracic movement sensors), and pulse oximetry. Bulbocavernosus–ischiocavernosus activity, penile blood flow, and snoring sounds are sometimes recorded. Usually, two penile circumference channels are recorded, with one gauge being placed at the penile base and the other at the coronal sulcus. Dual-channel SRE recording offers several advantages compared with a single gauge placed at mid shaft, including greater reliability and improved sensitivity to erectile anomalies.

Airflow, respiratory effort, and pulse oximetry are recorded in diagnostic practice because studies find that men with erectile dysfunction often have comorbid obstructive sleep apnea (OSA).[46] In a study of more than 1000 patients referred to our laboratory for SRE testing,[47] 20% had moderate to severe sleep apnea (>15 apneic events per hour of sleep). Men complaining of erectile problems also have a high prevalence of periodic limb movement disorder (previously called nocturnal myoclonus); therefore, leg movement activity should routinely be recorded.[48] Fifty-four percent of 768 patients referred for SRE testing had 15 or more leg movement events per hour of sleep. Breathing and leg movement data channels provide information that helps the clinician interpret SRE recordings. False-positive and false-negative conclusions due to sleep disorders and body movements can be avoided when the full complement of polysomnographic data channels are available for review. Furthermore, therapeutic intervention for diagnosed sleep disorders can normalize sleep and permit SRE interpretation.

Measures of penile circumference

SREs occur episodically, closely correlated with REM sleep. Each episode can be characterized as having a beginning, middle, and ending phase. The three phases are referred to as T_{up}, T_{max}, and T_{down} (the 'T' stands for 'tumescence'). The beginning phase is called T_{up} and is the time from the initial increase in circumference above baseline (≥ 2 mm) until the circumference reaches 75% of the night's overall maximum circumference increase (MCI). In healthy potent young adult men, T_{up} commences near the transition from non-REM (NREM) to REM sleep. Penile circumference increases rapidly, and penile pulsations (transient small increases in circumference) can be observed. During T_{up}, arterial inflow expands the penile girth and increases the cavernosal pressure. The point at which the increase in circumference first exceeds 75% of MCI is sometimes called the T_{max} point. The interval between an episode's initial T_{max} point and the last point before the circumference drops below the T_{max} point is called the T_{max} phase. Transient decreases below 75% of

MCI during the T_{max} phase are called fluctuations. During the T_{max} phase, the circumference remains roughly at a maximum plateau. The arterial inflow is thought to decline; however, the venous outflow is considerably restricted. The cavernosal pressure is increased, and in healthy potent men, the penile rigidity (see below) will exceed 1000 g. The T_{max} phase normally continues until the end of the REM sleep episode. Fluctuations can occur spontaneously or secondary to brief arousals from sleep. In cases where the penile circumference during an SRE episode fails to reach 75% of the overall nightly MCI, the T_{max} phase duration is scored as 1 minute centered around the episode's maximal circumference. The final phase of a SRE episode is called T_{down}. It is initiated by increased venous outflow coincident with changes in central and autonomic nervous system activity associated with the termination of REM sleep. Sympathetic activity increases, and the circumference declines rapidly to baseline (the T_{zero} point). The T_{down} phase spans the time from the end of the T_{max} phase until the T_{zero} point is reached. Detailed scoring rules are given in Ware and Hirshkowitz.[49]

SREs can be represented numerically in terms of frequency, magnitude, and duration. Frequency is indexed by the number of episodes, magnitude by the overall MCI and the mean MCI per episode, and duration by total tumescence time and the mean SRE episode duration. Also of interest is the SRE pattern, quantified by calculating the slope of the T_{up} phase, the slope of T_{down}, and the duration of T_{max}. These measures may be thought of as representing SRE architecture. Abnormal SRE architecture can provide insight into pathophysiology. For example, disparate expansion at the penile base and coronal sulcus should alert the clinician to probable vascular abnormalities. Continual fluctuations during T_{max} suggest a vascular problem, possibly a venous leak. Closer examination of erectile architecture is also possible. Microarchitectural SRE features include the rate of pulsation during the T_{up} and T_{max} phases and the number of fluctuations.

Coordination between SRE episodes and REM sleep provides a rich source of data. Additionally, basic dimensional measures (frequency, magnitude, and duration) can be normalized using sleep parameters (e.g., total tumescence time as a percentage of REM sleep duration) to provide measures with less between-subject variability. These sleep-normalized measures can be compared across individuals and aid interpretation with respect to normative values. SRE frequency, periodicity, and duration largely depend upon REM sleep. Sleep-stage information helps the clinician avoid misinterpreting as organic impotence SRE decreases secondary to insufficient REM sleep. Fluctuations that occur spontaneously are abnormal; however, fluctuations associated with brief awakenings can be normal (although the awakening may be pathological). Frequent NREM erections should alert the clinician to possible neurogenic problems. Detumescence occurring long before the end of a well-consolidated REM sleep episode suggests vascular problems. Delay between the onset of REM sleep and the beginning of the T_{up} phase, coupled with a slowly developing T_{up} phase, points toward an etiology involving impaired arterial inflow.

Measures of penile rigidity

Perhaps the most important procedure during SRE evaluation involves measuring penile rigidity. Penile buckling resistance indexes axial rigidity and is defined as the minimum amount of force applied to the glans capable of buckling the penile shaft. Adequate resistance to buckling is critical to the ability to achieve penetration. Circumference increase, although correlated with rigidity under normal circumstances, is not the crucial parameter. Moreover, it is well documented that some patients complaining of erectile dysfunction achieve erections with normal circumferential expansion but the erection is not firm.[50]

Rigidity measurement involves awakening the patient during a representative SRE and applying a calibrated force to the tip of the penis, parallel to the shaft. The applied force is increased rapidly up to a maximum of 1000 g. The force at which the penile shaft is observed to buckle approximately 30° is recorded as the rigidity. If no buckling occurs, the value 1000 g is assigned. Currently, electronic and spring-loaded force meters are used most often; however, the original measurement instruments were pressure-based devices with a range from 0 to 300 mmHg. Thus, pressure rigidity values in the older literature must be converted for comparison.

Over the years, procedures have evolved to meet a variety of needs. Our surgical colleagues requested that we photograph the penis in the erect state to help document penile size and shape. Therefore, we began photographing SREs immediately following rigidity measurement. For patients electing for penile prostheses, the photograph was sometimes helpful for size selection. Additionally, we found the photograph useful to record abnormal penile curvature associated with Peyronie's disease, and to our surprise found that some patients were completely unaware of its presence. The photograph also served to validate rigidity measures, and we decided to have the technologist who measured buckling resistance also rate the erection for its percentage of a full erection. The technologist and patient estimates of the percent-of-full erection present at the time of rigidity measurement usually concord within a 20% range. However, sometimes a patient will vastly underestimate erectile quality compared with the technician and our judgment from examining the photograph. At first, we thought that this was a confusion produced by the patient being awakened from sleep; however, it later became apparent that some patients have a peculiar type of body dysmorphia. Even upon examining the photograph the next day, some men will judge a full erection with 1000 g rigidity as less than 25% of full. In cases such as these, therapeutic intervention will clearly need to address the misperception.

In an intriguing study by Schwartz,[51] the awakening procedure with rigidity measurement and patient self-estimate of erectile adequacy were found to be critical for differential diagnosis. This was particularly the case for patients who did not have seriously diminished maximum circumference increase. Of particular interest was a finding among men with probable psychogenic impotence. Apparently, patients being confronted by a full erection during the awakening procedure had some therapeutic benefit. According to the report, 'Nine of these 12 patients reported that after their NPT test they were able to have reproducibly satisfying erections during intercourse with their wives.' In contrast, among patients with symptoms suggesting organic or drug-related impotence, no changes were found after SRE testing.

Measuring penile rigidity objectively indexes SRE quality. Patient and technician percentage-of-full erection ratings estimate subjective erectile quality.

Diagnostic use of sleep-related erections

Forty years ago, the differential diagnosis of impotence relied mainly on self-report. Very few objective techniques were available to examine erectile competency. In cases where there existed no history of vascular, neurologic, or genitourinary disease, and no obvious abnormality was found on physical examination, diagnosis defaulted to psychogenic impotence.[52] The epidemiologic understanding of the time derived from the work of Kinsey et al,[53] who found approximately 2% of men by age 40, 6.7% of men aged 55, 18.4% of men aged 60, and 75% aged 80 years were impotent. Moreover, it was axiomatic that 90% of erectile failure was psychogenic.[54] Current prevalence estimates for male impotence are considerably higher than previously thought. Our recognition of the role of organic etiologies in erectile failure has improved, as our assessment techniques have become more sophisticated. Furthermore, the majority of etiologies are now believed to be organic.

The development of SRE testing to differentiate psychogenic from organic impotence was fueled by the desire to establish an objective, reliable diagnostic technique. As surgical interventions developed for treating erectile failure, the need for a biologic marker to rule out psychogenic impotence became crucial. In the past, one

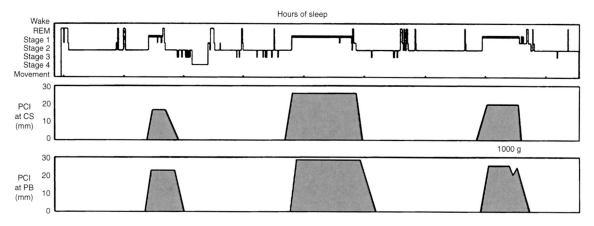

Figure 4.1   Sleep histogram and penile circumference increase (PCI) recorded at the coronal sulcus (CS) and penile base (PB) in a man with psychogenic erectile dysfunction. This 43-year-old man had a normal pattern of sleep-related erections, with rigidity measuring >1000 g buckling force

approach that was used to objectively assess erectile function involved having patients engage in sexual fantasies or view sexually explicit videotapes. If these activities produced an adequate erection, physiologic capacity was established, and it was concluded that the impotence was psychogenic in origin. However, if fantasies or erotica failed to produce an adequate erection, the etiology could be either organic or psychogenic. Situational factors in the clinical setting can inhibit erection in some men, especially those with performance anxiety. Thus, when no erection occurs under such testing circumstances, etiology remains unknown.

Once it had been determined that SREs are not affected by daytime sexual behavior, are unaffected by presleep sexual stimulation, and persist throughout the lifespan, they became viable as a possible biologic marker for erectile function. The diminution of SREs in men with erectile dysfunction and medical comobidities strongly suspected of causing impotence (e.g., diabetes) helped validate SRE testing.

Just as with daytime fantasy or viewing erotica, the presence of a normal-sized penile erection with full rigidity during REM sleep establishes erectile capability. To rule out specific and uncommon organic etiologies, endocrine, genital neurovascular examination, and nerve conduction studies may

be needed. These tests help rule out the four organic conditions known to be associated with apparently normal SREs – specifically pelvic steal syndrome, Peyronie's disease, somatic nerve lesion or neuropathy, and acute androgen deficiency. In pelvic steal syndrome, during sexual activity, movement (particularly of the lower limbs) shunts blood away from the penis, thereby causing detumescence. However, during sleep, a normal SRE can occur, because of the lack of movements. Peyronie's disease is associated with abnormal penile curvature during erection that may prevent penetration; however, a normal increase in penile circumference may occur. Figure 4.1 illustrates sleep stages and SREs recorded from a patient with psychogenic impotence.

In contrast, below-normal SREs suggest organic impotence; however, the clinician must first consider integrity of sleep, drug effects, and patient comorbidity factors. REM sleep of adequate duration and consolidation must be present to allow accurate interpretation of diminished SREs. As previously mentioned, this is an important issue, because sleep apnea and periodic limb movement disorder are common in men referred for evaluation of impotence.[47,48] Figure 4.2 illustrates sleep stages and SREs in a man with organic impotence.

Many drugs adversely affect REM sleep; therefore, a complete medication inventory is essential.

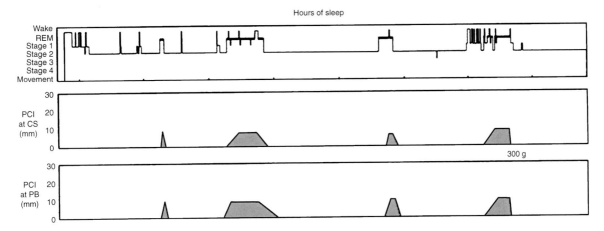

Figure 4.2   Sleep histogram and penile circumference increase (PCI) recorded at the coronal sulcus (CS) and penile base (PB) in a man with organic erectile dysfunction. This 58-year-old man with diabetes and hypertension had an abnormal pattern of sleep-related erections. The maximum rigidity measured on the final erection was only 300 g buckling force, which is considered inadequate to achieve vaginal penetration

Most antidepressant medications adversely affect SREs. This change is sometimes secondary to REM sleep suppression; however, it can also reflect a direct influence on the mechanisms underlying sexuality. Antidepressants with pronounced anticholinergic properties are particularly problematic. Selective serotonin reuptake inhibitors (SSRIs) have also been associated with erectile dysfunction. In one study of 152 men and 192 women, greater erectile dysfunction and delayed orgasm were found with paroxetine than fluvoxamine, fluoxetine, or sertraline, and sexual dysfunction generally correlated with dose.[55] However, SRE changes have not been systematically researched.

Many drugs reportedly cause impotence;[56] antihypertensives (especially β-blockers) can be particularly problematic. Other reputed impotence-causing medications include antipsychotic medications (notably haloperidol and chlorpromazine), antiandrogens, cancer chemotherapeutic agents, cimetidine, digoxin, disulfiram, and atropine.

Often the single most telling measure obtained during SRE testing is penile rigidity. With respect to diagnosis, this serves as a *functional erectile capacity index*. The rationae for this derives directly from studies. Female volunteers performing vaginal insertions with variously sized lubricated Lucite

rods needed an average minimum force of 500 g to achieve penetration.[57] During the SRE rigidity measurement procedure, men who were asked if their erections were adequate for intercourse indicated affirmatively when rigidity exceeded 500 g. Finally, rigidities in potent men average well above 500 g.[23] Thus, rigidities of 500–600 g are considered by many the *cutting score* below which organic impotence is diagnosed, assuming other validity conditions are met.

Advanced diagnostic practice – beyond dichotomization

Psychologic features in organic erectile dysfunction

An inability to volitionally attain a rigid erection can stem from psychogenic, organic, or a combination of these two causes. Regardless of etiology, the onset of erectile failure is usually distressing and can produce marital (or partner-related) problems, performance anxiety, and changes in mood. Psychometric indices may be elevated on these factors, even when the etiology is organic. In practice, we frequently find significant psychopathology in men whose impotence is clearly organic in origin. Thus, a positive result on psychosexual questionnaires or psychometric tests does not rule out organicity. In contrast, it is incorrect to assume that psychopathology will necessarily accompany psychogenic impotence. For example, a patient may not self-report accurately, and a completely normal profile may result. Alternatively, erectile failure arising from behavioral or relationship problems will be missed by tests whose scope is intra- rather than interpersonal.

For these and other reasons, initial successes using the Minnesota Multiphasic Personality Profile (MMPI) indices to differentiate psychogenic from organic impotence were followed by less reliable results.[58–60] More specific sex questionnaires have been developed, and appear to be more useful.[62–64] However, a positive finding for psychogenic impotence does not rule out possible underlying organic contributions. The presence of many comorbidities, the use of medications known to adversely affect erectile function, and the absence of dysfunction on a full range of psychogenic features (including behavioral, relationship, constitutional, conditioning, and religious) raise suspicion of impotence deriving from a biologic origin.

Subclinical organic contribution to psychogenic impotence

Although a penile rigidity of 500–600 g is often considered the *cutting score* for differentiating psychogenic from organic impotence, other factors should be considered. In the original study,[57] 500 g was the average minimum buckling resistance needed to achieve penetration during vaginal self-insertion under the best circumstances with lubrication. There were, however, between-subject differences. Therefore, partner-specific variables can alter the adequacy of an erection with 600 g rigidity for penetration. Furthermore, even though penile rigidity objectively addresses the issue of obtaining an erection, it does not address erectile maintenance. Assessing the ability to maintain an erection is better judged by examining the SRE profile and the coordination between SREs and REM sleep.

The duration of a sustained maximal erection (T_{max} phase) should continue throughout an REM sleep episode. When SRE episodes increase to normal magnitude but then terminate prematurely notwithstanding continued and uninterrupted REM sleep, a problem exists. Another pattern that we have noted is an increased number of fluctuations during the T_{max} phase that cannot be accounted for by sleep disruptions. When patients with such profiles complain primarily of problems maintaining erections, the SRE pattern concords with the symptom. Similarly, patients sometimes complain of intermittent difficulty obtaining erections and SRE testing reveals prolonged T_{up} duration or very few pulsations during T_{up}. All other SRE measures may be within normal limits, including rigidity. These SRE test findings are not sufficient by current standards to diagnose organic impotence; however, they clearly reflect physiologic compromise (Figure 4.3). We sometimes refer to this as evidence for *creeping organicity*. Specific pathophysiologies can sometimes be confirmed using invasive urologic techniques, but not in all cases.

One common marker for these subclinical changes is an increase in the variability of SREs and a decline, but not loss of, coordination between erections and REM sleep. Increased SRE variability goes hand-in-hand with intermittent erectile failure during sexual attempts. The SRE pattern seen in healthy young adult men is incredibly consistent, invariant, and robust. It varies as little as 10% per night, with erections commencing with REM sleep and continuing until REM sleep terminates. This invariant pattern gives way to a regular but more variable pattern where most erections meet normal criteria but some do not. The variability in erectile competence during sexual encounters may parallel the SRE changes and include instances where erectile failure occurs. However, the presence of even intermittent erectile failure can trigger another entire set of factors that lead to further deterioration of erectile function. Increased performance anxiety, increased interpersonal tension, depressed mood, and general concern may all be associated with increased sympathetic activation when attempting sexual activity. This may increase vasoconstriction and peripheral resistance, which can in turn interfere with the erectile process.

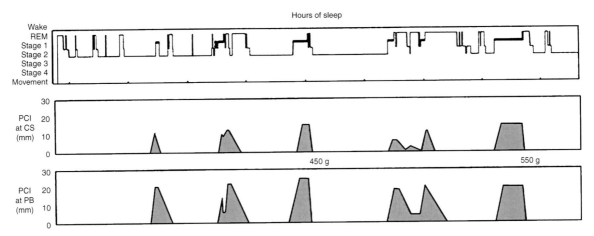

Figure 4.3 Sleep histogram and penile circumference increase (PCI) recorded at the coronal sulcus (CS) and penile base (PB) in a man with borderline erectile function. This 71-year-old man had a mixed pattern of sleep-related erections, with some episodes seemingly normal while others were diminished. The maximum rigidity measured on the two best episodes was only 450 and 550 g buckling force, which is considered marginal

The individual may also become avoidant, thereby increasing stress in the relationship. In such a manner, creeping organicity, while not the sole factor, makes a significant contribution to the overall clinical condition. In our experience, the patient is sometimes greatly relieved to find out that the problem is 'not entirely in his head' and at the same time is not 'irreversible organic impotence'. At that point, sex therapy can directly address taking maximum advantage of existing erectile capability, minimizing intra- and interpersonal problems, and adjusting expectations. SRE variability has also been demonstrated in men with depression.[65] It has been theorized that affective experience during the day accounts for some of the variability. In a study of 45 men with depression and 43 controls, daytime scores for affect intensity correlated with SRE duration and rigidity in the depressed group, but not in controls. REM sleep changes could account for some, but not all, of this relationship.

Our understanding of erectile dysfunction has greatly increased in the past 40 years. Public understanding and acceptance of impotence as a significant clinical problem that affects quality of life has increased the demand for services. Individuals who experience problems are more likely to seek help, and seek it sooner. Thus, in many clinics, the number of extreme and clear-cut cases of either organic or psychogenic impotence has declined in proportion to the total number of patients seeking care. The mixed organic–psychogenic etiology is more difficult to diagnose. Fortunately, a larger array of therapies is available. The traditional limited choice between psychotherapy and surgery is a thing of the past. SRE testing offers objective and highly refined information concerning the physiologic dynamics underlying a patient's erectile failure. This information can help the clinician and patient rationally formulate a realistic treatment plan.

SLEEP-RELATED PAINFUL ERECTIONS

Definition and description

Sleep-related painful erections (also known as penile pain syndrome) occurs when the normal, naturally occurring penile erections that non-volitionally occur during REM sleep in men are associated with intense pain that awakens the individual and disrupts sleep.[66] Erections occurring in sexual situations or at other times during the day are normal and not painful.

Although the etiology is not known, several theories have been proposed. Ferrini-Strambi et al[67] hypothesized that penile pain syndrome was an autonomic nervous system disorder. Based on their observation that vagal cardiac activity was reduced and there was possible hyperactive β-adrenergic activity during sleep, they tried β-blockers, which sometimes provided relief. Alternatively, endothelial dysfunction has been proposed, based on the fact that painful erections are sometimes produced by PGE_1 injections. Other candidate explanations have been suggested, including a bulbocavernosus–ischiocavernosus disorder and possible involvement of central dopamine agonists.[68]

Treatment

The sleep-related painful erection can be a very difficult condition to treat. A wide assortment of drug treatments has been used, with variable success. These include REM-suppressing antidepressants (e.g., tricyclics and monoamine oxidase inhibitors), β-blockers, and the atypical antipsychotic clozapine.[69] In very severe cases in which the patient will sacrifice potency for relief from the painful erections, medroxyprogesterone acetate and leuprolide acetate have been tried. Nonetheless, amitriptyline remains the first-line treatment and has the least side-effects.[70]

Special association with sleep

Sleep-related painful erection is classified as a parasomnia occurring during REM sleep. This disorder is mercifully very rare. In its severe form, a patient may awaken with erectile pain from every REM sleep episode, thereby producing profound REM sleep deprivation, hypersomnia, and impaired daytime function.

SLEEP AND THE MENSTRUAL CYCLE

Definition and description

Physiologic and in particular hormonal alterations occur in women's bodies in association with the menstrual cycle. This cycle serves reproductive functions and involves the production of an egg (ovum), its release, and (if it is not fertilized) its destruction and disposal. Individuals have varying responses to this process, which is marked by large swings in hormonal secretion. From the egg's viewpoint, the cycle timing is as follows.

Days 1–12 (before ovulation) is the time when menstruation (bleeding) occurs – usually for about 5 days. After menstruation, a new egg ripens in the ovary. Days 13–14 (egg release) is approximately when the egg is released and if it is fertilized, pregnancy occurs. During days 15–18 (after ovulation), if pregnancy has not occurred, the uterine wall lining breaks down and is shed during menstruation. The hormonal variations and the changes that occur in association with the menstrual cycle contribute to altered sleep quantity and quality.[71,72] Menstruation-associated sleep disorder has two different profiles, depending upon where in the cycle the problem occurs: premenstrual insomnia and premenstrual hypersomnia.

Treatment

Studies have revealed disturbances in the timing and coordination of sleep and other biologic rhythms. These include alterations in melatonin, temperature, cortisol, prolactin, and thyroid-stimulating hormone (TSH). In individuals predisposed to depressive and dysthymic disorders, these changes can provoke mood alterations.[73] Correcting the desynchronized rhythms is thought to serve as a viable treatment strategy to improve mood.[72] Symptomatic treatment can also be helpful.

Special association with sleep

Particular sleep problems are associated with each phase of the menstrual cycle. Tenderness and bloating during menstruation provoke insomnia in 50% of women according to the National Sleep Foundation Women and Sleep Poll. Premenstrual insomnia is characterized by difficulty in initiating or maintaining sleep, temporally associated with the week before onset of menses.[75–79] The sleeplessness difficulty is recurrent, and diagnostically it should have occurred for at least three consecutive cycles. Polysomnography shows decreased sleep efficiency, frequent arousals, prolonged periods of wakefulness, and, frequent sleep-stage transitions. In contrast, the premenstrual hypersomnia is marked by sleepiness occurring in association with the menstrual cycle, typically at days 19–21, when progesterone is at its peak level. Sleep studies have demonstrated normal duration and quality of nocturnal sleep; however, multiple sleep latency testing has objectively documented elevated physiologic sleepiness.

Estrogen and progesterone generally increase sleep (REM and NREM, respectively). When progesterone increases following ovulation, sleepiness or fatigue may ensue. When the bleeding begins, however, sleep quality usually declines. The deterioration in sleep coincides with the decrease in progesterone at the end of the cycle, during days 22–28 when premenstrual symptoms often occur (including bloating, headaches, cramps, and mood alterations).

REFERENCES

1. Weatherall M, Arnold T. Nocturia in adults: draft New Zealand guidelines for its assessment and management in primary care. NZ Med J 2006; 119: U1976.
2. Paick JS, Ku JH, Shin JW, Yang JH, Kim SW. Alpha-blocker monotherapy in the treatment of nocturia in men with lower urinary tract symptoms: a prospective study of response prediction. BJU Int 2006; 97: 1017–23.
3. Margel D, Shochat T, Getzler O, Livne PM, Pillar G. Continuous positive airway pressure reduces nocturia in patients with obstructive sleep apnea. Urology 2006; 67: 974–7.
4. Fitzgerald MP, Mulligan M, Parthasarathy S. Nocturic frequency is related to severity of obstructive sleep apnea, improves with continuous positive airways treatment. Am J Obstet Gynecol 2006; 194: 1399–403.
5. Nino-Murcia G, Keenan SA. Enuresis and sleep. In: Guilleminault C, ed. Sleep and its Disorders in Children. New York: Raven Press, 1987: 253–67.
6. Scharf MB, Pravda MF, Jennings SW, Kauffman R, Ringel J. Childhood enuresis: a comprehensive treatment program. Psychiatric Clin North Am 1987; 10: 655–74.
7. Glazener CM, Evans JH, Cheuk DK. Complementary and miscellaneous interventions for nocturnal enuresis in children. Cochrane Database Syst Rev 2005; (2): CD005230.
8. Glazener CM, Evans JH, Peto RE. Treating nocturnal enuresis in children: review of evidence. J Wound Ostomy Continence Nurs 2004; 31: 223–34.
9. Butler RJ, Gasson SL. Enuresis alarm treatment. Scand J Urol Nephrol 2005; 39: 349–57.
10. Lyon C, Schnall J. What is the best treatment for nocturnal enuresis in children? J Fam Pract 2005; 54: 905–6, 909.
11. Basha S, Bialowas C, Ende K, Szeremeta W. Effectiveness of adenotonsillectomy in the resolution of nocturnal enuresis secondary to obstructive sleep apnea. Laryngoscope 2005; 115: 1101–3.
12. Umlauf MG, Chasens ER. Sleep disordered breathing and nocturnal polyuria: nocturia and enuresis. Sleep Med Rev 2003; 7: 403–11.
13. Scott FB, Byrd GJ, Karacan I, et al. Erectile impotence treated with an implantable, inflatable prosthesis: five years of clinical experience. JAMA 1979; 241: 2609–12.
14. Fisher C, Gross J, Zuch J. Cycle of penile erection synchronous with dreaming (REM) sleep: preliminary report. Arch Gen Psychiatry 1965; 2: 29–45.
15. Fisher C. Dreaming and sexuality. In: Loewenstein RM, Newman LM, Schur M, Solnit AJ, eds. Psychoanalysis – A General Psychology. New York: International Universities Press, 1966: 537–69.
16. Karacan I. The effect of exciting presleep events on dream reporting and penile erections during sleep. Unpublished Doctoral Dissertation, Department of Psychiatry, Downstate Medical Center Library, New York University, Brooklyn, NY, 1965.
17. Snyder F. The phenomenology of dreaming. In: Madow L, Snow LH, eds. The Psychodynamic Implications of the Physiological Studies on Dreams. Springfield, IL: Charles C Thomas, 1970: 124–51.
18. McCarley RW, Hoffman E. REM sleep dreams and the activation–synthesis hypothesis. Am J Psychiatry 1981; 138: 904–12.
19. Ware JC, Hirshkowitz, M, Thornby J, et al. Sleep-related erections: effects of presleep sexual arousal. J Psychosom Res 1997; 42: 547–53.
20. Karacan I, Williams RL, Salis PJ. The effect of sexual intercourse on sleep patterns and nocturnal penile erections. Psychophysiology 1970; 7: 338.

21. Karacan I, Ware JC, Salis PJ, et al. Sexual arousal and activity: effect on subsequent nocturnal penile tumescence patterns. Sleep Res 1979; 8: 61.

22. Karacan I, Williams RL, Thornby JI, et al. Sleep-related penile tumescence as a function of age. Am J Psychiatry 1975; 132: 932.

23. Reynolds CF, Thase ME, Jennings JR, et al. Nocturnal penile tumescence in healthy 20- to 59 year olds: a revisit. Sleep 1989; 12: 368.

24. Schiavi RC, Schreiner Engel P, Mandeli J, Schanzer H, Cohen E. Healthy aging and male sexual function. Am J Psychiatry 1990; 147: 766–71.

25. Ware JC, Hirshkowitz M. Characteristics of penile erections during sleep recorded from normal subjects. J Clin Neurophysiol 1992; 9: 78.

26. Karacan I, Salis PJ, Ware JC, et al. Nocturnal penile tumescence and diagnosis in diabetic impotence. Am J Psychiatry 1978; 135: 191–7.

27. Hirshkowitz M, Karacan I, Rando KC, et al. Diabetes, erectile dysfunction, and sleep-related erections. Sleep 1990; 13: 53.

28. Fletcher EC, Martin RJ. Sexual dysfunction and erectile impotence in chronic obstructive pulmonary disease. Chest 1982; 81: 413.

29. Snyder S, Karacan I. Effects of chronic alcoholism on nocturnal penile tumescence. Psychosom Med 1981; 43: 423–9.

30. Halstead LS, Dimitrijevic M, Karacan I, et al. Impotence in spinal cord injury: neurophysiological assessment of diminished tumescence and its relation to supraspinal influences. Curr Concepts Rehab Med 1984; 1: 8.

31. Karacan I, Dervent A, Cunningham G, et al. Assessment of nocturnal penile tumescence as an objective method for evaluating sexual functioning in ESRD patients. Dialysis Transplant 1978; 7: 872–6, 890.

32. Hirshkowitz M, Karacan I, Gurakar A, et al. Hypertension, erectile dysfunction, and occult sleep apnea. Sleep 1989; 12: 223.

33. Karacan I, Salis PJ, Hirshkowitz M, et al. Erectile dysfunction in hypertensive men: sleep-related erections, penile blood flow, and musculovascular events. J Urol 1989; 142: 56–61.

34. Thase ME, Reynolds CF, Glanz LM, et al. Nocturnal penile tumescence in depressed men. Am J Psychiatry 1987; 144: 89.

35. Cunningham GR, Karacan I, Ware JC, et al. The relationships between serum testosterone and prolactin levels and nocturnal penile tumescence (NPT) in impotent men. J Androl 1982; 3: 241.

36. Cunningham GR, Hirshkowitz M, Korenman SG, et al. Testosterone replacement and sleep-related erections in hypogonadal men. J Clin Endocrinol Metab 1990; 70: 792.

37. Carani C, Granata AR, Bancroft J, Marrama P. The effects of testosterone replacement on nocturnal penile tumescence and rigidity and erectile response to visual erotic stimuli in hypogonadal men. Psychoneuroendocrinology 1995; 20: 743–53.

38. Bancroft J. Are the effects of androgens on male sexuality noradrenergically mediated? Some consideration of the human. Neurosci Biobehav Rev 1995; 19: 325–30.

39. Barry JM, Blank B, Boileau M. Nocturnal penile tumescence monitoring with stamps. Urology 1980; 15: 171.

40. Procci WR, Martin DJ. Preliminary observations of the utility of portable NPT. Archives of Sexual Behavior 1984; 13: 569–580.

41. Bradley WE. New techniques in evaluation of impotence. Urology 1987; 29: 383.

42. Imagawa, Kawanishi. 1986.

43. Morales A, Condra M, Reid K. The role of penile tumescence monitoring in the diagnosis of impotence: a review. J Urol 1990; 143: 441–4.

44. Allen R, Brendler CB. Snap-gauge compared to a full nocturnal penile tumescence study for evaluation of patients with erectile impotence. J Urol 1990; 143: 51.

45. Morales et al. 1983.

46. Schmidt HS, Wise HA. Significance of impaired penile tumescence and associated polysomnographic abnormalities in the impotent patient. J Urol 1981; 126: 348–52.

47. Hirshkowitz M, Karacan I, Arcasoy MO, et al. Prevalence of sleep apnea in men with erectile dysfunction. Urology 1990; 36: 232.

48. Hirshkowitz M, Karacan I, Arcasoy MO, et al. The prevalence of periodic limb movements during sleep in men with erectile dysfunction. Biol Psychiatry 1989; 26: 541.

49. Ware JC, Hirshkowitz M. Monitoring penile erections during sleep. In: Kryger MH, Roth T, Dement WC, eds. Principles and Practice of Sleep Medicine. Philadelphia, PA: WB Saunders, 1994: 967–77.

50. Wein AJ, Fishkin R, Carpiniello VL, Mallory TB. Expansion without significant rigidity during nocturnal penile tumescence: a potential source of misinterpretation. J Urol 1981; 126: 343–4.

51. Schwartz DT. Role of confrontation in performance and interpretation of nocturnal penile tumescence studies. Urology 1983; 22: 240–2.

52. Karacan I. Clinical value of nocturnal erection in the prognosis and diagnosis of impotence. Med Aspects Human Sexuality 1970; 4: 27.

53. Kinsey AC, Pomeroy WB, Martin CE. Sexual Behavior in the Normal Male. Philadelphia, PA: WB Saunders, 1948.

54. Masters WH, Johnson VE. Human Sexual Inadequacy. Boston, MA: Little Brown, 1970.

55. Montejo-Gonzalez AL, Llorca G, Izquerdo JA, et al. SSRI-induced sexual dysfunction: fluoxetine, paroxetine, sertraline, and fluvoxamine in a prospective, multicenter and descriptive clinical study of 344 patients. Sex Marital Ther 1997; 23: 176.

56. Segraves RT, Schoenberg HW, Segraves KAB. Evaluation of the etiology of erectile failure. In: Segraves RT, Schoenberg HW, eds Diagnosis and Treatment of Erectile Distrubances: A Guide for Clinicians. New York: Plenum, 1985: 165–95.

57. Karacan I, Moore CA, Sahmay S. Measurement of pressure necessary for vaginal penetration. Sleep Res 1985; 14: 269.

58. Beutler LE, Karacan I, Anch AM, et al. MMPI and MIT discriminators of biogenic and psychogenic impotence. J Consult Clin Psychol 1975; 43: 899–903.

59. Marshall P, Surridge D, Delva N. Differentiation of organic and psychogenic impotence on the basis of MMPI decision rules. J Consult Clin Psychol 1980; 48: 407–8.

60. Martin LM, Rodgers DA, Montague DK. Psychometric differentiation of biogenic and psychogenic impotence. Arch Sex Behav 1983; 12: 475–85.

61. Jefferson TW, Glaros A, Spevack M, Boaz TL, Murray FT. An evaluation of the Minnesota Multiphasic Personality Inventory as a discriminator of primary organic and primary psychogenic impotence in diabetic males. Arch Sex Behav 1989; 18: 117–26.

62. Hatch JP, De La Pena AM, Fisher JG. Psychometric differentiation of psychogenic and organic erectile disorders. J Urol 1987; 138: 781–3.

63. Seagraves KA, Segraves RT, Schoenberg HW. Use of sexual history to differentiate organic from psychogenic impotence. Arch Sex Behav 1987; 16: 125–37.

64. Geisser ME, Jefferson TW, Spevak M, et al. Reliability and validity of the Florida Sexual History Questionnaire. J Clin Psychol 1991; 47: 519–28.

65. Nofzinger EA, Schwartz RM, Reynolds CF 3rd, et al. Correlation of nocturnal penile tumescence and daytime affect intensity in depressed men. Psychiatry Res 1993; 49: 139–50.

66. Ferini-Strambi L, Oldani A, Zucconi M, et al. Sleep-related painful erections: clinical and polysomnographic features. J Sleep Res 1996; 5: 195–7.

67. Ferini-Strambi L, Montorsi F, Zucconi M, et al. Cardiac autonomic nervous activity in sleep-related painful erections. Sleep 1996; 19: 136–8.

68. Calvet U. Painful nocturnal erection. Sleep Med Rev 1999; 3: 47–57.

69. Steiger A, Benkert O. Examination and treatment of sleep-related painful erections – a case report. Arch Sex Behav 1989; 18: 263–7.

70. Karsenty G, Werth E, Knapp PA, et al. Sleep-related painful erections. Nat Clin Pract Urol 2005; 2: 256–60; quiz 261.

71. Ho A. Sex hormones and the sleep of women. In: Chase MH, Stern WC, Walter PL, eds. Sleep and Research. Brain Information Service/Brain Research Institute, Volume 1. Los Angeles: UCLA, 1972.

72. Billiard M, Guilleminault C, Dement WC. A menstruation-linked periodic hypersomnia. Kleine–Levin syndrome or new clinical entity? Neurology 1975; 25: 436–43.

73. Parry BL, Mendelson WB, Duncan WC, Sack DA, Wehr TA. Longitudinal sleep EEG, temperature, and activity measurements across the menstrual cycle in patients with premenstrual depression and in age-matched controls. Psychiatry Res 1989; 30: 285–303.

74. Parry BL, Martinez LF, Maurer EL, et al. Sleep, rhythms and women's mood. Part I. Menstrual cycle, pregnancy and postpartum. Sleep Med Rev 2006; 10: 129–44.

75. Moline ML, Broch L, Zak R, Gross V. Sleep in women across the life cycle from adulthood through menopause. Sleep Med Rev 2003; 7: 155–77.

76. Lee KA, Shaver JF, Giblin EC, Woods NF. Sleep patterns related to menstrual cycle phase and premenstrual affective symptoms. Sleep 1990; 13: 403–9.

77. Shibui K, Uchiyama M, Okawa M, et al. Diurnal fluctuation of sleep propensity across the menstrual cycle. Psychiatry Clin Neurosci 1999; 53: 207–9.

78. Chuong CJ, Kim SR, Taskin O, Karacan I. Sleep pattern changes in menstrual cycles of Women with premenstrual syndrome: a preliminary study. Am J Obstet Gynecol 1997; 177: 554–8.

79. ICSD – International Classification of Sleep Disorders: Diagnostic and Coding Manual. Diagnostic Classification Steering Committee, Thorpy MH, Chairman, Rochester, MN: American Sleep Disorders Association, 1990.

5

Sleep and depression: A functional neuroimaging perspective

Christoph Nissen, Eric A Nofzinger

INTRODUCTION

Mood disorders are a prevalent problem with serious consequences for individual and public health. Major depressive disorder itself causes functional impairments and reductions in quality of life similar to or greater than those for common medical disorders, such as coronary heart disease or diabetes mellitus.[1] Sleep disturbances are among the most common clinical symptoms in depression. Moreover, characteristic alterations of polysomnographic sleep patterns are among the most consistently replicated biologic alterations in depressed patients.[2] Studying sleep – as a window to the brain – may provide significant insights into the pathophysiology of depressive disorders, ultimately leading to better diagnosis and treatment.

The present chapter will give a brief summary of polysomnographic findings in depression, outline the idea and challenges of imaging the sleeping brain, and summarize the functional neuroanatomy of healthy sleep. This will provide the empirical and conceptual background for the subsequently described alterations measured by brain imaging techniques during sleep in depression. At the end of the chapter, we will try to integrate these findings into a sleep-neuroscience model of depression.

POLYSOMNOGRAPHIC STUDIES IN DEPRESSION

Sleep in patients with depression in comparison with healthy controls is mainly characterized by disturbed sleep continuity, enhanced rapid eye movement (REM) sleep, and reduced slow-wave sleep measures.[3] Figure 5.1 depicts these characteristics. The transient therapeutic effect of sleep deprivation in some patients[4] and the predictive value of sleep parameters for the response to antidepressant therapy[5,6] corroborate the clinical interest in the relationships between sleep and depression. Despite these reliable observations, polysomnography, as surface electrophysiology, has been of limited value in elucidating underlying changes in brain function.

Note as conceptual background that the observation of quantifiable changes in brain function during sleep in depression (e.g., in the form of reduced REM sleep latency) supports the view that brain-based activity represents a final pathway for the clinical manifestation of depression. It is, however, as important to see that the electroencephalographic (EEG) sleep results, as well as the imaging findings described below, are descriptive and correlational in nature, and do not provide direct information about causality in the complex development of depression.

(a) Healthy
   control

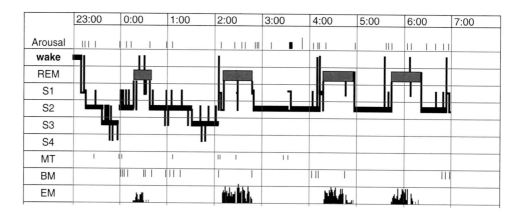

(3) Sleep continuity disturbances

(b) Depressed
   patient

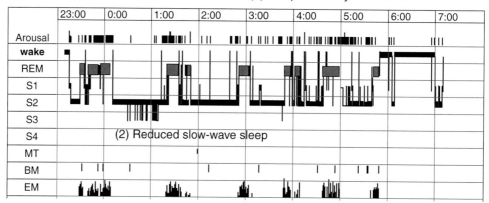

(2) Reduced slow-wave sleep

(1) Shortened REM sleep latency

Figure 5.1   Polysomnograms showing the characteristics of healthy sleep (a) in comparison with sleep in a depressed patient (b). (1) In depression, the period between sleep onset and the first occurrence of rapid eye movement (REM) sleep, shown in red, is markedly reduced (reduced REM latency). (2) The depressed patient spends less time in sleep stages 3 and 4 (reduced slow-wave sleep). (3) In depression, the number of awakenings and arousals is increased and the patient awakens early in the morning (disturbed sleep continuity). The sleep stages (REM and sleep stages 1–4 (S1–S4)) are given across the time. BM, body movement; EM, eye movement (See also color plate section.)

FUNCTIONAL NEUROIMAGING OF SLEEP

Recent advances in human brain imaging techniques may provide significant information regarding alternating brain activity during the sleep/wake rhythm in depression that is not accessible to surface electrophysiology. Various neuroimaging techniques have been developed to quantify physiologic processes of the brain, including blood flow (e.g., functional magnetic resonance imaging (fMRI) and $H_2^{15}O$ positron emission tomography

(PET), metabolism ([^{18}F]2-fluoro-2-deoxy-D-glucose ([^{18}F]FDG)-PET), and receptor binding (e.g., imaging of dopamine or acetylcholine receptors). Imaging sleep is particularly challenging: Many techniques, including fMRI and $H_2^{15}O$-PET, require that the subjects sleep in the scanner, with their head immobilized. These techniques can, therefore, only be performed on select subjects, and often only after a period of sleep deprivation to allow the occurrence of sleep in this adverse environment. Besides the burden on the subject, it is important to see that the physiologic integrity of sleep will be markedly affected by techniques that require sleeping in the scanner (for additional information, see reference 7).

The [^{18}F]FDG-PET method allows assessment of glucose brain metabolism during periods of more natural sleep.[8] Participants sleep in a comfortable sleep laboratory environment with polysomnographic monitoring. The [^{18}F]FDG tracer is administered intravenously, marking brain glucose metabolism during a 20-minute sleep period of interest. Subjects are subsequently awakened and transferred to the PET scanner unit. Due to the dynamics of [^{18}F]FDG uptake and metabolism, the preceding pattern of glucose metabolism during the sleep period can be quantified, without being significantly affected by postsleep procedures.

Note that current imaging modalities provide only limited information regarding small brain structures, such as the ventrolateral preoptic area, or faster neural events ultimately implicated in the regulation of sleep/wake rhythms.

FUNCTIONAL NEUROANATOMY OF HEALTHY SLEEP

In this section, brain processes that promote the physiologic rhythm of wakefulness and sleep are described. These processes include the wake-promoting function of the ascending arousal system, the initiation of sleep onset, and the physiologic changes during non-REM (NREM) and REM sleep. The preclinical body of evidence will be related to brain imaging findings in healthy humans. This will provide a means to understand the alterations in functional neuroanatomy during sleep in depression that will be described in the subsequent section.

The ascending arousal system

After the Second World War, Moruzzi and Magoun[9] suggested that there is an ascending arousal system originating from the brainstem that keeps the brain awake. Studies in the 1970s and 1980s clarified the anatomic and chemical nature of this pathway – known as the ascending reticular activating system (ARAS). Figure 5.2 illustrates the anatomic structures and cell types of the arousal system comprising a thalamic loop and a non-thalamic loop. The major input to the relevant nuclei of the thalamus originates from cholinergic cell groups in the pedunculopontine (PPT) and laterodorsal tegmental (LDT) nuclei in the upper pons. This cholinergic input is crucial to permit transmission between the thalamus and the cortex, which is important for the acquisition of information and wakefulness. The non-thalamic loop of the arousal system activates the cerebral cortex to facilitate the processing of inputs from the thalamus. The major input to this pathway originates from monoaminergic neurons in the upper brainstem and hypothalamus. The activating inputs include noradrenergic neurons from the locus ceruleus, serotonergic cells from the dorsal raphe nucleus, histaminergic projections from the tuberomammillary nucleus, orexinergic neurons from the lateral hypothalamus, dopaminergic inputs from the A10 area of the periaqueductal gray matter, and neurons in the basal forebrain that contain γ-aminobutyric acid (GABA) or acetylcholine. The combined high activity of the cholinergic and aminergic cell groups promotes the characteristics of wakefulness, including cortical activation, externally generated perception, voluntary movement, and logical thinking.

Sleep onset

During the 1990s, investigators began to reveal the crucial role of the ventrolateral preoptic nucleus (VLPO) for the onset of sleep. For sleep to begin, VLPO neurons containing galanin and GABA send inhibitory outputs to all of the major cell groups in the brainstem and hypothalamus that promote arousal. In turn, the VLPO also receives inhibitory afferents from each of the major cholinergic and monoaminergic systems. This reciprocal inhibitory circuit ('flip flop switch')[10] is under the control of orexinergic neurons that primarily reinforce the monoaminergic tone and stabilize wakefulness.

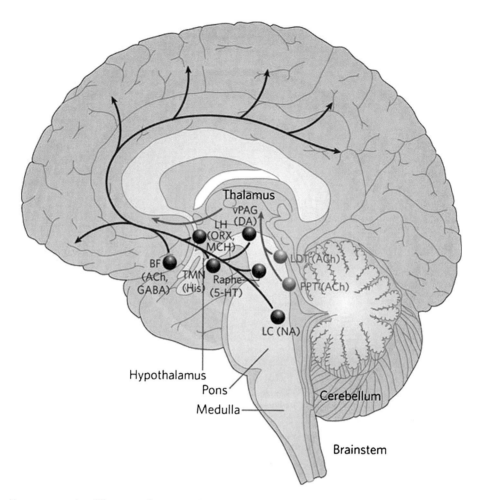

Figure 5.2 Key components of the ascending arousal system (ascending reticular activating system, ARAS). A major input to the thalamus (yellow pathway) originates from cholinergic (ACh) cell groups in the pons: the pedunculopontine (PPT) and laterodorsal tegmental (LDT) nuclei. These inputs facilitate thalamocortical transmission. A second, non-thalamic, pathway (red) activates the cerebral cortex to facilitate the processing of inputs from the thalamus. This pathway comprises neurons in monoaminergic cell groups, including the locus ceruleus (LC) containing norepinephrine (noradrenaline, NA), the raphe nucleus containing serotonin (5-hydroxytryptamine, 5-HT), the tuberomammillary nucleus (TMN) containing histamine (His), and neurons in the ventral periaqueductal gray matter (vPAG) containing dopamine (DA). This pathway also receives contributions from neurons in the lateral hypothalamus (LHA) containing orexin (ORX) or melanin-concentrating hormone (MCH), and from basal forebrain (BF) neurons containing γ-aminobutyric acid (GABA) or ACh (reprinted, by permission from Macmillan Publishers Ltd: Saper CB, Scammell TE, Lu J. Hypothalamic regulations of sleep and circadian rhythms. Nature 437:1257–63, Copyright 2005)[20] (See also color plate section.)

NREM sleep

During NREM sleep, the activity of the arousal-mediating cholinergic and aminergic cell groups diminishes to a minimum.[11] In healthy subjects, the transition from waking to NREM sleep is characterized by a global decline in whole-brain blood flow[12] and metabolism.[13] Brain activity decreases with greater depth of NREM sleep as assessed by glucose metabolism[14] and blood flow.[15] Glucose utilization during NREM sleep in comparison with waking is decreased by around 10% in stage 2[16] to 40% in stages 3 and 4.[17] However, the changes in glucose or blood oxygen use relative to waking are not equally distributed across the brain.

Regionally, greater reductions in glucose metabolism occur in the thalamus and broad regions of the frontal, parietal, temporal, and occipital cortex,[13,18,19] reflecting the attenuating excitatory input from the thalamic and non-thalamic loops of the ARAS to the cortex (Figure 5.3). It is interesting to note that the decline in activity from waking to NREM sleep reliably includes the dorsolateral prefrontal cortex (DLPFC), since this region will be of particular interest for the alterations observed in depression.

In contrast, relative increases in glucose metabolism during NREM sleep compared with waking were found bilaterally in the anterior hypothalamus, basal forebrain, and hippocampus.[13] This pattern of increased activity is consistent with preclinical findings suggesting hypothalamic and basal forebrain participation in the generation of NREM sleep.[20] Interestingly, this pattern is also consistent with the hypothesis of hippocampal–cortical reactivation processes during NREM sleep that may be implicated in the transition of initially unstable memory traces in the hippocampus into long-term memories in the cortex.[21]

REM sleep

Global cerebral energy metabolism during REM sleep is equal to or greater than that which occurs during waking and markedly greater than that during NREM sleep.[14,22] However, specific brain regions show distinct patterns of activity changes. Consistently, a high level of blood flow has been found in human REM sleep in the pontine brainstem.[12,23] This is consistent with the neurotransmitter changes during REM sleep, characterized by a maximally attenuated aminergic tone but – in contrast to NREM sleep – a high cholinergic tone arising from PPT and LDT activity in the brainstem. Imaging studies show, in addition to pontine brainstem activation, preferential activation of limbic and paralimbic regions of the forebrain in comparison with waking. More specifically, the REM sleep–associated activation comprises an extensive confluent region along the midline, including the lateral hypothalamic area, septal

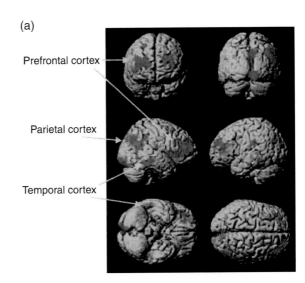

(a)

Prefrontal cortex

Parietal cortex

Temporal cortex

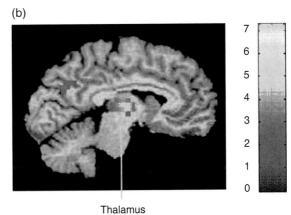

(b)

Thalamus

Figures 5.3 NREM sleep in healthy subjects. (a) Three-dimensional rendering of regions demonstrating significantly less relative metabolism during NREM sleep in relation to waking in healthy subjects. (b) Sagittal section showing regions of the thalamus demonstrating less relative metabolism during NREM sleep in relation to during waking (reproduced from Nofzinger EA et al. Brain 2002; 125:1105–15 by permission of Oxford University Press)[13] (See also color plate section.)

area, ventral striatum and substantia innominata, as well as the infralimbic, prelimbic, and orbitofrontal cortex (Figure 5.4). Importantly, the activation during REM sleep in comparison with waking in healthy subjects also includes the amygdala and the anterior cingulate cortex (ACC) – two regions that will be of particular interest for the alterations in depression.

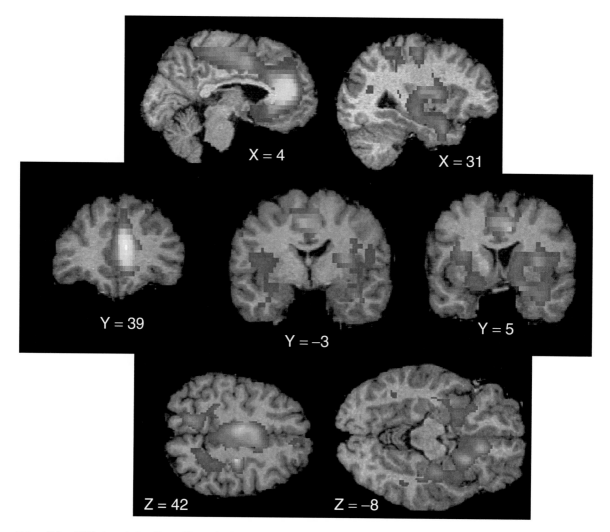

Figure 5.4   REM sleep in healthy subjects: brain structures where relative metabolism is greater in REM sleep than in waking in healthy subjects. This general pattern includes limbic and paralimbic structures, hippocampus, amygdala, ventral striatum, basal ganglia, supplementary motor area, anterior cingulate cortex, and medial prefrontal cortex (reprinted from Sleep Medicine Reviews, Vol 9, Nofzinger EA, Newimaging and sleep medicine, pp 157–72, Copyright © 2005, with permission from Elsevier)[7] (See also color plate section.)

Interestingly, the findings of specific brain activity patterns during different brain states relate, on a cognitive neuroscience level, to the subjective experiences that are characteristic of each brain state, with externally generated perception and logical thinking during waking, a decline in sensation and perception during deep NREM sleep, and a highly emotional, internally driven sensation during REM sleep. Note specifically that heteromodal association areas in the frontal and parietal cortex remain largely deactivated throughout REM and NREM sleep in comparison with waking. This deactivation in frontal and parietal cortical areas presumably relates to the lack of consciousness as a common hallmark of sleep, since activation in these areas is regarded as a necessary prerequisite for the emergence of conscious experience with its two main components[24] – wakefulness (level of consciousness) and awareness (content of consciousness).

The remarkable concordance of evidence emerging from different brain imaging techniques applied during healthy sleep indicates that the brain undergoes profound and specific changes in activity across the states of waking, NREM sleep, and REM sleep, and argues strongly for the basic validity of neuroimaging as a tool in sleep research.

FUNCTIONAL NEUROANATOMY OF SLEEP IN DEPRESSION

Recent neuroimaging studies show that the characteristic changes in brain activity across the brain states of waking, NREM sleep, and REM sleep differ between subjects with and without depression. These findings may help to understand the clinical complaints of poor sleep and the alterations revealed by polysomnography in depression on a level that is closer to basic neural processes implicated in the pathophysiology of depression. Functional neuroimaging, therefore, represents a potential link between cognitive, emotional, and behavioral symptoms in depression and neural processes, such as synaptic plasticity or gene–environment interaction, ultimately underlying the clinical symptomatology.

NREM sleep in depression

Like healthy controls, patients with depression show a reduction in activity in the thalamus and in the frontal, parietal, and temporal association cortex in NREM sleep in comparison with waking.[25] In spite of a similar overall pattern, depressed patients show less of a decline in activity than do healthy subjects in some brain regions and a greater decline in other regions.

Depressed patients show less of a decline in broad regions of the frontal, parietal and temporal cortex. Since this change is a relative measure referred to waking, it is important to see that the findings may reflect a change in brain function during either wakefulness or sleep, or an interaction between the two. Patients with depression reliably demonstrate reduced brain activity in frontal areas during waking ('hypofrontality') in the form of reduced glucose metabolism[26] or blood flow.[27] The integration of wake and sleep findings indicates that patients with depression show a hypofrontality during waking that does not further decline to the expected extent in NREM sleep (Figure 5.5). Given that prefrontal cortex function has repeatedly been implicated in the implementation of cognitive control, the hypofrontality observed in depressed patients may relate to the difficulties in organizing and guiding behavior toward the resolution of a conflict in depression.

This disturbed sleep/wake activity pattern may reflect disturbed NREM sleep processes, such as a lack in the depletion of glycogen stores[28] or an attenuated downscaling of synaptic plasticity,[29] resulting in waking hypofrontality. Alternatively, prefrontal cortex functioning during waking may be fundamentally attenuated in depression, resulting in less of a need for restorative processes during NREM sleep, which might explain the relative lack of deactivation in prefrontal brain areas during NREM sleep in depression. Further studies may elucidate the contributions of waking and NREM sleep processes for the alternated prefrontal activity pattern.

In addition, depressed patients show a greater decline than healthy subjects in brain structures that promote arousal and in ventral and posterior structures.[25] Secondary analyses, however, reveal hypermetabolism in these areas during waking that – in spite of a greater decline – persists during NREM sleep in depression. These areas comprise the arousal-promoting ARAS and the basal forebrain. The hyperactivity in these areas may relate to some typical clinical complaints, including increased arousal during waking and a disturbed continuity of sleep. The hypermetabolic areas also include the amygdala and the ACC. Preclinical and functional neuroimaging studies in humans have implicated these regions in the initial experience of emotions and in the automatic generation of emotional responses.[30] The amygdala and the ACC are closely connected to more caudal areas that promote arousal, including the brainstem and basal forebrain. Persistent hyperactivity in the amygdala

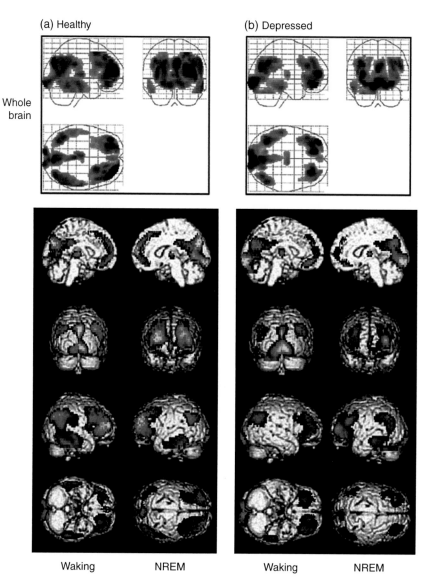

Figure 5.5   NREM sleep in depression, 'Glass brain' and 3-dimensional brain-rendering images showing regions with significant declines in relative metabolism from waking to NREM sleep, including the prefrontal cortex, cuneus, precuneus, and the temporoparietal cortex: (a) healthy subjects. (b) depressed subjects. Note that, despite a generally similar pattern of metabolism, depressed patients showed less frontal activity during waking ('hypofrontality') in comparison with healthy subjects and a relative lack of deactivation from waking to NREM sleep (reproduced from Nofzinger EA et al. Arch Ger Psychiatry 2005; 62:387–96. Copyright © 2005, American Medical Association. All rights reserved.)[25] (See also color plate section.)

and ACC throughout waking and NREM sleep may represent an emotional component of hyperarousal in depression.

The findings of a persistent hypoactivity in frontal areas implicated in the implementation of cognitive control and a persistent hyperactivity in systems that play a key role in the regulation of arousal and emotions throughout the sleep/wake cycle in depression will be further elaborated in a sleep-neuroscience model of depression at the end of this chapter.

REM sleep in depression

Depressed patients show different changes in brain activity from waking to REM sleep than do healthy controls. The main findings in depression can be summarized as stronger increases from waking to REM sleep in three brain areas: the brainstem reticular formation, the limbic and anterior paralimbic cortex, and parts of the executive cortex[31] (Figure 5.6).

The stronger increase in glucose metabolism in the brainstem reticular formation during REM sleep in depression may be driven by enhanced activity of cholinergic, REM sleep-generating neurons located in the LDT and PPT in the brainstem. This is consistent with the model of an elevated tone in cholinergic neurotransmission and an attenuated tone in monoaminergic neurotransmission that has been implicated in the pathophysiology of depression.[32]

Limbic *and* paralimbic areas that have demonstrated a more pronounced activity increase from waking to REM sleep in depression include the hippocampus, the basal forebrain/ventral pallidum, the ACC, and the medial prefrontal cortex. Given that these structures have the highest density of cholinergic receptors in the brain[33] and a high density of inhibitory 5-HT$_{1A}$ serotonergic receptors,[34] the described activity pattern may reflect the cholinergic/aminergic imbalance in limbic and paralimbic areas, in addition to that seen in the brainstem reticular formation. Cognitive neuroscience studies have implicated these limbic and paralimbic structures in the identification and production of affective states.[30] In depression, a high activation in these areas may be related to affective disturbances, including the experience of increased anxiety and depressed mood.[35]

The stronger relative increase in metabolism in the executive cortex, including the DLPFC, from waking to REM sleep in depression may also be driven by an unusually high cholinergic tone in depression. Note that hypoactivity in frontal brain areas and attenuated executive functions have been found in depression during waking. From the neurotransmission perspective, depression-associated reductions in aminergic neurotransmission may account for reductions in frontal cortex activity and executive function during waking. The specific neurotransmitter constellation during REM sleep in depression characterized by an unusually high cholinergic tone in a brain state when the aminergic tone is physiologically reduced to its minimum would, in this view, drive the stronger increase in activity in the executive cortex.

AFFECTIVE AND COGNITIVE NEUROSCIENCE OF DEPRESSION

It is of particular interest that many of the brain regions that undergo different changes in activity across the brain stages of waking, NREM sleep, and REM sleep in depressed patients in comparison with non-depressed controls are regions that have been implicated in the regulation of cognition and emotion. From a cognitive neuroscience perspective, it is plausible to assume that alterations in brain activity measured during the sleep/wake cycle relate to fundamental emotional and cognitive symptoms in depression. Note again that the plausible association does not directly inform whether the peculiarities in regional brain activity cause, reflect, or are bidirectionally interrelated with the clinical complaints in depression.

The following paragraphs provide an overview of the findings of affective and cognitive neuroscience studies on three brain regions and their interaction: the ACC, the DLPFC, and the amygdala. They are of particular interest since they demonstrate a different activity pattern across the sleep/wake cycle in patients with depression in comparison with healthy controls, and have been linked to cognitive and affective symptoms in depression.

The ACC, on the medial surface of the frontal lobe, is a highly differentiated structure. The caudal part of the dorsal ACC has been associated with conflict monitoring; for example, it is particularly active during conditions when one must arbitrate quickly between two likely responses.[36,37] As depression is associated with increased levels of conflict,

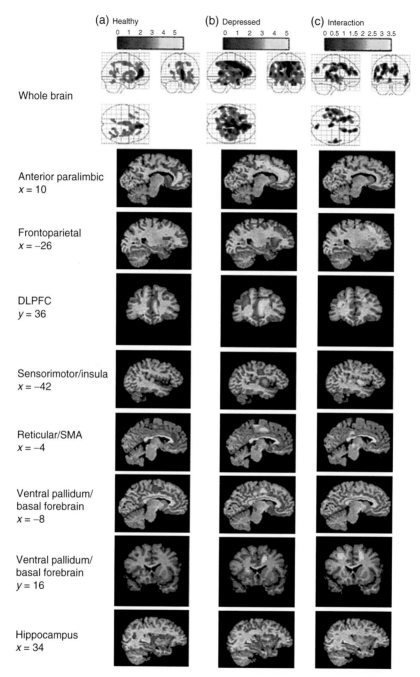

Figure 5.6 REM sleep in depression. Waking-to-REM sleep activations in healthy subjects (column a), depressed subjects (column b), and interactions showing regions where the depressed subjects' waking-to-REM activations are greater than those of healthy subjects (column c). Brain regions of greater activation from waking to REM sleep in depressed patients in comparison with healthy subjects include the brainstem reticular formation, the limbic and anterior paralimbic cortex, and parts of the executive cortex. DLPFC, dorsolateral prefrontal cortex; SMA, supplementary motor area; x and y are the Talairach x- and y-coordinates (reproduced from Nofzinger EA et al. Arch Ger Psychiatry 2004; 61:695–702. Copyright © 2005, American Medical Association. All rights reserved.)[31] (See also color plate section.)

manifested, for example, by intrusive thoughts, worry, self-doubt, and cognitive interference,[38] this region of the cingulate may be central to information processing disruptions. The rostral part of the ACC has been more strongly implicated in the evaluation of emotional information,[39] and the subgenual region has been associated specifically with mood reactivity.[40] Alterated activation has been reported in each region of the ACC in depressed individuals. Some authors have reported hypoactivation, others hyperactivation in depression (for an overview, see reference 41). As the ACC is a highly differentiated and one of the most frequently studied structures of the brain, a certain variability among findings can be expected. However, it is plausible that the supersensitive activation of the ACC in depressed patients seen in the waking-to-REM sleep neuroimaging probe corresponds to the abnormal affective responsivity seen in the aforementioned fMRI emotional and cognitive challenge studies.

In contrast to the ACC, which monitors performance, the prefrontal cortex seems to implement cognitive control – presumably as a second necessary component in the regulation of cognition.[42] Control in this context reflects how the brain finally executes higher functions, such as awareness, memory or language. Specifically, the dorsolateral part of the prefrontal cortex (the DLPFC) is active when sequences of items have to be held in working memory,[43] when dual tasks are performed rather than a single task,[44] or when the relevant task dimension switches.[45] This led to the hypothesis that DLPFC activation correlates with the relative difficulty of task demands and plays an important role in dealing with conflictual behavior and decision making. Hypofrontality, specifically associated with decreased DLPFC activity, has been repeatedly documented in depression,[26,27] and may underlie fundamental dysfunctions in organizing and guiding behavior toward the resolution of a conflict in depression.

From the results of previous studies, the amygdala plays an important role in directing attention to affectively salient stimuli and calling for further processing.[46] In depression, structural and functional abnormalities have been reported in the form of an enlargement of volume (in bipolar disorders[47] and temporal lobe epilepsy[48]) and increased functional activation during waking[49] and sleep.[31,50] Whereas the causal relations between these entities are still unknown, the hyperactivation described in depression may bias evaluation of and response to incoming information. Furthermore, the amygdala has been reported to be significantly involved in emotional learning,[51] leading to the hypothesis that increased amygdala activation during depressive episodes may favor the emergence of rumination based on an increased availability of emotionally negative memories.[52] For other important aspects of amygdala function that are beyond the scope of the present chapter see reference 41.

SLEEP-NEUROSCIENCE MODEL OF DEPRESSION

In this section, we shall try to integrate the polysomnographic, brain imaging, and cognitive/affective neuroscience findings presented above into a sleep-neuroscience model of depression.

Recent animal, human lesion, and functional neuroimaging studies have suggested that emotion perception – a process that includes the identification of the emotional significance of a stimulus, the generation of affective states, and the regulation of affective states – may depend upon the functioning of two neural systems: a ventral emotional system and a dorsal executive system.[30,35]

Following this conceptualization, the ventral system comprises the amygdala, insula, ventral striatum, and ventral regions of the ACC and prefrontal cortex. These brain regions are crucial for the initial identification of the emotional significance of a stimulus, the generation of affective states, and the automatic regulation of emotional responses. Hyperactivity of the ventral emotional system that persists throughout the sleep/wake cycle in patients with depression may be associated with affective disturbances characteristic of the disorder, such as increased anxiety and depressed mood. During sleep, the persistent hyperactivity of the ventral system may be related to the enhancement of REM sleep that has repeatedly been shown in patients with depression (Figure 5.7).

Whereas the ventral system has been implicated in the identification and early automatic processing of emotional stimuli, the dorsal neural system seems to be important for the performance of executive functions, such as selective attention, planning, and the effortful, non-automatic regulation of affective

states and subsequent behavior. The dorsal system comprises the hippocampus, the dorsal ACC, and the DLPFC. On a cognitive level, the hypoactivity in these regions ('hypofrontality') that persists throughout the sleep/wake rhythm in depression may be related to the difficulties of depressed patients in dealing with conflicting information and impairments of decision making. Given that the deactivation in frontal and prefrontal brain regions during sleep is a crucial component for the emergence of

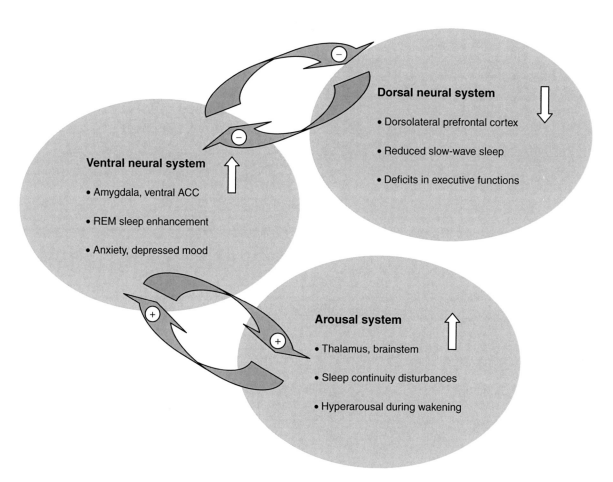

Figure 5.7 Sleep-neuroscience model of depression. The model aims to integrate findings from brain imaging studies, polysomnographic studies, and cognitive/affective neuroscience studies in depression. It proposes that three neural systems (arousal system, ventral emotional system, and dorsal executive system) are critically implicated in the pathophysiology of depression. The white arrows indicate the level of activity in each system in depressed patients in comparison with healthy controls. This level of activity is linked to polysomnographic characteristics and cognitive or affective symptoms in depression. The curved arrows reflect that the neural systems and their correlates on the polysomnographic and clinical levels are anatomically and functionally closely connected ('+' indicates functional enhancement. '−' indicates functional inhibition). REM, rapid eye movement; ACC, anterior cingulate cortex (See also color plate section.)

EEG slow-wave activity, alternated activity patterns in the dorsal system may relate to an attenuated generation of slow-wave sleep that has been found in depression.

The third system in the proposed model is the arousal system. As described above, the persistent hyperactivity in this system throughout the sleep/wake cycle in depression may be related to the experience of increased arousal during waking and disruptions of sleep continuity that include difficulties falling asleep, difficulties staying asleep, and early-morning awakenings.

The ventral emotional, dorsal executive, and arousal systems are anatomically and functionally closely connected. Evidence from studies examining the ventral and dorsal systems suggests that there is a reciprocal interaction between them.[30] Furthermore, the ventral emotional system is closely connected to the brainstem arousal system. Whereas these anatomic and functional relationships between the three neural systems can be plausibly linked to the alternated brain activity patterns, sleep peculiarities and clinical experience in depression, the causal relationships between the neural systems and the levels of assessment remain to be further elucidated.

SUMMARY AND PERSPECTIVES

The integration of preclinical and clinical evidence, including brain imaging studies throughout the sleep/wake cycle in depression, suggest functional neuroanatomic correlates for the characteristic EEG sleep alterations in depression, and led us to propose a sleep-neuroscience model of depression with three components:

- Hyperactivity in the brainstem arousal system persisting throughout the sleep/wake cycle is implicated in the experience of hyperarousal during waking and the disturbed continuity during sleep.

- Persistent hyperactivity in the ventral emotional system that includes the amygdala and the ventral ACC is related to affective disturbances,

such as depressed mood, and to the characteristic enhancement of REM sleep.

- Hypoactivity in the dorsal executive system that includes the DLPFC is implicated in the attenuation of executive functions and reduced slow-wave sleep in depression.

Future studies may focus on the dynamic interactions between the above-mentioned neural systems (e.g., connectivity analyses) and try to link the described alterations in depression to additional levels of organization, such as genetics (e.g., polymorphisms in genes of interest). To assess causality, it would be necessary to experimentally induce changes in specific neural systems (e.g., the ventral system in preclinical studies) or distinct clinical domains (e.g., executive functions via cognitive training in depressed patients) and measure the outcomes in the remaining systems/domains. Eventually, this approach may help to characterize brain processes and the clinical symptomatology in depression on an individual level, and may guide the development and individual application of therapy, including medications, psychotherapy, and other therapies.

REFERENCES

1. Spitzer RL, Kroenke K, Linzer M, et al. Health-related quality of life in primary care patients with mental disorders. Results from the PRIME-MD 1000 Study. JAMA 1995; 274: 1511–17.
2. Riemann D, Berger M, Voderholzer U. Sleep and depression – results from psychobiological studies: an overview. Biol Psychol 2001; 57: 67–103.
3. Benca RM, Obermeyer WH, Thisted RA, Gillin JC. Sleep and psychiatric disorders. A meta-analysis. Arch Gen Psychiatry 1992; 49: 651–68.
4. Wirz-Justice A, Van den Hoofdakker RH. Sleep deprivation in depression: What do we know, where do we go? Biol Psychiatry 1999; 46: 445–53.
5. Kupfer DJ, Frank E, McEachran AB, Grochocinski VJ. Delta sleep ratio. A biological correlate of early recurrence in unipolar affective disorder. Arch Gen Psychiatry 1990; 47: 1100–5.
6. Nissen C, Feige B, Konig A, et al. Delta sleep ratio as a predictor of sleep deprivation response in major depression. J Psychiatr Res 2001; 35: 155–63.

7. Nofzinger EA. Neuroimaging and sleep medicine. Sleep Med Rev 2005; 9: 157–72.

8. Nofzinger EA, Mintun MA, Price J, et al. A method for the assessment of the functional neuroanatomy of human sleep using FDG PET. Brain Res Brain Res Protoc 1998; 2: 191–8.

9. Moruzzi G, Magoun HW. Brain stem reticular formation and activation of the EEG. Electroencephalogr Clin Neurol 1949; 1: 455–73.

10. Saper CB, Chou TC, Scammell TE. The sleep switch: hypothalamic control of sleep and wakefulness. Trends Neurosci 2001; 24: 726–31.

11. Hobson JA, McCarley RW, Wyzinski PW. Sleep cycle oscillation: reciprocal discharge by two brainstem neuronal groups. Science 1975; 189: 55–8.

12. Braun AR, Balkin TJ, Wesenten NJ, et al. Regional cerebral blood flow throughout the sleep-wake cycle. An H$_2$^{15}O PET study. Brain 1997; 120: 1173–97.

13. Nofzinger EA, Buysse DJ, Miewald JM, et al. Human regional cerebral glucose metabolism during non-rapid eye movement sleep in relation to waking. Brain 2002; 125: 1105–15.

14. Maquet P. Sleep function(s) and cerebral metabolism. Behav Brain Res 1995; 69: 75–83.

15. Sutton JP, Caplan JB, Breiter HC, et al. Functional MRI study of human brain activity during NREM sleep. Soc Neurosci Abst 1997; 23: 21.

16. Maquet P, Dive D, Salmon E, et al. Cerebral glucose utilization during stage 2 sleep in man. Brain Res 1992; 571: 149–53.

17. Maquet P, Dive D, Salmon E, et al. Cerebral glucose utilization during sleep–wake cycle in man determined by positron emission tomography and [^{18}F]2-fluoro-2-deoxy-d-glucose method. Brain Res 1990; 513: 136–43.

18. Maquet P, Degueldre C, Delfiore G, et al. Functional neuroanatomy of human slow wave sleep. J Neurosci 1997; 17: 2807–12.

19. Hofle N, Paus T, Reutens D, et al. Regional cerebral blood flow changes as a function of delta and spindle activity during slow wave sleep in humans. J Neurosci 1997; 1712: 4800–8.

20. Saper CB, Scammell TE, Lu J. Hypothalamic regulation of sleep and circadian rhythms. Nature 2005; 437: 1257–63.

21. Buzsaki G. The hippocampo–neocortical dialogue. Cereb Cortex 1996; 6: 81–92.

22. Buchsbaum MS, Hazlett EA, Wu J, Bunney WE Jr. Positron emission tomography with deoxyglucose-F18 imaging of sleep. Neuropsychopharmacology 2001; 25(5 Suppl): S50–6.

23. Maquet P, Peters J, Aerts J, et al. Functional neuroanatomy of human rapid-eye-movement sleep and dreaming. Nature 1996; 383: 163–6.

24. Laureys S. The neural correlate of (un)awareness: lessons from the vegetative state. Trends Cogn Sci 2005; 9: 556–9.

25. Nofzinger EA, Buysse DJ, Germain A, et al. Alterations in regional cerebral glucose metabolism across waking and non-rapid eye movement sleep in depression. Arch Gen Psychiatry 2005; 62: 387–96.

26. Baxter LR Jr., Schwartz JM, Phelps ME, et al. Reduction of prefrontal cortex glucose metabolism common to three types of depression. Arch Gen Psychiatry 1989; 46: 243–50.

27. Mayberg HS, Lewis PJ, Regenold W, Wagner HN Jr. Paralimbic hypoperfusion in unipolar depression. J Nucl Med 1994; 35: 929–34.

28. Brown AM. Brain glycogen re-awakened. J Neurochem 2004; 89: 537–52.

29. Tononi G. The neuro-biomolecular basis of alertness in sleep disorders. Sleep Med 2005; 6 (Suppl 1): S8-12.

30. Phillips ML, Drevets WC, Rauch SL, Lane R. Neurobiology of emotion perception I: The neural basis of normal emotion perception. Biol Psychiatry 2003; 54: 504–14.

31. Nofzinger EA, Buysse DJ, Germain A, et al. Increased activation of anterior paralimbic and executive cortex from waking to rapid eye movement sleep in depression. Arch Gen Psychiatry 2004; 61: 695–702.

32. Janowsky DS, el Yousef MK, Davis JM, Sekerke HJ. A cholinergic-adrenergic hypothesis of mania and depression. Lancet 1972; ii: 632–5.

33. Mesulam MM, Hersh LB, Mash DC, Geula C. Differential cholinergic innervation within functional subdivisions of the human cerebral cortex: a choline acetyltransferase study. J Comp Neurol 1992; 318: 316–28.

34. Tsukada H, Kakiuchi T, Nishiyama S, Ohba H, Harada N. Effects of aging on 5-HT$_{1A}$ receptors and their functional response to 5-HT$_{1A}$ agonist in the living brain: PET study with [carbonyl-^{11}C] WAY-100635 in conscious monkeys. Synapse 2001; 42: 242–51.

35. Phillips ML, Drevets WC, Rauch SL, Lane R. Neurobiology of emotion perception II: Implications for major psychiatric disorders. Biol Psychiatry 2003; 54: 515–28.

36. Botvinick M, Nystrom LE, Fissell K, Carter CS, Cohen JD. Conflict monitoring versus selection-for-action in anterior cingulate cortex. Nature 1999; 402: 179–81.

37. Carter CS, Braver TS, Barch DM, et al. Anterior cingulate cortex, error detection, and the online monitoring of performance. Science 1998; 280: 747–9.

38. Schwartzer R. Thought control of action. In: Sarason IG, Pierce GR, Sarason BR, eds. Cognitive Interference. New York: Erlbaum, 1996: 90–115.

39. Whalen PJ, Bush G, McNally RJ, et al. The emotional counting Stroop paradigm: a functional magnetic resonance imaging probe of the anterior cingulate affective division. Biol Psychiatry 1998; 44: 1219–28.

40. Drevets WC, Frank E, Price JC, et al. PET imaging of serotonin 1A receptor binding in depression. Biol Psychiatry 1999; 46: 1375–87.

41. Davidson RJ, Pizzagalli D, Nitschke JB, Putnam K. Depression: perspectives from affective neuroscience. Annu Rev Psychol 2002; 53: 545–74.

42. MacDonald AW III, Cohen JD, Stenger VA, Carter CS. Dissociating the role of the dorsolateral prefrontal and anterior cingulate cortex in cognitive control. Science 2000; 288: 1835–8.

43. Cohen JD, Perlstein WM, Braver TS, et al. Temporal dynamics of brain activation during a working memory task. Nature 1997; 386: 604–8.

44. Courtney SM, Petit L, Maisog JM, Ungerleider LG, Haxby JV. An area specialized for spatial working memory in human frontal cortex. Science 1998; 279: 1347–51.

45. Konishi S, Nakajima K, Uchida I, et al. Transient activation of inferior prefrontal cortex during cognitive set shifting. Nat Neurosci 1998; 1: 80–4.

46. Holland PC, Gallagher M. Amygdala circuitry in attentional and representational processes. Trends Cogn Sci 1999; 3: 65–73.

47. Altshuler LL, Bartzokis G, Grieder T, Curran J, Mintz J. Amygdala enlargement in bipolar disorder and hippocampal reduction in schizophrenia: an MRI study demonstrating neuroanatomic specificity. Arch Gen Psychiatry 1998; 55: 663–4.

48. Tebartz van Elst, Woermann FG, Lemieux L, Trimble MR. Amygdala enlargement in dysthymia – a volumetric study of patients with temporal lobe epilepsy. Biol Psychiatry 1999; 46: 1614–23.

49. Drevets WC, Videen TO, Price JL, et al. A functional anatomical study of unipolar depression. J Neurosci 1992; 12: 3628–41.

50. Ho AP, Gillin JC, Buchsbaum MS, et al. Brain glucose metabolism during non-rapid eye movement sleep in major depression. A positron emission tomography study. Arch Gen Psychiatry 1996; 53: 645–52.

51. Ferry B, Roozendaal B, McGaugh JL. Role of norepinephrine in mediating stress hormone regulation of long-term memory storage: a critical involvement of the amygdala. Biol Psychiatry 1999; 46: 1140–52.

52. Drevets WC. Neuroimaging and neuropathological studies of depression: implications for the cognitive–emotional features of mood disorders. Curr Opin Neurobiol 2001; 11: 240–9.

6

Sleep alterations in schizophrenia

Matcheri S Keshavan

INTRODUCTION

Schizophrenia is one of the most disabling of all mental illnesses. It is characterized by disordered thinking, perceptual disturbances such as hallucinations, and delusional beliefs (positive symptoms), as well as deficits in motivation, socialization, and affect (negative symptoms). The illness begins in adolescence or early adulthood and leads to a marked decline in occupational and interpersonal function.

It has long been held that impaired sleep reflects a troubled mind. This view and the phenomenologic similarity between hallucinations and dreams have led to an increasing interest in sleep studies in schizophrenia. A vast literature has accumulated in regard to sleep abnormalities in schizophrenic illness. Impairments are seen in subjective quality of sleep,[1] as well as objective measures of sleep architecture, as measured by sleep polysomnographic studies. Notable findings include reductions in total sleep, impaired sleep continuity, rapid eye movement (REM) sleep latency, and amounts of slow-wave sleep (SWS). The amounts of REM sleep have been variably reduced in schizophrenia. There are some data suggesting alterations in the sleep–wake cycle as well.

Sleep disturbance is of considerable clinical importance, since it is related to impaired coping and perceived quality of life.[2] Impaired sleep also predicts symptomatic relapse with antipsychotic discontinuation.[3] The nature of such polysomnographic abnormalities and their relationship to the neurobiologic underpinnings of schizophrenia has remained poorly understood. In this chapter, we will briefly review the nature of SWS and REM sleep, the current state of knowledge with regard to the alterations in sleep architecture, the relation between antipsychotic medications and sleep, and the neurobiology of such impairments in schizophrenia.

NATURE OF SWS AND REM SLEEP

In recent years, there has been an increasing understanding of the possible functions of SWS and REM sleep. SWS is characterized by large-amplitude, low-frequency electroencephalographic (EEG) rhythms mainly occurring during the early part of sleep. The slow waves in SWS are associated with a large-scale spatiotemporal synchrony across the neocortex, and are thought to be generated predominantly in the prefrontal cortex.[4,5] SWS has been considered to reflect the overall synaptic density in the human cerebral cortex, in particular that of the prefrontal cortex. Deficits in SWS have therefore been thought to reflect parallel prefrontal cortical dysfunction. Sleep deprivation in normal subjects appears to cause impairments in sustained attention that closely resemble prefrontal cortical dysfunction.[5] SWS may be involved in a restorative activity reversing the 'wear and tear' caused during wakefulness; there is evidence for increased protein synthesis during this sleep phase.[6,7]

REM sleep is characterized by low-amplitude, relatively fast EEG rhythms, saccadic eye movements, and decreased muscle tone. In contrast to SWS, REM sleep is associated with an increased activity in phylogenetically old limbic and paralimbic regions such as the amygdala, hippocampus, cingulated, and entorhinal cortices.[8] On the other hand, the dorsolateral prefrontal and parietal cortices, as well as the posterior cingulate cortex and precuneus, are the least active brain regions during REM sleep. These observations are significant in view of the cognitive functions mediated by the prefrontal and limbic brain regions, as will be discussed later.

ALTERATIONS IN SLEEP ARCHITECTURE IN SCHIZOPHRENIA

Alterations of REM sleep

Early sleep polysomnographic studies examined the hypothesis that schizophrenia is a 'spillover' of the dream state into wakefulness. While no evidence thus far directly supports this prediction, subtle alterations in the architecture of REM sleep have been described.[9] REM latency was found to be decreased in several early studies;[10] this may result either from a deficit in SWS in the first non-REM (NREM) period leading to a passive advance, or from early onset of the first REM period or from 'REM pressure'. Amounts of REM sleep have been reported to variably increase, decrease, or not change.[10,11] Treatment-naive schizophrenia patients show no increases in REM sleep:[12,13] the increases in REM sleep observed in previously treated subjects may reflect effects of medication withdrawal and/or changes related to the acute psychotic state.[13] It is unlikely that the observed decreases in REM latency in some schizophrenia patients result from primary abnormalities in REM sleep.

Sleep deprivation provides a naturalistic, physiologic challenge for dynamic manipulation of sleep processes, and can help clarify the primary nature

of sleep abnormalities. An intriguing reduction in REM rebound following REM sleep deprivation has been described in several studies in acute schizophrenia, but a normal or exaggerated REM rebound has been found in remitted schizophrenic patients.[10] This rebound failure in acute schizophrenia has been attributed to a possible 'leakage' of phasic REM events from REM sleep into NREM sleep, although no systematic investigation has supported this hypothesis.

Alterations of slow-wave sleep

SWS is of particular interest with regard to schizophrenia because of the involvement of the prefrontal cortex in the generation of SWS as well as the cognitive deficits.[14,15] Several studies have shown a reduction of SWS in schizophrenic patients; SWS deficits have been seen in acute and chronic, as well as remitted states; and in never-medicated and neuroleptic-treated, as well as unmedicated patients.[10] However, not all studies show these deficits. Studies which failed to find differences in SWS have generally used conventional visual scoring. On the other hand, studies that reported quantified sleep EEG parameters revealed reductions in SWS. Ganguli et al[12] observed no change in visually scored SWS, but instead, a significant reduction in delta-wave counts in drug-naive schizophrenic patients, suggesting that visually scored SWS may not be sensitive enough, and automated counts may be a better marker of SWS deficiency in schizophrenia. Other groups have described similar reductions in delta counts. SWS deficits have been demonstrated in early-course schizophrenia using sensitive approaches such as spectral analysis.[16]

Reductions in low-frequency power may be associated with alterations in high-frequency EEG activity (HFA) (>20 Hz) as well. HFA is associated with feature binding and attention. Tekell et al[17] reported that schizophrenic patients showed significantly greater HFA than healthy controls in all sleep stages. Elevated HFA during sleep in unmedicated patients is associated with positive symptoms of illness.

Sleep-deprivation studies can also help clarify whether SWS abnormalities in schizophrenia are secondary to pathology in neuronal circuits in this disorder, or whether they reflect primary homeostatic disruption in sleep processes. There is evidence that following total sleep deprivation recovery of stage 4 sleep is diminished in schizophrenia.[18] SWS deprivation is known to consistently cause impaired attention, prolonged reaction time, verbal learning, and vigilance similar to what is seen in frontal lobe dysfunction and schizophrenia.[19] A defect in SWS recovery might be consistent with impairments in critical cognitive processes such as psychomotor vigilance observed in schizophrenia. Such a defect might also suggest impairment in restorative processes in schizophrenia.

Circadian sleep abnormalities

In addition to alterations in sleep architecture, some studies suggest that schizophrenia may be associated with a disturbance in rest–activity timing.[20] The question of whether these disturbances are secondary to antipsychotic medications or whether they are primary to the illness, however, remains to be clarified.[21] Circadian alterations appear to be correlated with poor cognitive functioning in schizophrenia.[22]

RELATION BETWEEN SLEEP ABNORMALITIES AND CLINICAL MEASURES IN SCHIZOPHRENIA

Research during the past two decades has focused increasingly on the positive and negative syndromes, a conceptual distinction of particular importance to the pathophysiology of schizophrenia. Several studies have examined the association between REM sleep parameters and clinical parameters. Tandon et al[13] reported an inverse association between REM latency and negative symptoms. While no association has been seen between sleep abnormalities and depressive symptoms,[13] there is some evidence that increased REM sleep may correlate with suicidal behavior in schizophrenia.[23,24]

In order to elucidate the significance of sleep abnormalities for pathophysiology, it is important to understand their longitudinal nature in schizophrenia: stage 4 sleep does not improve while other sleep stages change following 3–4 weeks of conventional antipsychotic treatment.[25] In a longitudinal polysomnographic study, SWS deficits remained stable at 1 year, but the REM sleep reductions appeared to improve. These observations suggest the possible trait-related nature of SWS deficits in schizophrenia.[26] Consistent with this view, SWS abnormalities correlate with negative symptoms[12] and with impaired outcome at 1 and 2 years.[27]

Attentional impairment appears to correlate with SWS deficits in early studies of schizophrenia.[28] The thalamus, the main 'switchboard' for information processing pathways in the brain, plays a crucial role in attention and gating of information because it is the major relay station receiving input from the reticular activating system and limbic and cortical association areas. A defect in the thalamus therefore could explain alterations in SWS and the psychopathology of schizophrenia. In a recent study, impairments in visuospatial memory were positively correlated with reduction in the amount of SWS and in sleep efficiency.[29] These results point to a functional interrelationship between regulation of SWS and performance in visuospatial memory in schizophrenia.

Schizophrenia patients have deficits mastering procedural learning. Procedural learning seems to be dependent on sleep. Manoach et al[30] tested the hypothesis that patients with schizophrenia have a deficit in sleep-dependent procedural learning. Patients failed to show overnight improvement and differed significantly from control subjects, who showed a significant 11% improvement. This suggests that sleep abnormalities may contribute, at least in part, to the cognitive impairments in schizophrenia.

RELATION BETWEEN SLEEP FINDINGS AND NEUROBIOLOGY IN SCHIZOPHRENIA

Studies of the ontogeny of sleep during normal adolescence are of significance to our understanding of the pathophysiology of SWS deficits, in the context of a neurodevelopmental framework for schizophrenia. Adolescence is characterized by a substantial reorganization of human brain function: a marked decline in synaptic density in the prefrontal cortex and pronounced reductions in cortical gray matter volume and regional cerebral metabolism have been seen during adolescence. In parallel, polysomnographic studies show robust SWS decreases across the age span from childhood to late adolescence.[31] The time courses for maturational changes in SWS, cortical metabolic rate, and synaptic density are strikingly similar. It has been suggested that the maturational processes in sleep EEG, cortical synaptic density and regional cerebral metabolism might reflect a common underlying biologic change (i.e., a large-scale programmed synaptic elimination).[32]

Do the polysomnographic abnormalities in schizophrenia relate to the brain maturational changes discussed above? In addition to SWS deficits, consistent alterations in the structure and function of cortical and subcortical brain regions have been observed in schizophrenia. Studies of the correlations between such alterations and sleep can help us better understand the pathophysiologic substrate underlying schizophrenia.

Altered brain structure

Schizophrenia is associated with widespread reductions in cortical gray matter, notably in the frontal and temporal cortex, as well as the thalamus.[33] The relationship between alterations in these brain structures and SWS is interesting, since SWS is generated by a complex neural system involving the anterior brain regions and the thalamus. SWS is inversely correlated with anterior horn ratio, a measure of frontal lobe size,[34] and positively correlated with lateral ventricular size.[35]

These correlations may result from reductions in subcortical structures such as the thalamus, which forms a substantial part of the ventricular boundaries.

Altered brain metabolism

SWS may result from several neurochemical processes involved in neural inhibition, excitation, and EEG synchrony. Activation of the cholinergic system facilitates arousal and enhances REM sleep. Cholinergic hyperfunction postulated to underlie schizophrenia, therefore, could account for SWS and REM latency reduction in schizophrenia sleep.[36] Interestingly, schizophrenia is associated with supersensitive REM sleep induction with the cholinergic agonist R5 86,[37] suggesting cholinergic hyperfunction. Nicotinic receptors may also be involved: sensory gating deficits as evidenced by P50 event-related potentials, which are possibly related to central nicotinergic system alterations, are reversed following sleep in schizophrenia.[38] Disturbances in catecholaminergic mechanisms may also underlie SWS deficits in schizophrenia. Serotonergic abnormalities may also be involved: an inverse correlation is seen between serotonin metabolites in the cerebrospinal fluid (CSF) and SWS in schizophrenia.[39] Noradrenergic and serotoninergic neurotransmission, which are presumed to be abnormal in schizophrenia, are inhibitory to REM; therefore, it is plausible that cholinergic and monoaminergic abnormalities mediate the constellation of reduced REM latency and SWS deficit without increases in REM sleep amounts in schizophrenia.[36]

Hormonal substances may also be related to delta sleep alterations. Adenosine, an amino acid neuromodulator, has attracted increasing interest in recent years as a possible endogenous sleep-promoting agent, as it tends to accumulate during waking hours.[40] Adenosine agonists such as dipyridamole, which increase delta sleep, have been suggested as having possible therapeutic benefits in schizophrenia.[41]

Altered physiology

There is evidence for decreased frontal lobe metabolism ('hypofrontality') in schizophrenia from a variety of physiologic imaging techniques. It may be instructive to examine SWS deficits in the context of such physiologic alterations. An association has been demonstrated in schizophrenia between SWS deficits and reduced frontal lobe membrane phospholipid metabolism as examined by ^{31}P magnetic resonance spectroscopy (MRS).[42] It has been suggested that membrane phospholipid alterations are related to loss of synaptic neuropils (i.e., decreased synaptic density), postulated to underlie schizophrenia. Conceivably, this could result in reduced SWS by decreased membrane surface (fewer dendrites per neuron), causing a smaller voltage response to the synchronizing stimulus, thereby leading to decreased SWS.

Single-cell recordings in cats have shown that slower (<1 Hz) synchronized oscillations originate mainly in the neocortex,[43] whereas delta waves (1–4 Hz) arise primarily from activity of thalamocortical neurons. A finer analysis of these oscillations may clarify the nature of pathophysiology in schizophrenia. Preliminary analysis of this question using period amplitude analyses suggested more prominent deficits in the <1 Hz range in schizophrenia, pointing to a thalamocortical dysfunction.[16] This finding deserves further study and application.

EFFECTS OF ANTIPSYCHOTIC DRUGS ON SLEEP

Studies of the acute effects of neuroleptics have consistently shown improvements in sleep continuity, as reflected by reduced sleep latencies, improved sleep time, greater sleep efficiency, and prolongation of REM latency;[10] however, changes in SWS have been less consistent. Studies that have examined the sedative effect of conventional neuroleptics have reported either no effects or modest increases in SWS.

Studies have begun to examine the effect of atypical antipsychotics on sleep. One study showed a robust increase in SWS with olanzapine following acute administration.[44] Olanzapine-induced increases in delta sleep may predict better treatment response.[45] On the other hand, clozapine increases stage 2 sleep, but may actually decrease stage 4 sleep.[46] In normal subjects, quetiapine increases total sleep time, sleep efficiency, percentage of stage 2 sleep, and subjective sleep quality.[47] These studies have frequently used small sample sizes; few studies have examined sleep variables in relation to acute versus long-term treatment with neuroleptics in a longitudinal design.

Attempts to examine polysomnographic characteristics of schizophrenia have to consider potential effects of neuroleptic discontinuation on sleep EEG. Neylan et al[48] reported significant worsening of REM and NREM sleep in a series of schizophrenic patients undergoing controlled neuroleptic discontinuation. Patients experiencing relapse have greater impairments in sleep. The effects of neuroleptic discontinuation continued to worsen from 2 to 4 weeks of a neuroleptic-free condition, and did not correlate with clinical change.[49] These suggest it is important to control for medication state in the investigation of EEG sleep in schizophrenia.

CONCLUSIONS AND FUTURE DIRECTIONS

In summary, sleep disturbances are pervasive, and cause substantial subjective distress as well as disability in schizophrenia. The emerging literature pointing to the relation between sleep alterations and neurobiologic changes in this illness suggest that sleep abnormalities may represent a window into the pathophysiology of schizophrenia. New knowledge of brain mechanisms of sleep is likely to open new avenues to explore such relationships. First, functional brain imaging studies suggest distinct patterns of regional brain activation in SWS and REM sleep; such studies can provide clues to the pathophysiology of schizophrenia, especially when used in conjunction with physiologic perturbation paradigms such as sleep deprivation.[50] Second, sleep architecture changes dramatically during development; sleep studies during development in health and disease can shed considerable light on developmentally mediated neuropsychiatric disorders.[51] Finally, sleep changes are often the earliest signs of disturbance, and may even represent trait-related vulnerability markers for psychiatric disorders; sleep studies of individuals at risk for schizophrenia are likely to be fruitful.[52]

REFERENCES

1. Ritsner M, Kurs R, Ponizovsky A, Hadjez J. Perceived quality of life in schizophrenia: relationships to sleep quality. Qual Life Res 2004; 3: 783–91.
2. Hofstetter JR, Lysaker PH, Mayeda AR. Quality of sleep in patients with schizophrenia is associated with quality of life and coping. BMC Psychiatry 2005; 5: 13.
3. Chemerinski E, Ho BC, Flaum M, et al. Insomnia as a predictor for symptom worsening following antipsychotic withdrawal in schizophrenia. Compr Psychiatry 2002; 43: 393–6.
4. Horne J. Human slow-wave sleep and the cerebral cortex. J Sleep Res 1992; 1: 122–4.
5. Horne JA. Human sleep, sleep loss and behavior. Implications for the prefrontal cortex and psychiatric disorder. Br J Psychiatry 1993; 162: 413–19.
6. Ramm P, Smith CT. Rates of cerebral protein synthesis are linked to slow wave sleep in the rat. Physiol Behav 1990; 48: 749–53.
7. Nakanishi H, Sun Y, Nakamura RK, et al. Positive correlations between cerebral protein synthesis rates and deep sleep in Macaca mulatta. Eur J Neurosci 1997; 9: 271–9.
8. Maquet P, Laureys S, Peigneux P, et al. Experience dependent changes in cerebral activation during human REM sleep. Nat Neurosci 2000; 3: 831–6.
9. Poulin J, Daoust AM, Forest G, Stip E, Godbout R. Sleep architecture and its clinical correlates in first episode and neuroleptic-naive patients with schizophrenia. Schizophr Res 2003; 62: 147–53.
10. Zarcone VP Jr, Benson KL. Sleep and schizophrenia. In: Kryger MH, Roth T, Derment WT, eds. Principles and Practice of Sleep Medicine. Philadelphia, PA: WB Saunders, 1994: 105–214.
11. Benca RM, Obermeyer WH, Thisted RA, Gillin JC. Sleep and psychiatric disorders. A meta-analysis. Arch Gen Psychiatry 1992; 49: 651–68.
12. Ganguli R, Reynolds CF 3rd, Kupfer DJ. Electroencephalographic sleep in young, never-medicated schizophrenics. A comparison with delusional and nondelusional depressives and with healthy controls. Arch Gen Psychiatry 1987; 44: 36–44.
13. Tandon R, Shipley JE, Taylor S, et al. Electroencephalographic sleep abnormalities in schizophrenia. Relationship to positive/negative symptoms and prior neuroleptic treatment. Arch Gen Psychiatry 1992; 49: 185–94.
14. Keshavan MS, Anderson S. Pettegrew JW. Is schizophrenia due to excessive synaptic pruning in the prefrontal cortex? The Feinberg hypothesis revisited. J Psychiatr Res 1994; 28: 239–65.
15. Werth E, Achermann P, Borberly AA. Front-occipital EEG power gradients in human sleep. J Sleep Res 1997; 6: 102–12.
16. Keshavan MS, Reynolds CF 3rd, Miewald MJ, et al. Delta sleep deficits in schizophrenia: evidence from automated analyses of sleep data. Arch Gen Psychiatry 1998; 55: 443–8.
17. Tekell JL, Hoffmann R, Hendrickse W, et al. High frequency EEG activity during sleep: characteristics in schizophrenia and depression. Clin EEG Neurosci 2005; 36: 25–35.
18. Benson KL, Sullivan EV, Lim KO, et al. The effect of total sleep deprivation on slow wave recovery in schizophrenia. Sleep Res 1993; 22: 143.
19. Horne J. Neuroscience. Images of lost sleep. Nature 2000; 403: 605–6.
20. Wirz-Justice A, Cajochen C, Nussbaum P. A schizophrenic patient with an arrhythmic circadian rest–activity cycle. Psychiatry Res 1997; 73: 83–90.
21. Wirz-Justice A, Haug HJ, Cajochen C. Disturbed circadian rest-activity cycles in schizophrenia patients: an effect of drugs? Schizophr Bull 2001; 27: 497–502.
22. Martin J, Jeste DV, Caligiuri MP, et al. Actigraphic estimates of circadian rhythms and sleep/wake in older schizophrenia patients. Schizophr Res 2001; 47: 77–86.
23. Keshavan MS, Reynolds CF, Montrose D, et al. Sleep and suicidality in psychotic patients. Acta Psychiatr Scand 1994; 89: 122–5.
24. Lewis CF, Tandon R, Shipley JE, et al. Biological predictors of suicidality in schizophrenia. Acta Psychiatr Scand 1996; 94: 416–20.
25. Maixner S, Tandon R, Eiser A, et al. Effects of antipsychotic treatment on polysomnographic

measures in schizophrenia: a replication and extension. Am J Psychiatry 1997; 155: 1600–2.

26. Keshavan MS, Reynolds CF 3rd, Miewald JM, et al. A longitudinal study of EEG sleep in schizophrenia. Psychiatry Res 1996; 59: 203–11.

27. Keshavan MS, Pettegrew JW, Reynolds CF 3rd, et al. Slow wave sleep deficits in schizophrenia: pathophysiologic significance. Psychiatry Res 1995; 57: 91–100.

28. Orzack MH, Hartmann EL, Kornetsky C. The relationship between attention and slow-wave sleep in chronic schizophrenia. Psychopharmacol Bull 1977; 13: 59–61.

29. Goder R, Boigs M, Braun S, et al. Impairment of visuospatial memory is associated with decreased slow wave sleep in schizophrenia. J Psychiatr Res 2004; 38: 591–9.

30. Manoach DS, Cain MS, Vangel MG, et al. A failure of sleep-dependent procedural learning in chronic, medicated schizophrenia. Biol Psychiatry 2004; 56: 951–6.

31. Smith JR, Karacan I, Yang M. Ontogeny of delta activity during human sleep. Electroencephalogr Clin Neurophysiol 1977; 43: 229–37.

32. Feinberg I. Schizophrenia: caused by a fault in programmed synaptic elimination during adolescence. J Psychiatr Res 1982/83; 17: 319–34.

33. Andreasen NC, Arndt S, Swayze V 2nd, et al. Thalamic abnormalities in schizophrenia visualized through magnetic resonance image averaging. Science 1994; 266: 294–8.

34. Keshavan MS, Reynolds CF 3rd, Ganguli R, et al. Electroencephalographic sleep and cerebral morphology in functional psychoses: a preliminary study with computed tomography. Psychiatry Res 1991; 39: 293–301.

35. van Kammen DP, van Kammen WB, Peters J, et al. Decreased slow-wave sleep and enlarged lateral ventricles in schizophrenia. Neuropsychopharmacology 1988; 1: 265–71.

36. Keshavan MS, Tandon R. Sleep abnormalities in schizophrenia: pathophysiological significance. Psychol Med 1993; 23: 831–5.

37. Reimann D. Cholinergic REM induction test: muscarinic supersensitivity underlies polysomnographic findings in both depression and schizophrenia. J Psychiatric Res 1994; 28: 195–210.

38. Griffith JM, O'Neill JE, Petty F, et al. Nicotinic receptor desensitization and sensory gating deficits in schizophrenia. Biol Psychiatry 1998; 44: 98–106.

39. Benson KL, Faull KF, Zarcone VP Jr. Evidence for the role of serotonin in the regulation of slow wave sleep in schizophrenia. Sleep 1991; 14: 133–9.

40. Porkka-Heiskanen T, Strecker RE, Thakkar M, et al. Adenosine: a mediator of the sleep-inducing effects of prolonged wakefulness. Science 1997; 276: 1265–8.

41. Ferre S. Adenosine–dopamine interactions in the ventral striatum. Implications for the treatment of schizophrenia. Psychopharmacology (Berl) 1997; 133: 107–20.

42. Keshavan MS, Reynolds CF, Miewals J, et al. Slow-wave sleep deficit and outcome in schizophrenia and schizoaffective disorder. Acta Psychiatr Scand 1995; 91: 291–2.

43. Steriade M. Brain electrical activity and sensory processing during waking and sleep states. In: Kryger MH, Roth T, Dement WC, eds. Principles and Practice of Sleep Medicine. Philadelphia, PA: WB Saunders, 1994: 205–14.

44. Salin-Pascual RJ, Herrera-Estrella M, Galicia-Polo L, et al. Olanzapine acute administration in schizophrenic patients increases delta sleep and sleep efficiency. Biol Psychiatry 1999; 46: 141–3.

45. Salin-Pascual RJ, Herrera-Estrella M, Galicia-Polo L, Rosas M, Brunner E. Low delta sleep predicted a good clinical response to olanzapine administration in schizophrenic patients. Rev Invest Clin 2004; 56: 345–50.

46. Hinze-Selch D, Mullington J, Orth A, et al. Effects of clozapine on sleep: a longitudinal study. Biol Psychiatry 1997; 42: 260–6.

47. Cohrs S, Rodenbeck A, Guan Z, et al. Sleep-promoting properties of quetiapine in healthy subjects. Psychopharmacology (Berl) 2004; 174: 421–9.

48. Neylan TC, van Kammen DP, Kelley ME, et al. Sleep in schizophrenic patients on and off haloperidol thereby. Clinically stable vs relapsed patients. Arch Gen Psychiatry 1992; 49: 643–9.

49. Nofzinger EA, van Kammen DP, Gilbertson MW, et al. Electroencephalographic sleep in clinically stable schizophrenic patients: two-weeks versus six-weeks neuroleptic-free. Biol Psychiatry 1993; 33: 829–35.

50. Drummond SP, Brown GG, Gillin JC, et al. Altered brain response to verbal learning following sleep deprivation. Nature 2000; 403: 655–7.

51. Dahl RE. The development and disorders of sleep. Adv Pediatr 1998; 45: 73–90.

52. Lauer CJ, Schreiber W, Holsboer F, et al. In quest of identifying vulnerability markers for psychiatric disorders by all-night polysomnography. Arch Gen Psychiatry 1995; 52: 145–53.

7

Sleep and neurologic disorders

Sheldon Kapen, Jacob L Gordon

INTRODUCTION

Most neurologic diseases affecting the brain are accompanied by sleep disruptions or specific sleep disorders that contribute significantly to morbidity and mortality. Although this is also true of many non-neurologic conditions, their effects on sleep are usually indirect, via pain, discomfort, or metabolic aberrations (arthritis, respiratory diseases, congestive heart failure, etc.), in contrast to central nervous system (CNS) diseases, which directly impact mechanisms and neuroanatomic structures that control the sleep–wake cycle (brainstem, thalamus, and basal ganglia). This chapter reviews the association of abnormal sleep and pathologic sleepiness with neurologic diseases. Because the effect of these conditions on sleep is ubiquitous, it is necessary to prioritize the discussion within the space available. This chapter includes three major conditions that are most illustrative of the influence of sleep in CNS disorders: Parkinson's disease, stroke, and traumatic brain injury. Other conditions are considered briefly at the end of the chapter.

SLEEP IN PARKINSON'S DISEASE

Sleep problems in Parkinson's disease (PD) patients can be divided into three categories (Table 7.1): sleep disruption and sleep disorders, parasomnias, and excessive daytime sleepiness.

Sleep disruption and sleep disorders

In a national survey of 220 PD patients conducted in England, Lees et al[1] found that sleep complaints were practically universal, with immobility and nocturia being the most disturbing factors. Tandberg et al[2] carried out a community-based epidemiologic study in Norway that included 245 patients with PD who were compared with 100 patients with diabetes and another 100 healthy elderly people. Sixty percent of the PD subjects had sleep problems (considered moderate to severe in one-third), compared with 46% and 33% of the diabetic and healthy groups, respectively. Hypnotic medications were used by approximately 40% of the PD group, which is significantly higher than the other groups. Sleep problems were correlated with symptoms of depression and with the duration of L-dopa (levodopa) treatment. Happe et al[3] also highlighted the importance of depression when they reported higher ratings on the Zung Depression Scale for 56 PD patients compared with an age-matched control group. Depression was correlated with the duration of disease.

In an early polysomnographic study, Kales et al[4] reported greater difficulties with sleep initiation and with sleep maintenance in PD compared with an elderly control group. Factor et al[5] found that sleep maintenance was the major problem: 72% of PD patients who completed a questionnaire had two or more awakenings per night compared with

Table 7.1   List of sleep-related conditions associated with Parkinson's disease

Sleep disorders
   Insomnia
   Obstructive sleep apnea
   Central sleep apnea
   Restless legs syndrome
   Periodic leg movements of sleep
   Dystonia
   Bradykinesia
Parasomnias
   REM behavior disorder
   Somnambulism
   Night terrors
Excessive daytime sleepiness
   Hypersomnolence secondary to sleep disorder
   Idiopathic hypersomnia?
   Narcolepsy?

46.5% for an elderly control group. van Hilten et al[6] used actigraphy to record 89 PD and 83 age-matched control subjects, and reported a greater degree of nocturnal activity (more disturbed sleep) in PD. The degree of sleep disruption significantly increased with the dose of dopaminergic medications. Significantly poor sleep was also reported by Kumar et al[7] and Pal et al.[8] Most of these studies were based on questionnaires and interviews, rather than on electrophysiology.

Specific sleep disorders might contribute to nocturnal sleep problems in PD patients. For instance, the motor disability of PD might affect various muscles of respiration, including those of the upper airway. Conflicting conclusions regarding the prevalence of obstructive sleep apnea (OSA) in idiopathic PD make it unclear whether to ascribe a major role to this disorder in the sleep disruption of PD patients over and above that expected in normal aging and obesity. An early study found no evidence of sleep apnea in a group of idiopathic PD patients compared with a control group unless autonomic disturbances were present.[9] A subsequent

letter reported a greater number of respiratory events during sleep, particularly in more advanced disease, although the severity was mild (a total of 48.5 events for the entire night in the latter group, compared with 10 in the controls).[10] More recently, 15 PD subjects and 15 controls were studied with polysomnography, revealing that patients had a greater apnea–hypopnea index (AHI) than controls and more severe changes in oxygen saturation. Sixty percent of the patients had OSA based on AHI > 5 and one patient had central sleep apnea.[11] In a series of 86 patients completing a sleep questionnaire from Braga Neto et al,[12] 71.8% acknowledged snoring, which was related significantly to excessive daytime sleepiness (EDS). Finally, Diederich et al[13] reported polysomnographic data for 49 patients in a case–control study. Twenty-one (43%) had an AHI ≥ 5, one-third of whom had an AHI > 30. The patients had less oxygen desaturation during the night than controls who were matched for AHI. The patients had mostly central apneas, while events in controls were mainly obstructive.

Restless legs syndrome (RLS) is present in about 20% of the PD population, as opposed to 5–10% of non-PD individuals.[14,15] RLS may interfere with sleep onset and is often associated with periodic limb movements of sleep (PLMS), which may impair sleep maintenance.[16] Four criteria for the diagnosis of RLS have been identified by the International Restless Legs Syndrome Study Group (IRLSSG):[16] (1) an urge to move the legs, often accompanied by an unpleasant sensation; (2) relief of the symptoms by moving the legs; (3) exacerbation of the symptoms when lying down; and (4) a peak of symptoms in the late evening as part of a diurnal rhythm.

The prevalence of RLS seems to be higher in studies of PD than in non-PD controls, although there are exceptions. In a movement disorders clinic survey, Ondo et al[17] found RLS in 20.8% of PD patients. The incidence was lower in a study reported from India, but still significantly greater than matched controls (7.9% vs 0.8%).[18] Notably, Tan et al[19] could find no difference between patients and controls in Singapore (0.8% vs 0.6% in the general population and 0.1% in a clinic sample). RLS seems to be less common in Asia than in the Western world. The association between RLS and PD is strengthened by the finding of Banno et al[20] that during a 5-year period, 17.5% of a cohort of 218 male patients with RLS developed movement disorders, compared with only 0.2% of 872 matched controls; for female patients, the corresponding figure was 23.5%. Periodic limb movement disorder (PLMD) is also more frequent in PD. One report found a PLM index of 68.3, compared with 13.9 in matched controls.[21] Hogl et al[14] reported a mean PLM index of 34.9 in 15 PD patients, which decreased to 6.7 during treatment with cabergoline.

Parasomnias

Although parasomnias such as somnambulism and night terrors have received passing mention in the literature in relation to PD,[22] rapid eye movement (REM) behavior disorder (RBD) is by far the most frequent associated parasomnia and has received the most investigation. RBD is characterized by excessive motor activity, usually in response to imperatives of a REM sleep dream narrative that is often threatening and leads to defensive maneuvers (e.g., protecting oneself or one's spouse from an attacker).[23] RBD is seen primarily in older men; the etiology is felt to be the loss of REM-associated muscle atonia due to an anatomic or functional lesion of the motor control pathways in the upper brainstem.[23] Indeed, the appearance of excessive phasic or tonic submental muscle discharge is often a prodrome to development of the full syndrome years later.[24] Periodic leg movements are also commonly present for a long period of time prior to the appearance of frank RBD.[25]

In a group of 33 PD patients, 33% had polysomnographic criteria for RBD (increased muscle tone during REM sleep and complex motor activity).[24] Fifty-eight percent had REM sleep without atonia (RSWA) (defined as increased tonic or phasic activity occupying at least 20% of

REM sleep time), while among 16 controls only 1 had this finding. A prevalence of 24% for RSWA and 16% for RBD was reported in a survey of 45 PD patients, 15 of whom had never been treated and another 10 of whom had undergone previous treatment but were drug-free for 2 weeks.[26] Those with REM sleep abnormalities had a longer duration of disease, a higher Hoehn–Yahr Score, and higher doses of dopaminergic drugs (when treated). Eisensehr et al[27] studied 292 consecutive patients with sleep disorders, of whom 19 had PD, and found that 47% of the PD group had RBD, compared with 1.8% of those without PD. Thus, RBD is commonly seen in PD. Boeve et al[28,29] presented evidence that RBD is highly selective for synucleinopathies (PD, multiple system atrophy (MSA), or diffuse Lewy body disease (DLBD)), as opposed to tauopathies such as Alzheimer's disease. (Synuclein is a marker for these diseases, since it is contained in Lewy bodies.[30]) Conflicting evidence exists on this point, since RBD has been reported in patients with progressive supranuclear palsy (PSP),[31] a non-synucleinopathy, and in PD caused by the *Parkin* mutation (in which there are few or no Lewy bodies).[32]

Once the diagnosis of RBD has been made, treatment with small to moderate doses of clonazepam (0.5–1.0 mg prior to bedtime) is usually effective.[33] It is important to recognize and treat RBD, because it frequently causes serious injuries such as fractures and hematoma.[34]

Excessive daytime sleepiness

Excessive daytime sleepiness (EDS) is found in up to 76% of PD patients, compared with 47% in matched control subjects.[35] The Canadian Movement Disorders Group reported EDS in 51% of a group of 638 parkinsonian subjects evaluated by questionnaire.[36] Excessive daytime sleepiness is associated with nocturnal sleep disturbances but in PD, correlation with obstructive sleep apnea is not always found.[9] Arnulf et al[37] emphasized the similarity of sleepiness in PD to that of narcolepsy because of such features as sleep-onset REM periods (SOREMPs) during daytime naps and the high incidence of hallucinatory phenomena in sleepy PD patients. In their study of 54 treated patients referred for evaluation of sleepiness, the mean Epworth Sleepiness Scale (ESS)[38] Score was 14 (>10 is considered significant – the maximum is 24, and narcoleptics often have a score ≥18). Thirty-nine percent of the patients had two or more SOREMPs during the Multiple Sleep Latency Test (MSLT), a finding typical of narcolepsy.[39] Those with SOREMPs were objectively sleepier than those without (mean sleep latency on the MSLT 4.6 minutes vs 7.4 minutes). Arnulf et al[37] concluded that the sleepiness was related to the pathology of Parkinson's disease. Rye and Jankovic[40] emphasized the role of dopaminergic mechanisms in the control of the sleep–wake cycle and as a possible factor contributing to sleepiness in PD.

Drouot et al[41] found hypocretin-1 levels in ventricular cerebrospinal fluid (CSF) to be much lower in advanced PD patients than in controls, but another study found normal hypocretin-1 in the CSF of three sleepy parkinsonians.[42] (In narcoleptics, hypocretin-1 is almost universally low or absent.[43]) Also, HLA-DR2 and -DQ1 alleles, seen in over 90% of narcoleptics,[44] are no more frequent in PD patients with SOREMPs, hallucinations, and RBD than in patients without these phenomena.[45] Thus, sleepiness in parkinsonism has similarities to narcolepsy,[37] but is not identical to it.

Frucht et al[46] directed attention to a side-effect of dopaminergic agents termed 'sleep attacks' and defined as a sudden onset of sleep without warning signs, particularly while driving. They emphasized the newer D2–D3 dopaminergic agonists as the main culprit in nine patients (eight taking pramipexole and one taking ropinirole) who had automobile crashes due to falling asleep at the wheel. Since then, much data have been gathered about the phenomenon of 'sleep attacks' and have cast doubt on its validity. Rather, the general impression is that most patients taking dopaminergic agonists who fall asleep have excessive daytime sleepiness and that, with few exceptions, episodes of sudden sleep onset are preceded by the same inability to resist

sleep as seen in sleep deprivation or narcolepsy[35,36,47–71] (Table 7.2). The most predictive factors are the ESS Score and the dose of levodopa/carbidopa.[35,53] Also, most investigators found no difference between levodopa/carbidopa and dopaminergic agonists, which seem similar in their sleepiness-inducing qualities. The role of dopaminergic agents in producing sleepiness or alertness is complex. The effects may be dose-related: smaller doses may stimulate presynaptic autoreceptors and reduce alertness, whereas larger doses may stimulate postsynaptic dopaminergic receptors.

PD patients must be questioned carefully about their nocturnal sleep and the presence of daytime sleepiness. If symptoms suggest the possibility of sleep disorders such as RLS or OSA, polysomnography is indicated. Attention should be paid to factors such as insufficient sleep, impaired sleep hygiene, alcohol intake, etc., and corrective steps should be taken as appropriate. Some patients may respond to simple interventions such as a well-timed cup of coffee or a strategically placed nap. Others may require stimulant medication, with modafinil being the most studied for PD.[62,72–75] Adler et al[72] reported a double-blind, placebo-controlled, crossover study of 21 PD patients with baseline ESS Score ≥10. Modafinil led to a decrease in ESS Score (17.8 to 14.4) during a treatment period of 3 weeks, whereas ESS Score did not improve (16.0 to 17.0) with placebo administration. Four other studies of modafinil in PD also reported improvement in daytime sleepiness.[62,73–75]

SLEEP AND STROKE

The association of OSA with ischemic hemispheric stroke was first described in 1990,[76] and was confirmed in subsequent studies.[77–80] Since OSA is also a risk factor for hypertension,[81] coronary heart disease, and myocardial infarction,[82] the association with stroke is not surprising. Yet, the association is stronger than that for heart disease,[82,83] and perhaps even hypertension, prompting special attention to the effects of OSA on the cerebral circulation

Table 7.2 Reports in peer-reviewed publications of effects of dopaminergic medications in Parkinson's disease patients on sleepiness and 'sleep attacks'. Abbreviations: EDS; excessive daytime sleepiness, ESS; Epworth Sleepiness Scale, HLA; human leukocyte antigen, MSLT; multiple sleep latency test, N/A; not applicable, PBO; placebo, PD; Parkinson's disease, PSQI; Pittsburgh Sleep Quality Inventory, SOREMP; sleep onset REM period, SOS; sudden onset of sleep

Authors	Year	Number of patients	Medication	Methods	Observations
Nausieda PA, et al[60]	1982	100 PD	L-dopa	Survey	Insomnia and EDS; increasing severity with time on drug
Frucht S, et al[46]	1999	8 PD	Pramipexole and ropinirole	Case reports	"Sleep attacks"
Hauser RA, et al[61]	2000	1 PD	Pramipexole	Case report. ESS	Modafinil was effective
Hauser RA, et al[62]	2000	40 PD. In double-blind phase, 22 on pramipexole and 18 PBO. Extension phase, 37 PD	Pramipexole	Clinical trial. PSG	Greater EDS with pramipexole than with PBO. In extension phase, 57% reported EDS (38% moderate or severe). Some fell asleep at wheel
Olanow CW, et al[63]	2000	N/A	N/A	N/A	Viewpoint
Schapira AH, et al[56]	2000	N/A	N/A	N/A	Review
Happe S, et al[47]	2001	111 PD	Various	Questionnaire	EDS in 9–12% on medications, 4.5% on no drugs. EDS increased in those who discontinued drugs. EDS increased to 25% in patients newly started on dopaminergic medications
Tracik F, et al[65]	2001	1 PD	Sinemet, agonists, entacapone	PSG (24 hours)	60 seconds from wakefulness to stage 2 during "sleep attacks"
Arnulf I, et al[37]	2002	54 PD	L-dopa. 50% on agonists	PSG. MSLT	ESS 14.3% 2 or more SOREMPs in 39%. EDS was correlated weakly with L-dopa dose
Fabbrini G, et al[66]	2002	25 new PD. 50 treated PD. 25 controls	Various	ESS. PSQI	ESS and PSQI were higher in treated patients
Ferreira JJ, et al[48]	2002	20 normals	Ropinirole	MSLT	Decreased sleep latency with the drug

Continued...

Table 7.2   Continued...

Authors	Year	Number of patients	Medication	Methods	Observations
Hobson DE, et al[36]	2002	638 PD	Various	ESS and ISCS ("inappropriate sleep composite score")	EDS in 51%. 3.8% had SOS, only 0.7% without warning. No difference between agonists. ESS and ISCS predicted SOS
Homann CN, et al[51]	2002	N/A	N/A	N/A	Review
Moller JC, et al[67]	2002	47 PD, of whom 17 had SOS. 6 of latter had battery of tests	Pramipexole and ropinirole	PSG. MSLT. ESS. Driving simulator. HLA typing.	SOS patients had EDS on MSLT and ESS. Erratic on simulator
Rye DB, et al[40]	2002	N/A	N/A	N/A	Review
Tan EK, et al[57]	2002	201 PD	Various	Questionnaire	13.9% had "sleep attacks". L-dopa dose and longer duration of disease predicted sleep attacks as did ESS over 10
Ulivelli M, et al[58]	2002	1 PD	Pergolide and L-dopa	PSG	4 "sleep attacks" on pergolide, SOREMPs on 3 of them
Brodsky MA, et al[35]	2003	101 PD	Various	Questionnaire. ESS	76% had EDS. Falling asleep at wheel predicted by ESS and L-dopa dose
Contin M, et al[68]	2003	2 PD	L-dopa	L-dopa challenge	L-dopa precipitated sleep
Homann CN, et al[50]	2003	N/A	N/A	N/A	Review
Paus S, et al[55]	2003	2952 PD	Various	Phone interview	6% had SOS, 50% of whom without warning. 75% had ESS more than 10. 37% over 15. Of the medications, L-dopa was least associated with SOS, combination of L-dopa and agonists the most

Continued...

Table 7.2 Continued...

Authors	Year	Number of patients	Medication	Methods	Observations
Roth T, et al[69]	2003	24 PD with ESS over 10 (16 with sleep attacks, 8 without)	Various	PSG/MSLT	42% had mean MSLT under 5. EDS not different with or without sleep attacks. No difference between agonists
Schlesinger I, et al[70]	2003	70 PD	Agonists	Survey	34% had sleep attacks. Those with attacks were younger than those without. 79% of them had attacks while driving (3 crashes). EDS was risk factor. Pramipexole was most associated with sleep attacks
Zesiewicz TA, et al[59]	2003	N/A	N/A	N/A	Review
Korner Y, et al[52]	2004	12,000 PD (6620 responded)	Various	Questionnaire	42% had SOS, 10 of whom had no warning. Those on therapy were at risk; other risk factors: age, male gender, longer duration of disease, sleep disturbance
Kaynak D, et al[71]	2005	15 PD	Various	PSG	Treatment associated with higher ESS, decreased latency on MSLT. Higher dose of dopaminergic drug was predictive

and brain. In all studies so far, approximately 75% of ischemic hemispheric stroke patients have an AHI ≥ 10,[77–80] while 50% have an AHI ≥ 20 (a severity that correlates with cardiovascular morbidity and mortality)[84] (Figure 7.1). Following an acute stroke, patients with OSA have longer hospitalizations and a worse functional outcome.[85–87] Epidemiologic evidence from more recent longitudinal studies indicates that OSA is an independent risk factor for stroke. Arzt et al[88] showed a correlation between baseline AHI and incidence of stroke, and other investigators confirmed this finding even when controlling for obesity, age, hypertension, smoking, alcohol intake, and other risk factors.[89] Even small changes in AHI increase the odds ratio for future stroke.[83]

OSA is also related in a complex way to the more well-known risk factors for stroke such as hypertension, obesity, age, male gender, and metabolic syndrome. Thickening of the carotid arterial wall, a marker of atherosclerotic plaques, is more severe in OSA patients than in controls.[90,91] Harbison et al[92] found more periventricular angiomatosis (also called leukoaraiosis, a condition known to indicate white matter ischemia) in acute stroke patients with higher AHI, although another report revealed no significant difference for leukoaraiosis between OSA and non-OSA patients without stroke.[93]

Sleep apnea (or hypopnea) can be divided into *obstructive*, with impaired air flow despite continued ventilatory effort, and *central*, with decreased or absent air flow due to decreased ventilatory effort. Both types of apnea occur in cerebrovascular disease, but one study described a different time course between central and obstructive events.[80] In the acute stage, both central and obstructive apneic events were seen. After several months, central events subsided, but obstructive events remained.[80] This suggested that central apneas resulted from direct effects of the stroke, while persistence of obstructive events indicated that OSA was present prior to the stroke and pointed to its importance as a risk factor. Another form of central apnea is Cheyne–Stokes breathing, a not-infrequent accompaniment of acute stroke.[94] Naughton and Bradley[95] reported increased mortality in congestive heart failure patients with Cheyne–Stokes breathing, so a study of mortality in stroke patients with this breathing pattern would be important. Although the present discussion focuses on hemispheric lesions, it should be emphasized that brainstem strokes are often associated with central sleep apnea.[96]

The most effective treatment for OSA is continuous positive airway pressure (CPAP), which acts as a splint for the upper airway, increases lung volume, and decreases upper airway compliance.[97] CPAP reduces excessive daytime sleepiness (the most common behavioral manifestation of OSA), lowers blood pressure (particularly in patients with hypertension), and improves cardiac function.[98] CPAP reduces the deleterious consequences of OSA in stroke patients. After 18

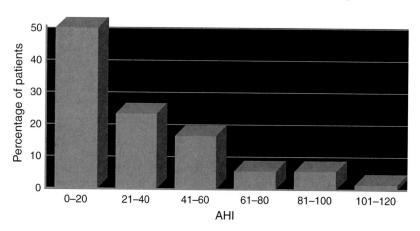

Figure 7.1 Percentage of 61 ischemic stroke patients (at various times since the stroke) with different values of apnea–hypopnea index (AHI) (unpublished data)

months' follow-up, Martinez-Garcia et al[99] reported less stroke recurrence with CPAP in OSA (AHI ≥ 20; $n = 15$) compared with patients who did not tolerate CPAP ($n = 36$) (odds ratio 5.09). Marin et al[100] divided 1651 subjects without previous stroke into five groups: healthy controls, simple snorers, untreated mild-to-moderate OSA patients, untreated severe OSA patients, and OSA patients treated with CPAP. Multivariate analysis after a mean follow-up of 10.1 years showed that the untreated severe OSA group had odds ratios of 2.87 for fatal cardiac and cerebrovascular events and 3.17 for non-fatal events compared with healthy controls. Untreated severe patients also had significantly worse results than the remaining three patient groups. Finally, Doherty et al[101] followed 168 patients with OSA for a mean of 7.5 years and compared the treated patients ($n = 107$) with those intolerant of CPAP, finding a 14.8% incidence of fatal cardiovascular disease (including stroke) in the untreated group compared with 1.9% in the CPAP group. No significant difference was reported for non-fatal cardiac or stroke events. Overall, the data strongly support the role of OSA as a risk factor for stroke, and underscore the necessity of diagnosing and treating OSA patients to prevent a first or recurrent stroke.

Although OSA is the most important sleep disorder in stroke patients, sleep is rarely normal even when OSA is absent.[102] Insomnia is common and is associated with low sleep efficiency, long sleep latency, and elevated wake time after sleep onset. One case of periodic leg movements in association with stroke was reported[103] and one case of restless legs syndrome,[104] but the true incidence of these disorders after a stroke is unknown. Finally, polysomnographic studies of recovering stroke patients have shown reduced sleep spindles[105] and other sleep architectural changes.[106–108]

SLEEP AND TRAUMATIC BRAIN INJURY

Traumatic brain injury and disordered sleep are linked reciprocally, although causation is not always clear. The injury may have been caused by a sleep disorder (such as OSA) that was present at the time of the traumatic event.[109] Conversely, sleep disturbance commonly develops after brain injury, involving three primary symptoms: hypersomnolence, insomnia, and disruption of sleep timing and circadian rhythms.

Clinchot et al[110] surveyed sleep disturbances in 86 patients with traumatic brain injury. Fifty percent exhibited sleep difficulties: 64% reported early awakening, 25% described sleeping more than usual, and 45% described problems initiating sleep. Sleep complaints correlated with the presence of fatigue. Patients with more severe injury (as measured by the Glasgow Coma Scale) were less likely to report sleep problems, due presumably to decreased insight. Haboubi et al[111] reported initial sleeping problems in 300 of 639 minor head injury patients: sleep problems persisted in 232 out of 300 at 2 weeks and 81 of 111 after 6 weeks.

Hypersomnolence after brain injury

The earliest observations of hypersomnolence after brain injury were recorded before widespread acceptance of standardized measures of sleepiness such as the MSLT[112] and the ESS.[113] Using polysomnography, Guilleminault et al[114] reported severity data on 20 patients with brain injury who were referred for evaluation of EDS. Eighteen had objective evidence of daytime somnolence and eight had significant sleep apnea. In a subsequent report of 184 patients,[115] skull fracture, coma for more than 24 hours, and immediate neurosurgical intervention were more likely to involve higher scores on quantitative sleepiness measures. Brain injury patients who developed sleep apnea were more likely to have concurrent neck injury. Masel et al[116] evaluated 71 consecutive brain injury inpatient admissions, and found hypersomnolence in 33 patients (12 with and 21 without sleep apnea). Twelve patients had elevated periodic limb movement indices. Borgaro et al[117] found that ability to function without a daytime nap was the best indicator of fatigue in 47 brain injury patients compared with controls, highlighting the difficulty of separating sleepiness from other aspects of fatigue. Thus, in all cases of post-traumatic hypersomnolence, it is important to identify risk factors (e.g., obesity) and aspects of the sleep history (e.g., snoring and movement during sleep) that will yield a sleep differential diagnosis and management plan.

Post-traumatic narcolepsy is a specific cause of hypersomnolence after brain injury.[118–120] Lankford et al[121] reported nine patients with EDS and mild-to-moderate neuropsychologic impairment: five had cataplexy, five had sleep paralysis, and five had hallucinations. Three patients had all four symptoms. All had SOREMPs and shortened mean sleep latencies. HLA typing revealed three patients with DR2 and one patient with DQw1, suggesting that patients were genetically predisposed and that brain injury had unmasked their narcolepsy. In a study of 44 consecutive traumatic brain injury patients, Baumann et al[122] found low CSF hypocretin levels in 95% of those with moderate to severe injury, possibly reflecting hypothalamic damage.[123]

Insomnia after brain injury

Insomnia has been examined in brain injury patients with regard to demographics, injury characteristics, coexisting conditions, and psychosocial variables.[124] Fichtenberg et al[125] reported insomnia in 30% of 50 consecutive brain injury patients. A score of 14 or more on the Beck Depression Scale and initial emergency room Glasgow Coma Score were the most important components of a logistic regression model that predicted insomnia (as reflected by the Pittsburgh Sleep Quality Index) in 91 consecutive postacute brain injury patients – self-report of pain and litigation status were also important.[126] Kemp et al[127] reported preliminary evidence for efficacy of melatonin and amitriptyline in both initiation and maintenance insomnia after brain injury. Beetar et al[128] found significantly more insomnia in traumatic brain injury patients than in patients with non-traumatic neurologic disorders. The presence of pain increased insomnia twofold, and insomnia was more likely with mild

than with moderate or severe injury. Identification of insomnia and related psychiatric and psychosocial conditions should be a part of rehabilitation care for brain injury patients in the post-acute phase.

Circadian rhythm disorders after brain injury

Steele et al[129] found no significant differences between ten brain injury patients and controls in dim light melatonin onset or morningness–eveningness. Delayed sleep phase syndrome (DSPS) has been reported after brain injury.[130,131] Smits and Nagtegaal[132] found moderate to large improvements with melatonin administration in 16 patients with DSPS and chronic whiplash syndrome. Dagan[133] reported an irregular ('disorganized') sleep–wake pattern after head trauma. Head injuries incurred during car crashes or boxing were reported as etiologic possibilities in patients who developed episodic hypersomnolence along with hyperphagia, behavioral disturbance, and sexual disinhibition – the Kleine–Levin syndrome.[134,135]

Effective treatment of traumatic brain injury patients requires analysis of any identified specific nighttime sleep disorders in the context of overall daytime neuropsychologic functioning.[136]

SLEEP AND OTHER NEUROLOGIC DISORDERS

Sleep and neuromuscular disorders

Impaired control of the airway during sleep is a major mechanism for sleep disturbance in neuromuscular disease.[137] Quera Salva et al[138] studied 20 consecutive myasthenia gravis patients who were assessed clinically to have intact daytime neuromuscular function and were on stable medication doses. An overall Respiratory Disturbance Index (RDI) ≥ 5 events per hour was found in 11 patients, and all of these had dramatic increases in RDI during REM sleep. Breathing events during REM sleep were associated with disturbed nocturnal sleep, a sensation of breathlessness, and daytime somnolence, and were of the 'diaphragmatic' rather than obstructive type. Barber et al[139] noted the difficulty in distinguishing muscle weakness from lack of central drive in patients with Duchenne muscular dystrophy.[140,141] Patients with myotonic dystrophy had more objective sleepiness by MSLT, longer sleep times, and more sleep fragmentation than controls.[142] Significant sleep apnea is not found in myotonic dystrophy,[143] and sleep abnormalities may be related to associated cerebral abnormalities.

Ferguson et al[144] compared 18 patients with amyotrophic lateral sclerosis (ALS) with 10 age-matched controls and found more arousals, shorter sleep time, and more sleep-disordered breathing, although breathing events showed a muscle weakness pattern and were not obstructive. Kimura et al[145] found significant sleep-disordered breathing in 3 of 11 patients with bulbar involvement in ALS despite absence of breathing complaints or subjective sleep disturbance symptoms. Monitoring of apnea and hyperpnea events, especially during REM sleep, may provide indicators for early intervention in ALS.[146] Nocturnal bilevel positive airway pressure is a standard component of care for patients with ALS, but should be part of a comprehensive plan of care that incorporates end-of-life decision making.[147,148] Bourke et al[149] found improvements in survival and quality of life in ALS patients randomized to non-invasive ventilation rather than standard care.

Sleep and epilepsy

Sleep is one of the important physiologic states modulating abnormal electrical brain activity and seizures. Sleep facilitates seizures through activity in thalamocortical circuits.[150,151] In most epileptic syndromes, interictal epileptiform discharges are more likely seen during non-REM (NREM) sleep than during REM sleep.

The differential diagnosis of behavioral and motor disturbances during sleep[152] includes seizure as well as non-epileptic disorders such as RBD, primary disorders of arousal such as sleep terrors, and psychogenic episodes. The stereotyped motor attacks of nocturnal paroxysmal dystonia (NPD) are responsive to carbamazepine and are probably epileptic, despite a lack of EEG abnormalities.[153,154] Multiple generalized and partial epileptic syndromes are associated with sleep.[152] Frontal lobe seizures are more common during sleep than wakefulness, and frontal epilepsy can be nocturnal and related to a genetic mutation.[155] Sleep deprivation can worsen seizures and is used to provoke epileptiform discharges in clinical EEG protocols.

Sleep and multiple sclerosis

Many patients with multiple sclerosis (MS) experience fatigue,[156] and often report it as their most disabling symptom.[157] The relationship of MS fatigue to intact or disordered sleep and to depression is complex and is possibly mediated by immunopathologic and neurohormonal mechanisms[158] and by axonal damage.[159] Attarian et al[160] studied controls and MS patients with and without fatigue using sleep logs, the ESS[38,161] and actigraphy. Of 15 MS patients with fatigue, 12 had disordered sleep (10 had sleep disruption and 2 had delayed sleep phase), whereas 12 of 15 non-fatigued MS patients had normal sleep cycles without disruption.

Sleep in pediatric neurologic disorders

Grigg-Damberger[162] reviewed multiple central and peripheral neurologic disorders with disordered sleep as a significant manifestation. Brain-injured children can have circadian rhythm disorders due to deficits in biologic clock entrainment. Attention deficit hyperactivity disorder in children can be secondary to OSA or RLS. Anticonvulsants, stimulants, and sympathomimetics can all produce sleep disturbance in children.

SUMMARY AND FUTURE DIRECTIONS

Neurologic disorders produce disturbances of sleep and wakefulness by direct negative influences on brain structures, as well as indirect influences such as pain and primary medical, psychologic, and social derangements. Recognition that specific sleep disorders often accompany neurologic disease should lead to more careful history-taking, including attention to circadian patterns and sleep-related behaviors. Appropriate use of sleep medicine techniques such as quantification of sleepiness and sleep quality, polysomnography, and actigraphy can facilitate diagnosis of sleep disorders accompanying neurologic disease and can lead to identification of therapeutic interventions. Newer concepts, such as the role of the hypocretin system,[123,163–165] and newer imaging techniques,[166] show promise for better elucidation of the pathophysiologic mechanisms of disordered sleep in neurologic disease. More complete insight into these mechanisms will allow a better choice of pharmacologic and other treatments.

REFERENCES

1. Lees AJ, Blackburn NA, Campbell VL. The nighttime problems of Parkinson's disease. Clin Neuropharmacol 1988; 11: 512–19.

2. Tandberg E, Larsen JP, Karlsen K. A community-based study of sleep disorders in patients with Parkinson's disease. Mov Disord 1998; 13: 895–9.

3. Happe S, Schrodl B, Faltl M, et al. Sleep disorders and depression in patients with Parkinson's disease. Acta Neurol Scand 2001; 104: 275–80.

4. Kales A, Ansel RD, Markham CH, Scharf MB, Tan TL. Sleep in patients with Parkinson's disease and normal subjects prior to and following levodopa administration. Clin Pharmacol Ther 1971; 12: 397–406.

5. Factor SA, McAlarney T, Sanchez-Ramos JR, Weiner WJ. Sleep disorders and sleep effect in Parkinson's disease. Mov Disord 1990; 5: 280–5.

6. van Hilten JJ, Weggeman M, van der Velde EA, et al. Sleep, excessive daytime sleepiness and fatigue in Parkinson's disease. J Neural Transm Park Dis Dement Sect 1993; 5: 235–44.

7. Kumar S, Bhatia M, Behari M. Sleep disorders in Parkinson's disease. Mov Disord 2002; 17: 775–81.

8. Pal PK, Thennarasu K, Fleming J, et al. Nocturnal sleep disturbances and daytime dysfunction in patients with Parkinson's disease and in their caregivers. Parkinsonism Relat Disord 2004; 10: 157–68.

9. Apps MC, Sheaff PC, Ingram DA, Kennard C, Empey DW. Respiration and sleep in Parkinson's disease. J Neurol Neurosurg Psychiatry 1985; 48: 1240–5.

10. Hardie RJ, Efthimiou J, Stern GM. Respiration and sleep in Parkinson's disease. J Neurol Neurosurg Psychiatry 1986; 49: 1326.

11. Maria B, Sophia S, Michalis M, et al. Sleep breathing disorders in patients with idiopathic Parkinson's disease. Respir Med 2003; 97: 1151–7.

12. Braga-Neto P, da Silva-Junior FP, Sueli Monte F, de Bruin PF, de Bruin VM. Snoring and excessive daytime sleepiness in Parkinson's disease. J Neurol Sci 2004; 217: 41–5.

13. Diederich NJ, Vaillant M, Mancuso G, Lyen P, Tiete J. Progressive sleep 'destructuring' in Parkinson's disease. A polysomnographic study in 46 patients. Sleep Med 2005; 6: 313–18.

14. Hogl B, Rothdach A, Wetter TC, Trenkwalder C. The effect of cabergoline on sleep, periodic leg movements in sleep, and early morning motor function in patients with Parkinson's disease. Neuropsychopharmacology 2003; 28: 1866–70.

15. Ohayon MM, Roth T. Prevalence of restless legs syndrome and periodic limb movement disorder in the general population. J Psychosom Res 2002; 53: 547–54.

16. Earley CJ. Clinical practice. Restless legs syndrome. N Engl J Med 2003; 348: 2103–9.

17. Ondo WG, Vuong KD, Jankovic J. Exploring the relationship between Parkinson disease and restless legs syndrome. Arch Neurol 2002; 59: 421–4.

18. Krishnan PR, Bhatia M, Behari M. Restless legs syndrome in Parkinson's disease: a case-controlled study. Mov Disord 2003; 18: 181–5.

19. Tan EK, Lum SY, Wong MC. Restless legs syndrome in Parkinson's disease. J Neurol Sci 2002; 196: 33–6.

20. Banno K, Delaive K, Walld R, Kryger MH. Restless legs syndrome in 218 patients: associated disorders. Sleep Med 2000; 1: 221–9.

21. Wetter TC, Collado-Seidel V, Pollmacher T, Yassouridis A, Trenkwalder C. Sleep and periodic leg movement patterns in drug-free patients with Parkinson's disease and multiple system atrophy. Sleep 2000; 23: 361–7.

22. Thorpy MJ. Sleep disorders in Parkinson's disease. Clin Cornerstone 2004; 6(Suppl 1A): S7–15.

23. Schenck CH, Mahowald MW. REM sleep behavior disorder: clinical, developmental, and neuroscience perspectives 16 years after its formal identification in SLEEP. Sleep 2002; 25: 120–38.

24. Gagnon JF, Bedard MA, Fantini ML, et al. REM sleep behavior disorder and REM sleep without atonia in Parkinson's disease. Neurology 2002; 59: 585–9.

25. Schenck CH, Bundlie SR, Mahowald MW. Delayed emergence of a parkinsonian disorder in 38% of 29 older men initially diagnosed with idiopathic rapid eye movement sleep behaviour disorder. Neurology 1996; 46: 388–93.

26. Wetter TC, Trenkwalder C, Gershanik O, Hogl B. Polysomnographic measures in Parkinson's disease: a comparison between patients with and without REM sleep disturbances. Wien Klin Wochenschr 2001; 113: 249–53.

27. Eisensehr I, v Lindeiner H, Jager M, Noachtar S. REM sleep behavior disorder in sleep-disordered patients with versus without Parkinson's disease: Is there a need for polysomnography? J Neurol Sci 2001; 186: 7–11.

28. Boeve BF, Silber MH, Ferman TJ, Lucas JA, Parisi JE. Association of REM sleep behavior disorder and neurodegenerative disease may reflect an underlying synucleinopathy. Mov Disord 2001; 16: 622–30.

29. Boeve BF, Silber MH, Parisi JE, et al. Synucleinopathy pathology and REM sleep behavior disorder plus dementia or parkinsonism. Neurology 2003; 61: 40–5.

30. Mouradian MM. Recent advances in the genetics and pathogenesis of Parkinson disease. Neurology 2002; 58: 179–85.

31. Arnulf I, Merino-Andreu M, Bloch F, et al. REM sleep behavior disorder and REM sleep without atonia in patients with progressive supranuclear palsy. Sleep 2005; 28: 349–54.

32. Kumru H, Santamaria J, Tolosa E, et al. Rapid eye movement sleep behavior disorder in parkinsonism with parkin mutations. Ann Neurol 2004; 56: 599–603.

33. Schenck CH, Bundlie SR, Patterson AL, Mahowald MW. Rapid eye movement sleep behavior disorder. A treatable parasomnia affecting older adults. JAMA 1987; 257: 1786–9.

34. Schenck CH, Milner DM, Hurwitz TD, Bundlie SR, Mahowald MW. A polysomnographic and clinical report on sleep-related injury in 100 adult patients. Am J Psychiatry 1989; 146: 1166–73.

35. Brodsky MA, Godbold J, Roth T, Olanow CW. Sleepiness in Parkinson's disease: a controlled study. Mov Disord 2003; 18: 668–72.

36. Hobson DE, Lang AE, Martin WR, et al. Excessive daytime sleepiness and sudden-onset sleep in Parkinson disease: a survey by the Canadian Movement Disorders Group. JAMA 2002; 287: 455–63.

37. Arnulf I, Konofal E, Merino-Andreu M, et al. Parkinson's disease and sleepiness: an integral part of PD. Neurology 2002; 58: 1019–24.

38. Johns MW. A new method for measuring daytime sleepiness: the Epworth Sleepiness Scale. Sleep 1991; 14: 540–5.

39. Aldrich MS. Diagnostic aspects of narcolepsy. Neurology 1998; 50(2 Suppl 1): S2–7.

40. Rye DB, Jankovic J. Emerging views of dopamine in modulating sleep/wake state from an unlikely source: PD. Neurology 2002; 58: 341–6.

41. Drouot X, Moutereau S, Nguyen JP, et al. Low levels of ventricular CSF orexin/hypocretin in advanced PD. Neurology 2003; 61: 540–3.

42. Overeem S, van Hilten JJ, Ripley B, et al. Normal hypocretin-1 levels in Parkinson's disease patients with excessive daytime sleepiness. Neurology 2002; 58: 498–9.

43. Mignot E, Lammers GJ, Ripley B, et al. The role of cerebrospinal fluid hypocretin measurement in the diagnosis of narcolepsy and other hypersomnias. Arch Neurol 2002; 59: 1553–62.

44. Rogers AE, Meehan J, Guilleminault C, Grumet FC, Mignot E. HLA DR15 (DR2) and DQB1*0602 typing studies in 188 narcoleptic patients with cataplexy. Neurology 1997; 48: 1550–6.

45. Onofrj M, Luciano AL, Iacono D, et al. HLA typing does not predict REM sleep behaviour disorder and hallucinations in Parkinson's disease. Mov Disord 2003; 18: 337–40.

46. Frucht S, Rogers JD, Greene PE, Gordon MF, Fahn S. Falling asleep at the wheel: motor vehicle mishaps in persons taking pramipexole and ropinirole. Neurology 1999; 52: 1908–10.

47. Happe S, Berger K. The association of dopamine agonists with daytime sleepiness, sleep problems and quality of life in patients with Parkinson's disease – a prospective study. J Neurol 2001; 248: 1062–7.

48. Ferreira JJ, Galitzky M, Thalamas C, et al. Effect of ropinirole on sleep onset: a randomized, placebo-controlled study in healthy volunteers. Neurology 2002; 58: 460–2.

49. Garcia-Borreguero D, Larrosa O, Bravo M. Parkinson's disease and sleep. Sleep Med Rev 2003; 7: 115–29.

50. Homann CN, Wenzel K, Suppan K, Ivanic G, Crevenna R, Ott E. Sleep attacks – facts and fiction: a critical review. Adv Neurol 2003; 91: 335–41.

51. Homann CN, Wenzel K, Suppan K, et al. Sleep attacks in patients taking dopamine agonists: review. BMJ 2002; 324: 1483–7.

52. Korner Y, Meindorfner C, Moller JC, et al. Predictors of sudden onset of sleep in Parkinson's disease. Mov Disord 2004; 19: 1298–305.

53. Meindorfner C, Korner Y, Moller JC, et al. Driving in Parkinson's disease: mobility, accidents, and sudden onset of sleep at the wheel. Mov Disord 2005; 20: 832–42.

54. Moller JC, Rethfeldt M, Korner Y, et al. Daytime sleep latency in medication-matched Parkinsonian patients with and without sudden onset of sleep. Mov Disord 2005; 20: 1620–2.

55. Paus S, Brecht HM, Koster J, et al. Sleep attacks, daytime sleepiness, and dopamine agonists in Parkinson's disease. Mov Disord 2003; 18: 659–67.

56. Schapira AH. Sleep attacks (sleep episodes) with pergolide. Lancet 2000; 355: 1332–3.

57. Tan EK, Lum SY, Fook-Chong SM, et al. Evaluation of somnolence in Parkinson's disease: comparison with age- and sex-matched controls. Neurology 2002; 58: 465–8.

58. Ulivelli M, Rossi S, Lombardi C, et al. Polysomnographic characterization of pergolide-induced sleep attacks in idiopathic PD. Neurology 2002; 58: 462–5.

59. Zesiewicz TA, Hauser RA. Sleep attacks and dopamine agonists for Parkinson's disease: What is currently known? CNS Drugs 2003; 17: 593–600.

60. Nausieda PA, Weiner WJ, Kaplan LR, Weber S, Klawans HL. Sleep disruption in the course of chronic levodopa therapy: an early feature of the levodopa psychosis. Clin Neuropharmacol 1982; 5: 183–94.

61. Hauser RA, Gauger L, Anderson WM, Zesiewicz TA. Pramipexole-induced somnolence and episodes of daytime sleep. Mov Disord 2000; 15: 658–63.

62. Hauser RA, Wahba MN, Zesiewicz TA, McDowell Anderson W. Modafinil treatment of pramipexole-associated somnolence. Mov Disord 2000; 15: 1269–71.

63. Olanow CW, Schapira AH, Roth T. Waking up to sleep episodes in Parkinson's disease. Mov Disord 2000; 15: 212–15.

64. Schapira AH. Excessive daytime sleepiness in Parkinson's disease. Neurology 2004; 63(8 Suppl 3): S24–7.

65. Tracik F, Ebersbach G. Sudden daytime sleep onset in Parkinson's disease: polysomnographic recordings. Mov Disord 2001; 16: 500–6.

66. Fabbrini G, Barbanti P, Aurilia C, et al. Excessive daytime sleepiness in de novo and treated Parkinson's disease. Mov Disord 2002; 17: 1026–30.

67. Moller JC, Stiasny K, Hargutt V, et al. Evaluation of sleep and driving performance in six patients with Parkinson's disease reporting sudden onset of sleep under dopaminergic medication: a pilot study. Mov Disord 2002; 17: 474–81.

68. Contin M, Provini F, Martinelli P, et al. Excessive daytime sleepiness and levodopa in Parkinson's disease: polygraphic, placebo-controlled monitoring. Clin Neuropharmacol 2003; 26: 115–18.

69. Roth T, Rye DB, Borchert LD, et al. Assessment of sleepiness and unintended sleep in Parkinson's disease patients taking dopamine agonists. Sleep Med 2003; 4: 275–80.

70. Schlesinger I, Ravin PD. Dopamine agonists induce episodes of irresistible daytime sleepiness. Eur Neurol 2003; 49: 30–3.

71. Kaynak D, Kiziltan G, Kaynak H, Benbir G, Uysal O. Sleep and sleepiness in patients with Parkinson's disease before and after dopaminergic treatment. Eur J Neurol 2005; 12: 199–207.

72. Adler CH, Caviness JN, Hentz JG, Lind M, Tiede J. Randomized trial of modafinil for treating subjective daytime sleepiness in patients with Parkinson's disease. Mov Disord 2003; 18: 287–93.

73. Happe S, Pirker W, Sauter C, Klosch G, Zeitlhofer J. Successful treatment of excessive daytime sleepiness in Parkinson's disease with modafinil. J Neurol 2001; 248: 632–4.

74. Hogl B, Saletu M, Brandauer E, et al. Modafinil for the treatment of daytime sleepiness in Parkinson's disease: a double-blind, randomized, crossover, placebo-controlled polygraphic trial. Sleep 2002; 25: 905–9.

75. Nieves AV, Lang AE. Treatment of excessive daytime sleepiness in patients with Parkinson's disease with modafinil. Clin Neuropharmacol 2002; 25: 111–14.

76. Kapen S, Maas C, Nichols C. Obstructive sleep apnea is a major risk factor for stroke. Neurology 1990; 39: 76.

77. Bassetti C, Aldrich MS. Sleep apnea in acute cerebrovascular diseases: final report on 128 patients. Sleep 1999; 22: 217–23.

78. Dyken ME, Somers VK, Yamada T, Ren ZY, Zimmerman MB. Investigating the relationship between stroke and obstructive sleep apnea. Stroke 1996; 27: 401–7.

79. Mohsenin V, Valor R. Sleep apnea in patients with hemispheric stroke. Arch Phys Med Rehabil 1995; 76: 71–6.

80. Parra O, Arboix A, Bechich S, et al. Time course of sleep-related breathing disorders in first-ever stroke or transient ischemic attack. Am J Respir Crit Care Med 2000; 161: 375–80.

81. Leung RS, Bradley TD. Sleep apnea and cardiovascular disease. Am J Respir Crit Care Med 2001; 164: 2147–65.

82. Schafer H, Koehler U, Ewig S, et al. Obstructive sleep apnea as a risk marker in coronary artery disease. Cardiology 1999; 92: 79–84.

83. Shahar E, Whitney CW, Redline S, et al. Sleep-disordered breathing and cardiovascular disease: cross-sectional results of the Sleep Heart Health Study. Am J Respir Crit Care Med 2001; 163: 19–25.

84. Partinen M, Jamieson A, Guilleminault C. Long-term outcome for obstructive sleep apnea syndrome patients. Mortality. Chest 1988; 94: 1200–4.

85. Cherkassky T, Oksenberg A, Froom P, Ring H. Sleep-related breathing disorders and rehabilitation outcome of stroke patients: a prospective study. Am J Phys Med Rehabil 2003; 82: 452–5.

86. Good DC, Henkle JQ, Gelber D, Welsh J, Verhulst S. Sleep-disordered breathing and poor functional outcome after stroke. Stroke 1996; 27: 252–9.

87. Kaneko Y, Hajek VE, Zivanovic V, Raboud J, Bradley TD. Relationship of sleep apnea to functional capacity and length of hospitalization following stroke. Sleep 2003; 26: 293–7.

88. Arzt M, Young T, Finn L, Skatrud JB, Bradley TD. Association of sleep-disordered breathing and the occurrence of stroke. Am J Respir Crit Care Med 2005; 172: 1447–51.

89. Yaggi HK, Concato J, Kernan WN, et al. Obstructive sleep apnea as a risk factor for stroke and death. N Engl J Med 2005; 353: 2034–41.

90. Nachtmann A, Stang A, Wang YM, Wondzinski E, Thilmann AF. Association of obstructive sleep apnea and stenotic artery disease in ischemic stroke patients. Atherosclerosis 2003; 169: 301–7.

91. Silvestrini M, Rizzato B, Placidi F, et al. Carotid artery wall thickness in patients with obstructive sleep apnea syndrome. Stroke 2002; 33: 1782–5.

92. Harbison J, Gibson GJ, Birchall D, Zammit-Maempel I, Ford GA. White matter disease and sleep-disordered breathing after acute stroke. Neurology 2003; 61: 959–63.

93. Davies CW, Crosby JH, Mullins RL, et al. Case control study of cerebrovascular damage defined by magnetic resonance imaging in patients with OSA and normal matched control subjects. Sleep 2001; 24: 715–20.

94. Nopmaneejumruslers C, Kaneko Y, Hajek V, Zivanovic V, Bradley TD. Cheyne–Stokes respiration in stroke: relationship to hypocapnia and occult cardiac dysfunction. Am J Respir Crit Care Med 2005; 171: 1048–52.

95. Naughton MT, Bradley TD. Sleep apnea in congestive heart failure. Clin Chest Med 1998; 19: 99–113.

96. Lassman AB, Mayer SA. Paroxysmal apnea and vasomotor instability following medullary infarction. Arch Neurol 2005; 62: 1286–8.

97. Sullivan CE, Issa FG, Berthon-Jones M, Eves L. Reversal of obstructive sleep apnoea by continuous positive airway pressure applied through the nares. Lancet 1981; i: 862–5.

98. Kushida CA, Littner MR, Morgenthaler T, et al. Practice parameters for the indications for polysomnography and related procedures: an update for 2005. Sleep 2005; 28: 499–521.

99. Martinez-Garcia MA, Galiano-Blancart R, Roman-Sanchez P, et al. Continuous positive airway pressure treatment in sleep apnea prevents new vascular events after ischemic stroke. Chest 2005; 128: 2123–9.

100. Marin JM, Carrizo SJ, Vicente E, Agusti AG. Long-term cardiovascular outcomes in men with obstructive sleep apnoea-hypopnoea with or without treatment with continuous positive airway pressure: an observational study. Lancet 2005; 365: 1046–53.

101. Doherty LS, Kiely JL, Swan V, McNicholas WT. Long-term effects of nasal continuous positive airway pressure therapy on cardiovascular outcomes in sleep apnea syndrome. Chest 2005; 127: 2076–84.

102. Kapen S, Mohan KK, Sander AM. Sleep disturbances in patients with cerebrovascular disease. Sleep Res 1996; 25: 422.

103. Kim JS, Lee SB, Park SK, et al. Periodic limb movement during sleep developed after pontine lesion. Mov Disord 2003; 18: 1403–5.

104. Anderson KN, Bhatia KP, Losseff NA. A case of restless legs syndrome in association with stroke. Sleep 2005; 28: 147–8.

105. Hachinski VC, Mamelak M, Norris JW. Clinical recovery and sleep architecture degradation. Can J Neurol Sci 1990; 17: 332–5.

106. Gottselig JM, Bassetti CL, Achermann P. Power and coherence of sleep spindle frequency activity following hemispheric stroke. Brain 2002; 125: 373–83.

107. Muller C, Achermann P, Bischof M, et al. Visual and spectral analysis of sleep EEG in acute hemispheric stroke. Eur Neurol 2002; 48: 164–71.

108. Vock J, Achermann P, Bischof M, et al. Evolution of sleep and sleep EEG after hemispheric stroke. J Sleep Res 2002; 11: 331–8.

109. Teran-Santos J, Jimenez-Gomez A, Cordero-Guevara J. The association between sleep apnea and the risk of traffic accidents. Cooperative Group Burgos–Santander. N Engl J Med 1999; 340: 847–51.

110. Clinchot DM, Bogner J, Mysiw WJ, Fugate L, Corrigan J. Defining sleep disturbance after brain injury. Am J Phys Med Rehabil 1998; 77: 291–5.

111. Haboubi NH, Long J, Koshy M, Ward AB. Short-term sequelae of minor head injury (6 years experience of minor head injury clinic). Disabil Rehabil 2001; 23: 635–8.

112. Carskadon MA, Dement WC, Mitler MM, et al. Guidelines for the multiple sleep latency test (MSLT): a standard measure of sleepiness. Sleep 1986; 9: 519–24.

113. Johns MW. Daytime sleepiness, snoring, and obstructive sleep apnea. The Epworth Sleepiness Scale. Chest 1993; 103: 30–6.

114. Guilleminault C, Faull KF, Miles L, van den Hoed J. Posttraumatic excessive daytime sleepiness: a review of 20 patients. Neurology 1983; 33: 1584–9.

115. Guilleminault C, Yuen KM, Gulevich MG, et al. Hypersomnia after head–neck trauma: a medicolegal dilemma. Neurology 2000; 54: 653–9.

116. Masel BE, Scheibel RS, Kimbark T, Kuna ST. Excessive daytime sleepiness in adults with brain injuries. Arch Phys Med Rehabil 2001; 82: 1526–32.

117. Borgaro SR, Baker J, Wethe JV, Prigatano GP, Kwasnica C. Subjective reports of fatigue during early recovery from traumatic brain injury. J Head Trauma Rehabil 2005; 20: 416–25.

118. Good JL, Barry E, Fishman PS. Posttraumatic narcolepsy: the complete syndrome with tissue typing. Case report. J Neurosurg 1989; 71: 765–7.

119. Maccario M, Ruggles KH, Meriwether MW. Post-traumatic narcolepsy. Mil Med 1987; 152: 370–1.

120. Bruck D, Broughton RJ. Diagnostic ambiguities in a case of post-traumatic narcolepsy with cataplexy. Brain Inj 2004; 18: 321–6.

121. Lankford DA, Wellman JJ, O'Hara C. Posttraumatic narcolepsy in mild to moderate closed head injury. Sleep 1994; 17(8 suppl): S25–8.

122. Baumann CR, Stocker R, Imhof HG, et al. Hypocretin-1 (orexin A) deficiency in acute traumatic brain injury. Neurology 2005; 65: 147–9.

123. Baumann CR, Bassetti CL. Hypocretins (orexins) and sleep–wake disorders. Lancet Neurol 2005; 4: 673–82.

124. Ouellet MC, Savard J, Morin CM. Insomnia following traumatic brain injury: a review. Neurorehabil Neural Repair 2004; 18: 187–98.

125. Fichtenberg NL, Zafonte RD, Putnam S, Mann NR, Millard AE. Insomnia in a post-acute brain injury sample. Brain Inj 2002; 16: 197–206.

126. Fichtenberg NL, Millis SR, Mann NR, Zafonte RD, Millard AE. Factors associated with insomnia among post-acute traumatic brain injury survivors. Brain Inj 2000; 14: 659–67.

127. Kemp S, Biswas R, Neumann V, Coughlan A. The value of melatonin for sleep disorders occurring post-head injury: a pilot RCT. Brain Inj 2004; 18: 911–19.

128. Beetar JT, Guilmette TJ, Sparadeo FR. Sleep and pain complaints in symptomatic traumatic brain injury and neurologic populations. Arch Phys Med Rehabil 1996; 77: 1298–302.

129. Steele DL, Rajaratnam SM, Redman JR, Ponsford JL. The effect of traumatic brain injury on the timing of sleep. Chronobiol Int 2005; 22: 89–105.

130. Quinto C, Gellido C, Chokroverty S, Masdeu J. Posttraumatic delayed sleep phase syndrome. Neurology 2000; 54: 250–2.

131. Nagtegaal JE, Kerkhof GA, Smits MG, Swart AC, van der Meer YG. Traumatic brain injury-associated delayed sleep phase syndrome. Funct Neurol 1997; 12: 345–8.

132. Smits MG, Nagtegaal JE. Post-traumatic delayed sleep phase syndrome. Neurology 2000; 55: 902–3.

133. Dagan Y. Circadian rhythm sleep disorders (CRSD). Sleep Med Rev 2002; 6: 45–54.

134. Critchley M. Periodic hypersomnia and megaphagia in adolescent males. Brain 1962; 85: 627–56.

135. Will RG, Young JP, Thomas DJ. Kleine–Levin syndrome: report of two cases with onset of symptoms precipitated by head trauma. Br J Psychiatry 1988; 152: 410–12.

136. Kowatch RA. Sleep and head injury. Psychiatr Med 1989; 7: 37–41.

137. Bourke SC, Gibson GJ. Sleep and breathing in neuromuscular disease. Eur Respir J 2002; 19: 1194–201.

138. Quera-Salva MA, Guilleminault C, Chevret S, et al. Breathing disorders during sleep in myasthenia gravis. Ann Neurol 1992; 31: 86–92.

139. Barbe F, Quera-Salva MA, Agusti AG. Apnoea in Duchenne muscular dystrophy. Thorax 1995; 50: 1123.

140. Khan Y, Heckmatt JZ. Obstructive apnoeas in Duchenne muscular dystrophy. Thorax 1994; 49: 157–61.

141. Barbe F, Quera-Salva MA, McCann C, et al. Sleep-related respiratory disturbances in patients with Duchenne muscular dystrophy. Eur Respir J 1994; 7: 1403–8.

142. Giubilei F, Antonini G, Bastianello S, et al. Excessive daytime sleepiness in myotonic dystrophy. J Neurol Sci 1999; 164: 60–3.

143. van der Meche FG, Bogaard JM, van der Sluys JC, et al. Daytime sleep in myotonic dystrophy is not caused by sleep apnoea. J Neurol Neurosurg Psychiatry 1994; 57: 626–8.

144. Ferguson KA, Strong MJ, Ahmad D, George CF. Sleep-disordered breathing in amyotrophic lateral sclerosis. Chest 1996; 110: 664–9.

145. Kimura K, Tachibana N, Kimura J, Shibasaki H. Sleep-disordered breathing at an early stage of amyotrophic lateral sclerosis. J Neurol Sci 1999; 164: 37–43.

146. Aboussouan LS, Lewis RA. Sleep, respiration and ALS. J Neurol Sci 1999; 164: 1–2.

147. Miller RG, Rosenberg JA, Gelinas DF, et al. Practice parameter: the care of the patient with amyotrophic lateral sclerosis (an evidence-based review): report of the Quality Standards Subcommittee of the American Academy of Neurology: ALS Practice Parameters Task Force. Neurology 1999; 52: 1311–23.

148. Leigh PN, Abrahams S, Al-Chalabi A, et al. The management of motor neurone disease. J Neurol Neurosurg Psychiatry 2003; 74(Suppl 4): iv32–47.

149. Bourke SC, Tomlinson M, Williams TL, et al. Effects of non-invasive ventilation on survival and quality of life in patients with amyotrophic lateral sclerosis: a randomised controlled trial. Lancet Neurol 2006; 5: 140–7.

150. Steriade M, McCormick DA, Sejnowski TJ. Thalamocortical oscillations in the sleeping and aroused brain. Science 1993; 262: 679–85.

151. Steriade M, Contreras D, Amzica F. Synchronized sleep oscillations and their paroxysmal developments. Trends Neurosci 1994; 17: 199–208.

152. Malow BA. Sleep and epilepsy. Neurol Clin 2005; 23: 1127–47.

153. Provini F, Plazzi G, Lugaresi E. From nocturnal paroxysmal dystonia to nocturnal frontal lobe epilepsy. Clin Neurophysiol 2000; 111(Suppl 2): S2–8.

154. Tinuper P, Cerullo A, Cirignotta F, et al. Nocturnal paroxysmal dystonia with short-lasting attacks: three cases with evidence for an epileptic frontal lobe origin of seizures. Epilepsia 1990; 31: 549–56.

155. Scheffer IE, Bhatia KP, Lopes-Cendes I, et al. Autosomal dominant frontal epilepsy misdiagnosed as sleep disorder. Lancet 1994; 343: 515–17.

156. Krupp LB, Alvarez LA, LaRocca NG, Scheinberg LC. Fatigue in multiple sclerosis. Arch Neurol 1988; 45: 435–7.

157. Murray TJ. Amantadine therapy for fatigue in multiple sclerosis. Can J Neurol Sci 1985; 12: 251–4.

158. Gottschalk M, Kumpfel T, Flachenecker P, et al. Fatigue and regulation of the hypothalamo–pituitary–adrenal axis in multiple sclerosis. Arch Neurol 2005; 62: 277–80.

159. Tartaglia MC, Narayanan S, Francis SJ, et al. The relationship between diffuse axonal damage and fatigue in multiple sclerosis. Arch Neurol 2004; 61: 201–7.

160. Attarian HP, Brown KM, Duntley SP, Carter JD, Cross AH. The relationship of sleep disturbances and fatigue in multiple sclerosis. Arch Neurol 2004; 61: 525–8.

161. Johns MW. Sleepiness in different situations measured by the Epworth Sleepiness Scale. Sleep 1994; 17: 703–10.

162. Grigg-Damberger M. Neurologic disorders masquerading as pediatric sleep problems. Pediatr Clin North Am 2004; 51: 89–115.

163. Kilduff TS. Hypocretin/orexin: maintenance of wakefulness and a multiplicity of other roles. Sleep Med Rev 2005; 9: 227–30.

164. Bassetti CL. Narcolepsy: selective hypocretin (orexin) neuronal loss and multiple signaling deficiencies. Neurology 2005; 65: 1152–3.

165. Nishino S, Kanbayashi T. Symptomatic narcolepsy, cataplexy and hypersomnia, and their implications in the hypothalamic hypocretin/orexin system. Sleep Med Rev 2005; 9: 269–310.

166. Lovblad KO, Thomas R, Jakob PM, et al. Silent functional magnetic resonance imaging demonstrates focal activation in rapid eye movement sleep. Neurology 1999; 53: 2193–5.

8

Behavioral intervention for sleep disorders

Chien-Ming Yang, Arthur J Spielman

INTRODUCTION

Sleep disturbance is one of the most common health complaints in the general population. It is a symptom of various conditions of different pathogenesis. Some sleep disorders have clearly identified physiologic etiologies. Examples include breathing-related sleep disorders, narcolepsy, and sleep-related movement disorders.[1] Others are primarily caused by psychosocial or behavioral factors, such as stress-related transient insomnia (adjustment insomnia) or sleep disturbance associated with poor sleep hygiene. Moreover, sleep complaints in some other cases are associated with psychiatric or medical conditions. It has been estimated that about 40% of patients with insomnia and 47% of patients with hypersomnia carry one or more comorbid psychiatric diagnoses, with affective disorders, anxiety disorders, and substance abuse among the most prevalent.[2] Also, 16–82% of patients with chronic medical conditions, such as musculoskeletal and other painful disorders, heart disease, airway disease, and diabetes, have reported difficulty sleeping.[3–9] The sleep complaints in these cases are often assumed to be symptoms secondary to the primary conditions, or caused by the discomforts associated with these conditions. Ideally, the different aspects of sleep pathologies in a patient should be differentiated and treatment should be instituted accordingly. However, in clinical practice, the pathogenesis is usually multifaceted and the causal inferences among the factors are usually

difficult to tease apart. For example, a patient's sleep may be initially disrupted by the pain caused by a medical condition. The resulting worries over the consequences of sleeplessness may further worsen sleep and exacerbate the sleep problems. Also, in sleep disturbance associated with psychiatric disorders, the sleep problems may reciprocally feedback to aggravate, perpetuate, or predispose individuals to relapse of the psychiatric conditions. Evidence has shown that persistent insomnia may predispose to the development of psychiatric disorders, especially depression.[2,10] Furthermore, the neurophysiologic systems that regulate sleep and wake are impacted by psychologic and behavioral factors. Even in a physiologically based sleep disorder, such as mild sleep-related breathing disorder, anxiety over poor sleep and daytime functioning or inappropriate sleep practices can further disrupt the already fragile sleep. Therefore, behavioral intervention is beneficial not only in the treatment of sleep disorders of psychosocial origin, but also in the management of physiologically based sleep problems.

Many behavioral and psychologic interventions are effective in the treatment of sleep disorders, especially in the management of chronic insomnia.[11–13] Some of the behavioral techniques have also been applied to insomnia associated with medical or psychiatric disorders, with positive results.[11,14–17] In addition to improvements in sleep, psychiatric symptoms decreased.[18,19] Widely applicable, behavioral interventions have been used to enhance compliance with medical treatment in sleep-related breathing disorders.[20,21]

In this chapter, we will describe psychologic and behavioral influences on sleep, and the neurophysiologic mechanisms of normal sleep regulation. We will also provide a framework for the clinician to conceptualize the development of insomnia in individual patients. Further, we will review the behavioral techniques that are effective in the treatment of insomnia. Since there are some recent review articles on the treatment efficacy of cognitive–behavioral therapy (CBT) for insomnia,[22–24] this chapter will focus more on the conceptual rationales and practical aspects of cognitive–behavioral interventions. Lastly, we will briefly review behavioral interventions for specific sleep disorders other than insomnia.

PSYCHOSOCIAL AND BEHAVIORAL FACTORS AFFECTING SLEEP REGULATION

Sleep disturbances can be conceptualized as a disruption of the mechanisms that regulate normal processes of sleep. Thus, understanding the mechanisms of normal sleep control is important for the evaluation and treatment of sleep disorders. It is now recognized that human sleep is regulated by the interactions of three major systems: a homeostatic system that regulates the optimal level of sleep drive to maintain the internal balance between sleep and wakefulness, a circadian process that generates a biological rhythm of sleep and wake tendency over a day, and an arousal system that promotes wakefulness and opposes the sleep drive.[25,26]

The classical two-process model proposed that the propensity for sleep or wakefulness at a given time is a consequence of the interactions between the homeostatic and circadian processes.[27] The homeostatic sleep drive is determined by the amount of sleep acquired previously and the duration of prior wakefulness. Like other homeostatic systems, such as those that regulate body temperature, the system seeks

to maintain a set amount of sleep. Therefore, sleep deprivation is followed by enhanced sleep drive and extra recovery sleep. Satisfaction of sleep drive is, in contrast, followed by decreased sleep propensity and shorter or lighter sleep. In addition, increased physical activities may enhance homeostatic sleep drive. Empirical studies have documented that exercise leads to increased slow-wave sleep or slow-wave activity.[28]

The circadian system, on the other hand, generates a near 24-hour rhythm of sleep-and-wake tendency that is independent of prior amount of sleep. The tendency for sleeping and waking is determined by temporal factors associated with the phase of the endogenous circadian cycle. With the interactions of the two systems, the sleep propensity and amount of sleep obtained at a given time are determined by the accumulated sleep debt and the circadian sleep tendency at that time.

Studies with both animals and humans have identified the genetic determinants of the circadian sleep tendency.[29,30] The setpoint of the homeostatic regulation may also be genetically or biologically based. Also, exposure to environmental time cues, especially bright light, can stabilize or shift the endogenous circadian rhythm. It has been recognized that the endogenous circadian cycle in humans is slightly over 24 hours;[31,32] therefore, there is a natural tendency for the endogenous rhythm to drift later in time. Morning light exposure can advance the circadian sleep phase and maintain a 24-hour circadian period.[33,34]

Behavioral practices and environmental factors can optimize or disrupt the operations of these systems. Maladaptive behavioral practices, such as napping or sleeping late at weekends, may trigger and perpetuate sleep problems. These sleep episodes intrude into the typical waking period of the day and lead to insufficient sleep drive accumulated by bedtime. Furthermore, sleeping-in will prevent the morning light cue, which will permit a delay in the individual's endogenous circadian sleep tendency, making it difficult to fall asleep at night. Irregular sleep–wake habits may destabilize the endogenous circadian rhythm and produce fluctuations in the homeostatic sleep drive, both of which can interfere with a regular sleep–wake rhythm.

In addition to the homeostatic and circadian processes, the arousal system can be conceived of as reciprocal to the sleep processes, and may counteract sleep drive through the promotion of arousal and wakefulness. This system can be boosted by stress, and by emotional and environmental stimuli, leading to disruption of normal sleep processes. The arousal system is adaptive as a protective system that is intended to arouse the organism when it is at risk. However, when it is activated at bedtime, sleep disturbance may result. Several etiologic models addressing the role of arousal as a cause of insomnia have been proposed.[35,36] Characteristics of overactivation of the arousal system in insomniacs from either psychosocial or physiologic perspectives have been reported in previous research. Individuals with insomnia have been shown to have elevated indices of autonomic activity, such as higher metabolic rate, body temperature, heart rate, urinary cortisol and epinephrine (adrenaline) excretion, skin conduction, and muscle tension.[37,38] In addition, increased cognitive processing around sleep onset or during sleep was reflected by disturbing mental activity and faster electroencephalographic (EEG) frequencies.[39–41] The elevated high-frequency EEG power-spectral findings have been shown to be reduced after successful treatment with CBT for insomnia, but still maintained at a level that is higher than for good sleepers.[42] These results imply that the hyperarousal might in part be a predisposing trait, and in part aggravated in the course of chronic insomnia. One model proposed that the arousal state in chronic insomniacs might be learned through a process of classical conditioning.[43] In this model, transient sleep disturbance could be triggered by acute stressors. With repeated nights of waking and worrying in bed, the patient might soon associate the bedtime cues with waking and anxiety. As a result, the patient tends to become aroused when exposed to sleep-related cues and the insomnia becomes chronic even if the transient stressor that had triggered the sleep problem has been resolved.

Similar to homeostatic and circadian regulation, the arousal system is also highly susceptible to the effects of behavioral practices and psychologic status. Vigorous presleep activities and worries about sleep (e.g., watching the clock, counting the number of hours left for sleep, and the consequences of poor sleep), may activate the arousal system. Emotional arousal, such as feeling depressed over a loss or guilt, and anticipatory anxiety of challenges to come also lead to overactivation of the arousal system and further disrupt sleep processes. Both the behavioral practices and emotional arousal may be influenced by attitudes and beliefs concerning sleep. For example, a belief that one should obtain 8 hours of sleep can lead an insomnia sufferer to spend extra time in bed during the weekend. As discussed earlier, the consequent delayed wake-up time may lead to decreased homeostatic sleep drive at bedtime the next night and may delay the phase of endogenous circadian rhythms. Also, the failure to obtain 8 hours of sleep may lead to excessive worry that further aggravates the individual's sleep condition. Therefore, sleep cognition plays a major role in the pathogenesis of insomnia.[44–47] Changes in sleep cognition after treatment have also been found to be associated with sleep improvement.[45,48] Figure 8.1 shows the conceptual model of the interactions among the psychologic/behavioral factors and the neurophysiologic systems that regulate sleep. With this model in mind, the clinician can try to evaluate the patients' sleep problems by examining the functioning of the three neurophysiologic systems and the various factors that may have an impact on these systems.

As discussed above, the factors contributing to sleep disturbance in an individual are usually multi-dimensional. Organizing these contributions along the timeline of the development of the insomnia can be helpful in understanding the problem and formulation of a treatment plan. The factors contributing to insomnia can be classified into predisposing, precipitating, or perpetuating factors.[49] Predisposing factors are the individual traits that set the stage for the development of insomnia, but do not necessarily lead to insomnia. Examples include

Psychological/behavioral factors   Neurophysiologic systems

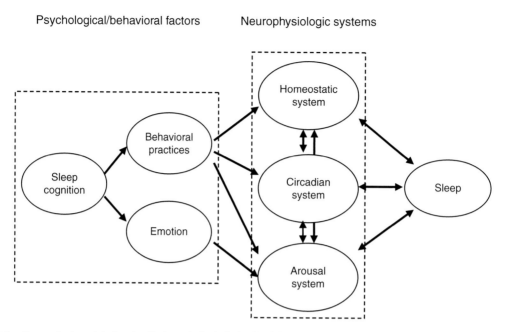

Figure 8.1   Conceptual model showing that psychologic/behavioral factors influence sleep mediated by the neurophysiologic systems for sleep regulation

arousal-prone personality styles, a hypersensitive physiologic arousal system, a rigid circadian system, and vulnerable sleep systems. The clinician may need to assess the patient's premorbid sleep pattern, sleep history at a younger age, and general personality style in order to identify these factors. Understanding the risk factors can help in establishing a realistic expectation of the patient's sleep and help them avoid getting into situations that may trigger a sleep problem. Precipitating factors are usually readily identified as the event or conditions that initiate the sleep disturbance. The most common precipitating factor is a major life stressor, such as loss, having a baby, change of working schedule, major illness, retiring, or any event that heightens arousal or leads to significant changes in daily life routines. In some cases, resolving the triggering event is the only treatment needed to address the sleeping problem. However, in many cases, the insomnia persists and becomes chronic over time. Common perpetuating factors include the conditioned association between anxiety and

bedtime cues, maladaptive sleep–wake habits intended to gain more sleep, strategies to minimize daytime deficits, and excessive worries over sleeplessness. In these cases, the perpetuating factors should then become the focus of the treatment.

To illustrate this model, take an individual with a high anxiety trait as an example. Their anxiety tendency predisposes them psychologically to worry about trivial matters and physiologically to be easily aroused. The trait alone may not ordinarily be sufficient to produce a persistent sleep disturbance, but may lead to occasional poor sleep. However, a life stressor (e.g, a break-up in a relationship) may boost the arousal system and precipitate the onset of insomnia. The individual starts tossing and turning in bed and ruminating over the conflicts in the relationship. Stress management to help the patient cope with the stressor by direct actions, or temporizing and allowing time to dampen these problems, may be the first therapeutic plan. However, in reacting to the insomnia, this individual may develop behavioral adaptations and thoughts that are counterproductive. For example, the patient may start to spend too much time in bed to 'get rest' or to 'make up for lost sleep'. These behaviors may strengthen the association between the bed and fretful tossing and turning, and lead to a conditioned insomnia. The patient may start to worry about not being able to fall asleep or to worry about job performance the next day. These worries further activate the arousal system and exacerbate the sleep difficulties. At this point in time, treatment should target the reduction of arousal, the changed view of sleep, and the elimination of maladaptive sleep practices. Without proper treatment, the individual may start to use hypnotic medication regularly and have difficulty stopping because of the rebound effects when withdrawing from the drug. At this point in the course of the insomnia, education about the effects of hypnotic use and withdrawal, as well as strategies to taper off medication, should be included as part of the treatment. Although all components of this model may not be present in a particular patient, it does provide a framework for the clinician to organize the multiple determinants and to formulate a comprehensive treatment plan. Table 8.1 shows the common contributing factors associated with the development of insomnia.

BEHAVIORAL INTERVENTIONS FOR INSOMNIA

Various behavioral techniques have been applied for the treatment of insomnia. Many of these techniques are effectively combined as a multicomponent approach that is usually referred to as CBT for insomnia. CBT for insomnia can be conducted in groups with a structured program or conducted individually with techniques selected that are tailored for an individual. Meta-analyses and review articles on the efficacy of individual behavior techniques as well as multicomponent CBT programs have shown moderate to large effect sizes on the major sleep parameters.[11,12,50,51] Furthermore, the treatment effects have been shown to be equal to or better than pharmacologic treatments at the end of treatment sessions and with long-term follow-up of up to 2 years.[13,22,52]

Before the initiation of a cognitive and behavioral intervention for insomnia, it is important to conduct a thorough evaluation to identify the contributing factors. Patients with sleep disturbances are often puzzled by their condition. The feeling of being out of control and the mystery of what is causing the problem often generates worries and anxiety that may further disrupt their sleep. Thus, sharing the formulation with the patient may be therapeutic by restoring some modicum of control and reducing unnecessary worry. Furthermore, the patient's grasp of the formulation will facilitate the understanding of treatment rationales and may motivate the patient to practice the behavioral techniques. In addition to the evaluation and etiologic formulation, providing the rationale and describing the treatment procedures comprise a comprehensive first treatment session.

Furthermore, it is useful for patients to know what to expect from treatment. For example, providing information that the behavioral techniques require a few weeks to have significant impact may prevent premature demoralization when improvement is not immediate. The patient needs to understand that reliably carrying out behavioral practices is crucial for the treatment to be effective. Change in sleep habits, daily life routines, and practice of some techniques are all likely to be required. A series of office visits or group sessions is then scheduled on a weekly or biweekly base, with sleep log recording and/or phone contacts in between sessions. For both individual and group CBT, the whole program usually takes 4–8 weeks. Lately, abbreviated, two-session CBT has also been reported to be effective in a primary care setting.[53] The following are the rationales and practical guidelines of the major CBT techniques for insomnia.

Sleep hygiene education

Sleep hygiene refers to practices of everyday living and sleep-related activities that promote

Table 8.1   Common contributing factors associated with the development of insomnia

Predisposing factors

Homeostatic process

- Abnormality or weakness of the neurophysiologic system that generates sleep

Circadian process

- Extreme circadian type – functioning better during late evening or early morning as an individual trait
- Less flexible circadian system

Arousal system

- Anxiety-prone and depressive personality traits and tendencies toward neuroticism and somatization lead to a higher level of emotional and physiologic arousal
- Personality traits associated with sustained level of arousal, such as perfectionism and excessive need for control
- Heightened or more sensitive physiologic arousal system

Precipitating factors

Homeostatic process

- Lack of or decrease of daytime activities, such as retirement

Circadian process

- Change of sleep–wake schedule, such as jet lag or starting a nightshift job

Arousal system

- Life stressors or events lead to emotional and physiologic distress

Perpetuating factors

Homeostatic process

- Increased resting in bed
- Discharge of the sleep drive by sleeping outside of the nocturnal sleep period, such as increased daytime naps or frequent dozing offs
- Reduced daytime activities

Circadian process

- Sleeping-in during weekends to catch up on sleep

Arousal system

- Dysfunctional beliefs and attitudes about sleep that lead to increased emotional arousals and worries over sleep loss
- Conditioning between bedtime cues and arousal

good-quality sleep or that make sleep more resistant to disruption. The objectives of sleep hygiene education are to improve basic knowledge about sleep and to modify counterproductive sleep practices.[54] Sleep hygiene education usually includes both a knowledge part and a practice part. Firstly, sleep hygiene education provides basic knowledge about sleep and sleep disorders, including

information about the homeostatic process and function of normal sleep, the influence of circadian rhythms on sleep, the influences of stress and emotion on sleep, the variability in sleep from night to night, developmental changes of sleep, the effect of daily activities on sleep, and the effect of sleep disturbances on daytime function. Understanding empowers the patient and eliminates unnecessary worry about the consequences of sleep loss. It also provides the rationale for sleep-promoting behavioral practices. Secondly, good sleep hygiene requires the patient to modify daily living practices that are counterproductive for sleep. The clinician reviews the lifestyle and sleep–wake habits with the patient and identifies a set of practices that are not consistent with good sleep hygiene. The patient is asked to refrain from maladaptive activities and, in some cases, to engage in sleep-promoting behaviors. Common behavioral practices that are incompatible with good sleep are listed in Table 8.2.

Sleep hygiene education is usually part of a more comprehensive treatment program. Sleep hygiene education alone has been shown to be less effective than the other behavioral treatments.[50] Many patients are aware of sleep hygiene practices, but do not believe that these will produce significant changes in their sleep. It is important to convey to such individuals that insomnia is the result of the interaction of a number of factors, and that an effective treatment should address multiple factors at the same time. Eliminating these habits may not solve the problem. However, a successful treatment result may be prevented or delayed due to poor sleep hygiene practices. Also, patients with chronic sleep problems may engage in counterproductive sleep practice, such as daytime napping, going to bed earlier, or staying in bed in the morning to catch up on sleep, as a way of coping with the consequences of their sleep problem. It is important to convey to the patient that these coping strategies may help in the short run, but they sacrifice robust sleep in the long term.

Cognitive therapy

Worrying about sleeplessness may promote arousal, and becomes a self-fulfilling prophecy that further exacerbates sleep difficulties. Misconceptions about sleep may also lead to sleep-disruptive behavioral practices. Faulty beliefs and attitudes about sleep have been shown to be associated with the symptoms of insomnia.[45,47,48] Common dysfunctional cognitions about sleep can be classified into five categories: misconceptions of the causes of insomnia; misattributions or amplifications of its consequences; unrealistic sleep expectations; diminished perceptions of control; and predictability of sleep.[49] Changes of dysfunctional thoughts can reduce the worries and therefore break the vicious cycle that leads to arousal. The disruptive cognitions about sleep may be corrected with sleep hygiene education. Relaxation training can also be helpful to distract patients from excessive worry and reduce the physical arousal. Cognitive restructuring, on the other hand, addresses the sleep-disturbing cognitions directly, and replaces the thoughts with more realistic thoughts and positive ideas.[44,49]

To institute cognitive restructuring, the clinician should discuss with the patient their beliefs regarding sleep in general and their sleep problems. Beliefs that lead to maladaptive behavioral practices or enhance worries about sleep should be identified. The clinician can provide correct information about sleep and the consequences of sleep loss to help the patient develop more positive and less disruptive ideas about their sleep problems. The Dysfunctional Beliefs and Attitudes Scale[49] can be utilized to help with the evaluation of patients' sleep cognitions. Also, a cognitive–behavioral strategy may be employed by enlisting the patient as a co-investigator to gather data that will address the validity of specific beliefs. For example, a patient who reported that poor sleep always make them perform poorly at work may be asked to rate job performance on daily sleep logs. In this way, data could be collected to disconfirm dysfunctional thoughts and beliefs regarding sleep.

Stimulus-control therapy

Stimulus-control therapy is designed to break the maladaptive association of bedtime cues with wakefulness and worrying. Patients are instructed to get out of bed if unable to fall asleep and return to bed when feeling ready to fall asleep. Over time, the repeated association of bedroom cues with

---

Table 8.2   Sleep-related habits and daily life practices that may interfere with sleep

Practices that reduce homeostatic drive at bedtime

Daily life behaviors

- Insufficient activities during the day
- Lying down to get rest during the day

Sleep-related habits

- Napping, nodding, and dozing off during the day or evening
- In a trance, semi-awake in the evening
- Spending too much time in bed
- Extra sleep during the weekends

Practices that disrupt circadian regularity

Daily life behaviors

- Insufficient morning light exposure, leading to a phase delay in circadian rhythm
- Early-morning light exposure, producing early-morning awakening due to a phase advance in circadian rhythm

Sleep-related habits

- Irregular sleep–wake schedule
- Sleeping-in in the morning during weekends

Practices that enhance the level of arousal

Daily life behaviors

- Excess caffeine consumption or caffeine later in the day
- Smoking in the evening
- Alcohol consumption in the evening
- Exercising in the late evening
- Late-evening meal or fluid (may cause frequent urination)
- Getting home late or not enough time to wind down

Sleep-related habits

- Evening apprehension of sleep
- Preparations for bed are arousing
- No regular presleep ritual
- Distressing pillow talk
- Watching TV, reading or engaging in other sleep-incompatible behaviors in bed before lights out, or falling asleep with TV or radio left on
- Trying too hard to sleep
- Clock-watching during the night
- Staying in bed during awakenings, or lingering in bed awake in the morning
- Poor sleep environment, such as bed-partner snoring, noises, direct morning sunlight, or pets in the bedroom

---

rapid sleep onset brings sleep under the stimulus control of the bedroom environment.[43] The specific instructions are as follows:

- Go to sleep only when feeling sleepy.

- Do not use the bed or bedroom for activities other than sleep (sexual activity is the only exception).

- If you do not fall asleep within about 20 minutes, get up and go into another room to do something relaxing.

- Go back to bed only when feeling sleepy again.

- Repeat the procedure of getting out of bed if you still cannot fall asleep rapidly.

● Get up at the same time each morning, regardless how much sleep you obtain.

These instructions are easy to understand but hard for some patients to carry out regularly. Initially, patients will spend considerable time out of bed and thus will suffer some sleep loss. It is important to motivate patients by letting them fully understand the rationale of this treatment procedure. Although daytime functioning and mood may be impaired temporarily, the partial sleep deprivation will foster both rapid sleep onset and increased sleep. The patient needs to be educated that short-term sacrifice will produce long-term gains. Also, some patients may worry that they do not know what to do when they are out of the bed during the night. The clinician may need to prescribe activities to perform during the night that are not too taxing or activating.

Sleep-restriction therapy

Sleep-restriction therapy was developed on the assumption that the homeostatic sleep process can self-correct when sleep disturbance leads to sleep loss. Sleep-restriction therapy promotes sleep by inducing a mild sleep loss initially and gradually increasing sleep time after sleep is stabilized. Like stimulus control therapy, this procedure can also prevent or break the maladaptive association between anxiety and bedtime cues by decreasing the chance of lying awake in bed.[55,56] The specific procedures are as follows:

1. Patients complete a sleep log that records the daily sleep pattern over a 2-week period.

2. The average total sleep time per night of this 2-week period is then prescribed as the time in bed for the following week. The time of rising from bed is set to the time when the patient is required to wake up or when the patient generally awakens, and the time of retiring is calculated accordingly. To avoid the effects of severe sleep deprivation, the minimum time in bed is never set below 4.5 hours. Lying down or napping outside of the scheduled bedtimes is not permitted.

3. Patients fill out a sleep daily log to record bedtimes and estimated total sleep time. Sleep efficiency (estimated total sleep time/time in bed $\times$ 100%) is evaluated every week.

4. The prescribed time in bed is adjusted by three criteria: (a) when the mean sleep efficiency is equal to or more than 90% (85% in older individuals), the subject's time in bed is increased by 15 minutes by setting the retiring time earlier; (b) if the mean sleep efficiency is less than 85% (80% in seniors), then the time in bed is decreased by 15 minutes; (c) when the sleep efficiency is between 85% and 90% (80% and 85% in seniors), the time in bed remains the same.

Some modified procedures to adjust time in bed have been proposed and utilized. One way is to increase time in bed progressively by 15 or 30 minutes each week until the patient is spending 7 hours in bed. Further changes of time in bed may be made based on daytime functioning, fatigue, and sleepiness.[57] Also, a sleep-compression procedure has been utilized to gradually reduce time in bed instead of curtailing it abruptly. As in the original procedure, mean total sleep time and time in bed are determined from the 2 weeks of baseline sleep log. The difference between mean total sleep time and mean time in bed is then divided by 5, and the prescribed time in bed is compressed by this amount weekly. By the end of the fifth session, time in bed has been gradually compressed to match the initial total sleep time. Like the original procedure, time in bed is increased by 15 minutes if the sleep efficiency surpasses 90%. This procedure has been found to be helpful for elderly patients with insomnia.[58]

As with stimulus control instructions, patients should be told to expect mild sleep loss and daytime deficits at the initiation of the treatment.

It should be stressed that this temporary worsening of daytime mood, performance, and energy will lead to deeper and more consolidated sleep after a few weeks of practicing this method. Patients may have difficulty resisting the temptation to spend more time in bed. Clinicians should encourage patients to continue following the instruction and to plan specific activities for their increased time in the evening before going to bed.

Relaxation training

As described earlier, thoughts and behaviors resulting in arousal may interfere with sleep. For the same reasons, activities reducing arousal may facilitate sleep. Various relaxation techniques have been developed to assist in the reduction of tension and anxiety. Examples include progressive muscle relaxation that reduces muscle tension by sequential tensing and relaxing of the main muscle groups,[59,60] autogenic training that produces somatic relaxation by inducing sensations of warmth and heaviness of the body,[60] and guided imagery that aims to channel mental processes into a vivid storyline.[61] Biofeedback has also been utilized to assist the mastering of relaxation techniques.[62,63] The relaxation training starts with demonstration of how it is done by the clinician. Patients are then instructed to practice the technique at home between sessions. The instructions for the relaxation procedures can be recorded during the session for patients to practice at home. Commercial relaxation training tapes are also available to facilitate the practice at home. The patient is asked to practice the relaxation protocol once or twice a day. The patient's level of relaxation should be assessed before and after each practice session with a simple subjective rating scale in order to monitor the progress of the training. It may take weeks for some individuals to develop the skill to relax on cue. Only after mastering the procedure, is the patient told to use it to facilitate falling asleep or returning to sleep following a nocturnal awakening. At the start of training, patients are often distracted and deflected from the tasks, and find themselves thinking and worrying about other things. They should be told to anticipate that their mind will wander and to avoid self-criticism. It is crucial to help motivate patients to continue practicing the technique and to help them deal with obstacles that they encounter.

BEHAVIORAL INTERVENTION FOR ADJUSTMENTS OF CIRCADIAN RHYTHM

Sleep disturbances can result from a mismatch between endogenous circadian phase and environmental time. In these cases, patients' sleep per se may not be problematic when they are allowed to choose their preferred sleep schedule. For example, individuals with a delayed endogenous circadian sleep–wake system tend to have difficulty falling asleep in the evening as well as experiencing difficulty getting up in the morning. However, when allowed to sleep at their preferred schedule, such as during the weekend or on extended vacations, they usually choose to go to bed late and to sleep-in in the morning without experiencing sleep disruption. This condition is more frequently seen in adolescents and young adults.[64,65] In contrast, patients with an advanced endogenous circadian rhythm usually have no problem initiating sleep, but complain of early-morning awakenings. This sleep pattern is more commonly reported by elderly individuals.[66,67] In clinical cases, mild phase-shifting of circadian rhythm may interact with other sleep pathologies and make evaluation and treatment more complicated.

Although the mechanisms responsible for circadian rhythms have been shown to include a number of genetic factors, particular neuroanatomic loci, and environmental time cues, bright light has also been shown to be quite effective in phase-shifting human circadian rhythms.[33,34] Light exposure can be used to treat sleep disturbances related to phase shifts of endogenous circadian rhythms. The influence of light on the phase of circadian rhythms depends on the timing, wavelength, and intensity of the light exposure. There is a relationship between the timing of light exposure and the size and direction of the phase shift induced. This relationship can be plotted as a phase response curve (PRC). Light exposure in late subjective night and early subjective day produces a phase advance in circadian rhythms; in contrast, light exposure in late subjective day and early subjective night induces a phase delay.[34] Therefore, for patients complaining of difficulty falling asleep in the evening and getting up in the morning, indicating possible delayed sleep phase, bright light administration upon awakening in the morning can advance their circadian rhythms to the desired time.[68] Bright light exposure in the evening has also been used to treat patients with advanced sleep phase who complain of early-evening sleepiness and early-morning awakening.[69,70] Since endogenous circadian oscillators are advanced in time in these individuals, bright light exposure in the evening should be applied to delay their circadian rhythms. Also, manipulation of light exposure during work hours and avoiding light exposure after work have also been shown to facilitate the adjustment to shiftwork.[71]

To institute light therapy for phase-shifting, patients complete a sleep log that records the daily sleep pattern over a 1–2-week period, in order to estimate their endogenous circadian phase. They should also identify an ideal sleep schedule as the goal of the phase-shifting. In the beginning, patients are asked to set a sleep–wake schedule that is close to the estimated endogenous sleep phase. As the treatment proceeds, the wake-up time is progressively shifted earlier for patients with a delayed circadian phase; in contrast, the retiring time is gradually shifted later for patients with an advanced sleep phase. With the help of light exposure, most patients can shift their circadian phase for over an hour each week with little difficulty. In terms of the light exposure, bright light exposure should be administered in the morning as close to the scheduled wake-up time as possible for patients

with delayed sleep–wake pattern, and administered in the early evening for patients with advanced sleep–wake pattern. The source of bright light can be artificial or natural outdoor sunlight. Illumination of approximately 2500 lux or more at eye level is usually required to obtain successful results. The optimal duration of exposure must be determined individually. A 1–2-hour period of treatment each day usually achieves an adequate effect. Patients with eye pathology should consult with an ophthalmologist before receiving light therapy.

Another behavioral intervention used for the treatment of delayed sleep phase is chronotherapy. Since the sleep–wake cycle in humans has a period length slightly greater than 24 hours,[31,32] it tends to be easier to delay the sleep–wake schedule than to advance the phase. Based on this observation, chronotherapy was devised as a treatment for individuals with delayed sleep phase by gradually shifting the sleep–wake schedule later until it reaches the desired schedule.[72] Again, the conduct of this procedure requires an estimate of baseline circadian phase by sleep log, with the initial sleep–wake schedule being set up accordingly. The patient is then instructed to delay retiring time and arising time by 2 or 3 hours each day until these match the desired sleep schedule. Once the desired schedule has been achieved, the patient should be told to avoid sleeping late in order to prevent relapse. The primary problem in carrying out chronotherapy is that it requires the patients to follow an unusual sleep–wake schedule for several days. There will be a number of days in a row in which the patient is sleeping during daylight hours and is awake during the night. Therefore, patients usually take several days off from work and must ensure that they are not disturbed while they sleep. The relapse rate for patients with delayed sleep phase syndrome is as high as 91.5%.[73] Therefore, clinicians need to emphasize the importance of following a strict sleep–wake schedule after patients have reached their desired schedule. Morning exposure to bright light can be instituted to assist the maintenance of a stable circadian phase.

BEHAVIORAL INTERVENTION FOR OTHER SLEEP DISORDERS

Behavioral techniques have also been used to assist in the treatment of other sleep disorders, although evidence of effectiveness is still preliminary. The behavioral intervention can be the primary treatment or a supplementary treatment combined with pharmacologic therapy and/or other medical procedures.

Behavioral intervention has been applied as a supplementary treatment to facilitate compliance with the use of continuous positive airway pressure (CPAP) in patients with sleep-related breathing disorders. The treatment usually includes psychologic support, education regarding sleep-related breathing disorders and the function of CPAP, modeling of CPAP use, and systematic desensitization to overcome the anxiety associated with CPAP use. Studies of the effects of education and support on CPAP compliance have generated mixed results. Some studies have shown a facilitation of CPAP use,[21,74,75] while others did not.[76,77] Evidence supporting the effects of systematic desensitization is also limited. So far, there has only been one case study reporting efficacy.[20]

Behavioral intervention has also been developed for the management of nightmares. The clinician has the patient recall and rehearse the content of nightmares and change the dream narrative ending to a more positive outcome. The patient is then instructed to rehearse the revised version of the dream while awake each day for a few days. Dream rehearsal has been found to be effective in reducing the frequency and intensity of nightmares, and in improving the sense of control. This technique has also been applied successfully to patients with post-traumatic stress disorder (PTSD). Patients showed improved sleep and reduction in PTSD symptoms.[19,78]

In addition to these specific techniques, the basic conceptual framework and behavioral intervention developed for insomnia may also be applied to optimize sleep in patients with other sleep disorders. Although their sleep pathologies may disrupt the normal process of sleep regulation, maximizing the sleep drive at bedtime, maintaining stable circadian rhythm, and reducing the interference from cognitive and emotional arousals can strengthen sleep and may make patients more resistant to the disruption by the primary sleep pathology.

CONCLUSIONS

Classical Western medicine favors a single explanation for a cluster of symptoms. However, in the case of sleep disorders, the sleep symptom is often a manifestation of an interaction among multiple contributing factors. Frequently, both physiologic and psychologic factors are involved in the production of the sleep disturbance. Clinicians should take a broad perspective and avoid viewing the problem from a single aspect. A careful evaluation of the patient's overall condition is often the key to successful treatment. The basic rationale of behavioral intervention for sleep disorders is to make an individual's lifestyle and sleep pattern more compatible with the nature of the systems that regulate sleep. It often requires patients to change daily life routines and to engage in specific behavioral practices. Patient motivation is another key for effective treatment.

Although effective behavioral techniques for sleep disorders are available, the percentage of patients seeking help remains relatively low. Survey studies have reported that only around 5% of patients with insomnia seek help specifically for their sleep problem[79] and only one-third of patients with sleep difficulties discuss their problems with a healthcare professional.[80] Public education is important to promote awareness of treatment options and the wisdom in seeking help at an early stage of the sleep problem. Also, inclusion of sleep medicine training is important to provide physicians, psychologists, and other medical professionals with sufficient knowledge and techniques to help patients with sleep problems.

REFERENCES

1. American Academy of Sleep Medicine (AASM). The International Classification of Sleep Disorders, 2nd edn. Westchester, IL: American Academy of Sleep Medicine.
2. Ford D, Kamerow D. Epidemiologic study of sleep disturbances and psychiatric disorders: an opportunity for prevention? JAMA 1989; 262: 1479–84.
3. Katz DA, McHorney CA. Clinical correlates of insomnia in patients with chronic illness. Arch Intern Med 1998; 158: 1099–107.
4. Smith MT, Perlis ML, Smith MS, Giles DE, Carmody TP. Sleep quality and presleep arousal in chronic pain. J Behav Med 2000; 23: 1–13.
5. Sridhar GR, Madhu K. Prevalence of sleep disturbances in diabetes mellitus. Diabetes Res Clin Pract 1994; 23: 183–6.
6. Klink M, Quan S, Kaltenborn W, Lobowitz M. Risk factors associated with complaints of insomnia in a general adult population. Arch Intern Med 1992; 152: 1634–7.
7. Gislason T, Reyrnisdotter H, Kritbjarnarson H, Benediktsdotter B. Sleep habits and sleep disturbances among the elderly: an epidemiological survey. J Intern Med 1993; 234: 31–9.
8. Janson C, Lindberg E, Gislason T, Elmasry A, Boman G. Insomnia in men: a 10-year prospective population based study. Sleep 2001; 24: 425–30.
9. Ohayon MM. Relationship between chronic painful condition and insomnia. J Psychiat Res 2005; 39: 151–9.
10. Breslau N, Roth T, Rosenthal L, Andreski P. Sleep disturbance and psychiatric disorders: a longitudinal epidemiological study of young adults. Biol Psychiat 1996; 39: 411–18.
11. Morin CM, Culbert JP, Schwartz SM. Nonpharmacological interventions for insomnia: a meta-analysis of treatment efficacy. Am J Psychiatry 1994; 151: 1172–80.
12. Murtagh DRR, Greenwood KM. Identifying effective psychological treatment for insomnia: a meta-analysis. J Consult Clin Psychol 1995; 63: 79–89.
13. Smith MT, Perlis ML, Park A, et al. Comparative meta-analysis of pharmacotherapy and behavior therapy for persistent insomnia. Am J Psychiatry 2002; 159: 5–11.
14. Lichstein KL, Wilson NM, Johnson CT. Psychological treatment of secondary insomnia. Psychol Aging 2000; 15: 232–40.
15. Perlis ML, Sharpe MC, Smith MT, Greenblatt DW, Giles DE. Behavioral treatment of insomnia: treatment outcome and the relevance of medical and psychiatric morbidity. J Behav Med 2001; 24: 281–96.
16. Rybarczyk B, Lopez M, Benson R, Alsten C, Stepanski E. Efficacy of two behavioral treatment programs for comorbid geriatric insomnia. Psychol Aging 2002; 17: 288–98.
17. Rybarczyk B, Stepanski E, Fogg L, et al. A placebo-controlled test of cognitive–behavioral therapy for comorbid insomnia in older adults. J Consult Clin Psychol 2005; 73: 1164–74.
18. Kuo T, Manber R, Loewy D. Insomniacs with comorbid conditions achieved comparable improvement in a cognitive behavioral group treatment program as insomniacs without comorbid depression. Sleep 2001; 24: A62.
19. Krakow B, Hollifield M, Johnston L, et al. Imagery rehearsal therapy for chronic nightmares in sexual assault survivors with posttraumatic stress disorder. JAMA 2001; 286: 537–45.
20. Edinger JD, Radtke RA. Use of in vivo desensitization to treat a patient's claustrophobia response to nasal CPAP. Sleep 1993; 16: 678–80.
21. Likar LL, Panciera TM, Erickson AD, Rounds S. Group education sessions and compliance with nasal CPAP therapy. Chest 1997; 111: 1273–7.
22. Morin CM, Colecchi C, Stone J, et al. Behavioral and pharmacological therapies for late-life insomnia. JAMA 1999; 281: 991–9.
23. Edinger JD, Means MK. Cognitive–behavioral therapy for primary insomnia. Clin Psychol Rev 2005; 25: 539–58.
24. Smith MT, Huang MI, Manber R. Cognitive behavior therapy for chronic insomnia occurring within the context of medical and psychiatric disorders. Clin Psychol Rev 2005; 25: 559–92.
25. Mignot E, Taheri S, Nishino S. Sleeping with the hypothalamus: emerging therapeutic targets for sleep disorders. Nat Neurosci 2002; 5: 1071–5.
26. Saper CB, Scammell TE, Lu J. Hypothalamic regulation of sleep and circadian rhythms. Nature 2005; 437: 1257–63.

27. Borbely AA. A two process model of sleep regulation. Hum Neurobiol 1982; 1: 195–204.

28. Youngstedt SD, O'Connor PJ, Dishman RK. The effects of acute exercise on sleep: a quantitative synthesis. Sleep 1997; 20: 203–14.

29. Wager-Smith K, Kay SA. Circadian rhythm generics: from flies to mice to humans. Nat Genet 2000; 26: 23–7.

30. Klei L, Reitz P, Miller M, et al. Heritability of morningness–eveningness and self-report sleep measures in a family-based sample of 521 Hutterites. Chronobiol Int 2005; 22: 1041–54.

31. Dijk DJ, Czeisler CA. Paradoxical timing of the circadian rhythm of sleep propensity serves to consolidate sleep and wakefulness in humans. Neurosci Lett 1994; 166: 63–8.

32. Wyatt JK, Ritz-De Cecco A, Czeisler CA, Dijk DJ. Circadian temperature and melatonin rhythms, sleep, and neurobehavioral function in humans living on a 20-h day. Am J Physiol 1999; 277: R1152–63.

33. Czeisler CA, Allan JS, Strogatz SH, et al. Bright light resets the human circadian pacemaker independent of the timing of the sleep–wake cycle. Science 1986; 233: 667–71.

34. Minors DS, Waterhouse JM, Wirz-Justice A. A human phase-response curve to light. Neurosci Lett 1991; 133: 354–61.

35. Bonnet MH, Arand DL. Hyperarousal and insomnia. Sleep Med Rev 1997; 2: 97–108.

36. Perlis ML, Giles DE, Mendelson WB, et al. Psychophysiological insomnia: the behavioral model and a neurocognitive perspective. J Sleep Res 1997; 6: 179–88.

37. Vgontzas AN, Tsigos C, Bixler EO, et al. Chronic insomnia and activity of the stress system: a preliminary study. J Psychosom Res 1998; 45: 21–31.

38. Bonnet MH, Arand DL. 24-hour metabolic rate in insomniacs and matched normal sleepers. Sleep 1995; 18: 581–8.

39. Freedman RR. EEG power spectra in sleep-onset insomnia. Electroencephalogn Clin Neurol 1986; 63: 408–13.

40. Merica H, Blois R, Gaillard J-M. Spectral characteristics of sleep EEG in chronic insomnia. Eur J Neurosci 1998; 10: 1826–34.

41. Perlis ML, Smith MT, Andrews PJ, et al. Beta/gamma EEG activity in patients with primary and secondary insomnia and good sleeper controls. Sleep 2001; 24: 110–17.

42. Jacobs GD, Benson H, Friedman R. Home-based central nervous system assessment of a multifactor behavioral intervention for chronic sleep-onset insomnia. Behav Ther 1993; 24: 159–74.

43. Bootzin RR. Stimulus control treatment for insomnia. Proc Am Psychol Assoc 1972; 7: 395–6.

44. Harvey AG, Tang NK, Browning L. Cognitive approaches to insomnia. Clin Psychol Rev 2005; 25: 593–611.

45. Morin CM, Stone J, Trinkle D, Mercer J, Remsberg S. Dysfunctional beliefs and attitudes about sleep among older adults with and without insomnia complaints. Psychol Aging 1993; 8: 463–7.

46. Fichten CS, Creti L, Amsel R, et al. Poor sleepers who do not complain of insomnia: myths and realities about psychological and lifestyle characteristics of older good and poor sleepers. J Behav Med 1995; 18: 189–223.

47. Edinger JD, Fins AI, Glenn DM, et al. Insomnia and the eye of the beholder: Are there clinical markers of objective sleep disturbances among adults with and without insomnia complaints? J Consult Clin Psychol 2000; 68: 586–93.

48. Harvey L, Inglis SJ, Espie CA. Insomniacs' reported use of CBT components and relationship to long-term clinical outcome. Behav Res Ther 2002; 40: 75–83.

49. Morin CM. Insomnia: Psychological Assessment and Management. New York: Guilford, 1993.

50. Lacks P, Morin CM. Recent advances in the assessment and treatment of insomnia. J Consult Clin Psychol 1992; 60: 586–94.

51. Morin CM, Hauri PJ, Espie CA, et al. Nonpharmacologic treatment of chronic insomnia. Sleep 1999; 22: 1–23.

52. Jacobs GD, Pace-Schott EF, Stickgold R, et al. Cognitive behavior therapy and pharmacotherapy for insomnia. Arch Intern Med 2004; 164: 1888–96.

53. Edinger JD, Sampson WS. A primary care 'friendly' cognitive behavioral insomnia therapy. Sleep 2003; 26: 177–82.

54. Hauri PJ. Sleep hygiene, relaxation therapy, and cognitive interventions. In: Hauri PJ, ed. Case Studies in Insomnia. New York: Plenum, 1991: 65–84.

55. Spielman AJ, Saskin P, Thorpy MJ. Treatment of chronic insomnia by restriction of time in bed. Sleep 1987; 10: 45–56.

56. Friedman L, Bliwise DL, Yesavage JA, et al. A preliminary study comparing sleep restriction and relaxation

treatments for insomnia in older adults. J Gerontol B Psychol Sci 1991; 46: 1–8.

57. Rubenstein ML, Rothenberg SA, Maheswaran S, et al. Modified sleep restriction therapy in middle-aged and elderly chronic insomniacs. Sleep Res 1990; 19: 276.

58. Lichstein KL, Riedel BW, Wilson NM, Lester KW, Aguillard RN. Relaxation and sleep compression for late-life insomnia: a placebo-controlled trial. J Consult Clin Psychol 2001; 69: 227–39.

59. Borkovec TD, Grayson JB, O'Brien GT, et al. Relaxation treatment of pseudoinsomnia and idiopathic insomnia: an electroencephalographic evaluation. J Appl Behav Anal 1979; 12: 37–54.

60. Nicassio P, Bootzin R. A comparison of progressive relaxation and autogenic training as treatment for insomnia. J Abnorm Psychol 1974; 83: 253–60.

61. Woolfolk RL, Carr-Kaffashan L, McNulty TF. Meditation training as a treatment for insomnia. Behav Ther 1976; 7: 359–65.

62. Haynes SN, Sides H, Lockwood G. Relaxation instructions and frontalis electromyographic feedback intervention with sleep-onset insomnia. Behav Ther 1977; 8: 644–52.

63. Hauri PJ. Treating psychophysiologic insomnia with biofeedback. Arch Gen Psychiatry 1981; 38: 752–8.

64. Weitzman ED, Czeisler CA, Coleman RM, et al. Delayed sleep phase syndrome: a chronobiological disorder with sleep-onset insomnia. Arch Gen Psychiatry 1981; 38: 737–46.

65. Thorpy MJ, Korman E, Spielman AJ, Glovinsky PB. Delayed sleep phase syndrome in adolescents. Health Care 1988; 9: 22–7.

66. Czeisler CA, Dumont M, Duffy JF, et al. Association of sleep–wake habits in older people with changes in output of circadian pacemaker. Lancet 1992; 340: 933–6.

67. Kramer CJ, Kerkhof GA, Hofman WF. Age differences in sleep–wake behavior under natural conditions. Pers Indiv Differ 1999; 27: 853–60.

68. Rosenthal NE, Joseph-Vanderpool JR, Levendosky AA, et al. Phase-shifting effects of bright morning light as treatment for delayed sleep phase syndrome. Sleep 1990; 13: 354–61.

69. Campbell SS, Murphy PJ, van den Heuvel CJ, Roberts ML, Stauble TN. Etiology and treatment of intrinsic circadian rhythm sleep disorders. Sleep Med Rev 1999; 3: 179–200.

70. Lack L, Wright H, Kemp K, Gibbon S. The treatment of early-morning awakening insomnia with 2 evenings of bright light. Sleep 2005; 28: 616–23.

71. Eastman CI, Boulos Z, Terman M, et al. Light treatment for sleep disorders: consensus report. VI. Shift work. J Biol Rhythms 1995; 10: 157–64.

72. Czeisler CA, Richardson GS, Coleman RM, et al. Chronotherapy: resetting the circadian clocks of patients with delayed sleep phase insomnia. Sleep 1981; 4: 1–21.

73. Dagan Y, Yovel I, Hallis D, Eisenstein M, Raichik I. Evaluating the role of melatonin in the long-term treatment of delayed sleep phase syndrome (DSPS). Chronobiol Int 1998; 15: 181–90.

74. Hoy CJ, Vennelle M, Kingshott RN, Engleman HM, Douglas NJ. Can intensive support improve continouous positive airway pressure use in patients with the sleep apnea/hypopnea syndrome? Am J Resp Crit Care 1999; 159: 1096–100.

75. Chervin RD, Theut S, Bassetti C, Aldrich MS. Compliance with nasal CPAP can be improved by simple interventions. Sleep 1997; 20: 284–9.

76. Hui DS, Chan JK, Choy DK, et al. Effects of augmented continuous positive airway pressure education and support on compliance and outcome in a Chinese population. Chest 2000; 117: 1410–16.

77. Fletcher EC, Luckett RA. The effect of positive reinforcement on hourly compliance in nasal continuous positive airway pressure users with obstructive sleep apnea. Am Rev Respir Dis 1991; 143: 936–41.

78. Krakow B, Johnston L, Melendrez D, et al. An open-label trial of evidence-based cognitive behavior therapy for nightmares and insomnia in crime victims with PTSD. Am J Psychiatry 2001; 158: 2043–7.

79. Sleep in America 1991. Princeton, NJ: Gallup Organization, 1991.

80. Sleep in America 1995. Princeton, NJ: Gallup Organization, 1995.

9

Medication effects on sleep

JF Pagel

INTRODUCTION

Sleep is a global state that can be defined both behaviorally and cognitively. The sleep state and its spectrum of electrophysiologic correlates are affected by almost all medications with behavioral or cognitive effects and/or side-effects. Historically, the effects that medications exert on sleep and alertness have been considered global and non-specific. In the last 20 years, however, the selective neurotransmitter effects of most sedative/hypnotic drugs have been defined. The field of sleep disorder medicine has matured into an increasingly complex field involved in the diagnosis and treatment of more than 90 conditions; each of these has clear diagnostic criteria, and many of them are treated with specific pharmacologic therapies. An even larger group of medical and psychiatric diseases produce mental or physical discomfort that can adversely affect sleep.

Sleep disorders can generally be divided into three large groups: (1) those producing insomnia (the complaint of difficulty falling asleep or staying asleep or of non-restorative sleep); (2) those with a primary complaint of daytime sleepiness; and (3) those associated with disruptive behaviors during sleep – the disorders of arousal.[1,2] There is a full range of medications used to treat these disorders, each with particular benefits as well as potential

for harm. Medications used to treat sleep disorders have a checkered history that includes limited efficacy, serious side-effects, addiction, and lethal toxicity in overdose. One of the significant advances in the development of sleep medicine as a medical specialty has been the development and use of efficacious medications to treat these disorders; medications with minimal side-effects, low addiction potential, and limited toxicity in overdose.

MEDICATIONS INDUCING DISORDERED SLEEP

Drug-induced sleepiness is perhaps the most commonly reported side-effect of pharmacologic agents active on the central nervous system (CNS): the 1990 Drug Interactions and Side Effect Index of the Physicians' Desk Reference lists drowsiness as a side-effect of 584 prescription or over-the-counter (OTC) preparations.[3] Unfortunately the terminology describing daytime sleepiness, generally considered to be 'the subjective state of sleep need', is poorly defined, interchangeably including such contextual terminology as sleepiness, drowsiness, languor, inertness, fatigue, and sluggishness. The results of questionnaires and cognitive and performance tests for daytime sleepiness correlate only loosely with the actual effects of sleepiness on

This chapter is an updated, rewritten version of a paper entitled Medications and their effects on sleep. Primary Care: Clin Office Pract 2005; 32: 491–509.

complex performance tasks such as the operation of a motor vehicle.[4]

Most medications affecting CNS functioning can induce insomnia in some patients. The neuronal systems modulating waking and sleep are contained within the isodendritic core of the brain, extending from the medulla though the brainstem and hypothalamus up to the basal forebrain. Multiple factors and systems are involved, with no single chemical neurotransmitter identified as necessary or sufficient for modulating sleep and wakefulness. Medications affecting neurotransmitters such as norepinephrine (noradrenaline), serotonin, acetylcholine, and dopamine often induce insomnia and/or sleepiness. Less commonly, agents such as antibiotics, antihypertensives, oral contraceptives, and thyroid replacements can induce insomnia in susceptible individuals (Table 9.1).[5] OTC medications may induce insomnia, including decongestants (including nose sprays), weight loss agents, ginseng preparations and high-dose vitamin B_1 (niacin). Finally, chronic and long-term sedative/hypnotic use to induce sleep may cause tolerance to the sedative effect, and can contribute to chronic insomnia.[1,6]

Diagnoses that lead to alternations in sleep and alertness are quite common. Obstructive sleep apnea (OSA), with its well described effect of daytime somnolence, affects 5–10% of the population. Some of these patients with OSA also have chronic insomnia, yet treatment of these patients with sedative/hypnotic medications can cause respiratory depression, increased apnea, and worsened sleep. Patients with narcolepsy often report improved sleep with daytime amfetamine use. Periodic limb movement disorder may respond positively to benzodiazepine treatment yet increase in intensity with the use of some antidepressants. Increased daytime alertness typifies a spectrum of common diagnoses including chronic insomnia, anxiety disorder, and post-traumatic stress disorder (PTSD). Such patients may demonstrate altered responses to medications inducing alertness and/or sleepiness, with unexpected results. Stimulants may induce sleepiness in some patients, while hypnotics may induce agitation and insomnia even when used in anesthetic settings and dosages.[7]

Table 9.1   Medication types known to cause insomnia

Adrenocorticotropin (ACTH) and cortisone

Antibiotics (quinolones)

Anticonvulsants

Antihypertensives (α-agonists, β-blockers, central-acting agents)

Antidepressants (SSRIs)

Antineoplastic agents

Appetite suppressants

β-Agonists

Caffeine

Decongestants

Diuretics

Dopamine agonists

Ephedrine and pseudoephedrine

Ethanol

Ginseng

Lipid- and cholesterol-lowering agents

Niacin

Oral contraceptives

Psychostimulants and amfetamines

Sedative/hypnotics

Theophylline

Thyroid preparations

MEDICATIONS FOR THE TREATMENT OF INSOMNIA

Sedative/hypnotics

Insomnia is an extremely common complaint. Transient insomnia (<2 weeks in duration) affects up to 80% of the population on a yearly basis.[8] Chronic insomnia affects 15% of the population.[1] In the 1990s in the USA, 2.6% of adults were using prescription sedative/hypnotic medications and 3.1% OTC sleep medications (primarily antihistamines).[9]

Historically, sedative/hypnotics have been some of the most commonly prescribed drugs. Many sedatives were initially utilized as anesthetics.

Chloral hydrate was the original 'Mickey Finn' slipped into the drinks of unsuspecting marks for the purposes of criminal activity. Unfortunately, the LD50 (potentially fatal dose) for chloral hydrate is quite close to the therapeutic dose, and murders rather than robberies were often the result. In the years leading up to the 1960s, barbiturates were commonly utilized for their sedative effects. Unfortunately, these medications can be drugs of abuse and have a significant danger of overdose. Marilyn Monroe, Elvis Presley, and Jimi Hendrix, among others, were celebrities who died during this era from overdoses that included sleeping pills. Barbiturates and barbiturate-like medications (methaqualone (Quaalude, Sopor) glutethimide (Doriden), ethchlorvynol (Placidyl), and methyprylon (Nodudar)) are still available, but are rarely used because of their limited efficacy, cognitive effects, potential for abuse, and lethal toxicity associated with overdose.[5,10]

In the 1970s, benzodiazepines became available for the treatment of insomnia. These drugs act at γ-aminobutyric acid (GABA) neuroreceptors, and have far less overdose danger and abuse potential than the barbiturate-like medications. The many drugs in this class are best viewed therapeutically based on their pharmacodynamics (Table 9.2). Rapid onset of action is characteristic of flurazepam (Dalmane) and triazolam (Halcion), indicating that both of these agents have excellent sleep-inducing effects. Flurazepam, like diazepam (Valium) and clorazepate (Tranzene), has the characteristic of having active breakdown products. This results in an extraordinarily long active half-life, which can approach 11 days. This prolonged effect in the elderly has been associated with increased automobile accidents and falls with hip fractures.[11,12] Withdrawal from these long-acting agents can be difficult, with an initial syndrome of insomnia followed by persistent anxiety that may extend beyond the half-life of the agent.

Benzodiazepines are rapid eye movement (REM) sleep-suppressant medications, and withdrawal often results in episodes of increased REM sleep (REM sleep rebound). REM sleep is known to have a role in learning and memory consolidation. For short-acting agents such as triazolem, this rebound occurs during the same night in which the medication was taken, and has been associated with daytime memory impairment, particularly at higher dosages.[13,14] Temazepam (Restoril) and estazolam (Prosom) have half-lives compatible with an 8-hour night of sleep. Temazepam, because of its slower onset of action, is less efficacious as a sleep-inducing agent than other drugs used as hypnotics in this class. All benzodiazepines can result in respiratory depression in patients with pulmonary disease and tend to lose sleep-inducing efficacy with prolonged use.[14,15]

Insomnia is commonly a symptom of nocturnal discomfort, whether psychologic, physical, or environmental. Medications, in general, can be safely utilized on a short-term basis for the treatment of transient insomnia. Chronic hypnotic medication use has been associated with the development of mood disorders (depression) and hypnotic-dependent disorders of sleep.[16] Therefore, the underlying reasons and diseases resulting in chronic insomnia should be addressed.

The newer hypnotics zolpidem (Ambien), zaleplon (Sonata), eszopiclone (Lunesta), and indiplon are benzodiazepine-like agents exerting effects at the same GABA receptors. Benzodiazepine withdrawal is not blocked by these agents. These agents have excellent efficacy, with minimal side-effects. Although any agent used to induce sleep can result in a dependence on that agent to induce sleep, the abuse potential of these agents is minimal. Idiosyncratic reactions of persistent daytime somnolence and/or memory loss have been reported in some patients. Tachyphylaxis is unusual, and these agents can be used on a long-term basis. Sleep is altered minimally, and REM sleep rebound is not associated with these agents (Table 9.2).[10,13] Zolpidem and eszopiclone have half-lives of 6–8 hours, while zaleplon is a shorter-acting (3–4 hours). Clinical comparison of these agents suggests that zolpidem and eszopiclone may have greater sleep-inducing efficacy and zaleplon fewer side-effects.

Table 9.2 Sedative/hypnotics

Class	Drug[a]	Sleep-stage effects[b]	Significant side-effects	Indication
Benzodiazepines		• Decreased amplitude in stages 3 and 4 • Increased stage 2	• Loss of effect with chronic use • Dependence	
Short onset, short half-life (<4 h)	Triazolem [Halcion]	• Shortened sleep latency • In-night REMS rebound	• Antegrade amnesia	• Transient insomnia
Short onset, medium half-life (8.5 h)	Estazolam [Prosom]	• Shortened sleep latency • Decreased REMS	• Daytime sleepiness	• Transient insomnia
Short onset, long half-life (50–110 h)	Flurazepam [Dalmane]	• Shortened sleep latency • Decreased REMS • Withdrawal REMS rebound	• Daytime sleepiness • Chronic build-up (car accidents, hip fractures)	• Transient insomnia • Anxiety
Medium onset, medium half-life (7–10 h)	Temazepam [Restoril] Clonazepam [Klonopin]	• Decreased REMS	• Daytime sleepiness • Poor sleep induction	• Transient insomnia • Anxiety (For others, see text)
GABA receptor agents				
Short onset, medium half-life	Zolpidem [Ambien]	• Shortened sleep latency	• Idiosyncratic	• Transient insomnia
Short onset, short half-life	Zaleplon [Sonata]	• Benzodiazepine-like effects with dose above that normally perscribed	• Daytime sleepiness or antegrade amnesia	• Chronic insomnia
Other agents				
Chloral hydrate	Chloral hydrate	• Short sleep latency • Decreased REMS • Withdrawal REMS rebound	• Low lethal dose • Loss of effect with chronic use	• Transient insomnia in controlled settings
Barbiturates and barbiturate-like agents	Phenobarbital etc., methaqualone, glutethimide, ethchlorvynol, methyprylon	• REMS supression • Short sleep latency • Decreased REMS • Withdrawal REMS rebound	• Addiction • Low lethal dose • Loss of effect with chronic use	• No sleep indication
Sedating antihistamines (H_1-blockers)	Diphenhydramine	• Decreased sleep latency in some patients	• Daytime sedation • Anticholinergic	• OTC insomnia
Melatonin receptor agonists	Ramelteon [Rozarem]	• Shortened sleep latency	• Neurohormonal interactions	• Sleep-onset insomnia

[a]Trade names in square brackets.
[b]REMS, rapid eye movement sleep.

Melatonin agonists

Melatonin is a neural hormone effective in resetting circadian rhythms of sleep and body core temperature through its actions on the suprachiasmatic nucleus. For individuals with insomnia secondary to disruptions in circadian rhythms, melatonin can act as a hypnotic and is a useful adjunct to treatment that often includes cognitive therapies, light exposure and other hypnotics. Ramelteon (Rozarem) is a melatonin receptor agonist indicated for the treatment of transient and chronic sleep-onset insomnia. The side-effect profiles of melatonin agonists are neurohormonal. These differ significantly from the side-effects associated with hypnotics affecting GABA.

Hypnotics – overview

In the last 30 years, although the drugs for treatment of insomnia have become safer, the number of sedative/hypnotics prescribed in the USA has declined. This decrease most likely reflects the public's and the medical community's concern about the side-effects, limitations, and cost of the available hypnotic drugs. Most hypnotic medications, in general, can be safely utilized on a short-term basis for the treatment of transient insomnia. For persistent chronic insomnia due to anxiety disorders, idiopathic insomnia (persistent lifelong insomnia without other sleep-associated diagnoses), postmenopausal insomnia, agitated depression, and other less common diagnoses associated with persistent insomnia, chronic hypnotic use with the newer non-benzodiazepine hypnotics can be justified and is indicated if medication use leads to improvement in waking performance.[13,17] Eszopiclone has been approved by the Food and Drug Administration (FDA) for extended use in patients with chronic insomnia.[18] For zolpidem in a sustained-release preparation (Ambien-CR) and ramelteon, long-term use is no longer contraindicated. These newer hypnotic agents are less likely to have deleterious side-effects than most OTC treatments for insomnia.[19,20]

Non-prescription sedating agents

Ethanol is probably the most widely used hypnotic medication. In patients with chronic insomnia, 22% of patients report using ethanol as a hypnotic.[17,21] Unfortunately, chronic use to induce sleep can result in tolerance, dependence, and diminished sleep efficiency and quality. When used in excess with other sedative/hypnotic agents, overdose can be fatal. Among drugs of abuse, marijuana has significant hypnotic effects. The central sedative effects of barbiturates, barbiturate-like agents, benzodiazepines, and opioids can induce fatal respiratory suppression at higher doses, particularly when abuse is coupled with ethanol.

OTC sleeping pills contain sedating antihistamines, usually diphenhydramine. These agents are varyingly effective, but may result in daytime sleepiness, cognitive impairment, and anticholinergic effects that persist into the day after use, affecting driving performance.[20,22] These agents are not recommended for use in the elderly.[23] Seizure thresholds can be lowered by their use in epileptic patients. Both ethanol and sedating antihistamines are associated with decreased performance on daytime driving tests and an increase in automobile accidents. Sedation is infrequent with H_2 antagonists (e.g., cimetidine, ranitidine, famotidine, and nizatidine), but somnolence as a side-effect is evidently reproducible in susceptible individuals. The side-effect profiles of the newer sedative/hypnotics are generally more benign that those of the sedating antihistamines.[22,24]

In addition to OTC melatonin supplements and the sedating antihistamines, a variety of non-prescription and herbal agents are marketed as hypnotics. Tryptophan has a history of known efficacy in the treatment of chronic insomnia. In the late 1980s, use of this agent was associated with severe eosinophilia that was lethally toxic in some cases. This agent was removed from the market, despite speculation that the toxicity was not secondary to the drug itself, but to deficiencies in the preparation process. Kava, considered a drug of abuse in some cultures, has been used for insomnia, but has shown potential for hepatic toxicity in some patients. The best data supporting the sedative effect of a herbal agent are for valerian.[25] Evidence supporting the hypnotic efficacy of other herbal agents, including chamomile, passionflower, and skullcap, is limited.

Antidepressants

Sedating antidepressants are often used to treat insomnia. A significant percentage of individuals with chronic insomnia and/or daytime sleepiness also have depressive symptoms. Chronic insomnia itself can predispose patients to develop depression.[26] Depression associated with insomnia is likely a different diagnostic entity than depression without insomnia, and treatment of the former with non-sedating antidepressants may produce no improvement in sleep even when the underlying depression resolves.[26] Use of antidepressants is limited by side-effects (anticholinergic effects, daytime hangover, etc.) and danger with overdose (particularly the tricyclic antidepressants (TCAs)).[4,27,28] Sedating antidepressants include the TCAs (amitryptyline, imipramine, nortryptyline, etc.), Trazadone (Deseryl), and the newer agents mirtazapine (Remeron) and nefazodone (Serzone) (Table 9.3). The selective serotonin reuptake inhibitors (SSRIs) have a tendency to induce insomnia; however, in some patients, paroxetine (Paxil) may induce mild sedation. Depression-related insomnia responds to sedating antidepressants more rapidly and with lower doses compared with other symptoms of depression.[29] In patients with insomnia and concomitant depression, antidepressants are often used in combination with the newer sedative/hypnotic medications.[30] Use of sedating antidepressants has been associated with declines in daytime performance and driving test performance, and an increased potential for involvement in motor vehicular accidents.[31]

DAYTIME SLEEPINESS

Excessive daytime sleepiness (EDS) is present in 5–15% of the population.[1,8,21] Many patients with EDS, particularly those who also complain of snoring, will require overnight sleep evaluation (polysomnography) because of the potential diagnosis of OSA. OSA is usually treated with continuous positive airway pressure (CPAP: a system that utilizes positive nasal pressure to maintain airway patency during sleep). Other treatment approaches for OSA include ear, nose, and throat surgery and dental mouthpieces. Symptoms of a mood disorder (depression), which is also a common cause of daytime sleepiness, can be difficult to distinguish from the symptoms of OSA.[21] Chronic sleep deprivation as a basis for daytime sleepiness is particularly common in the adolescent and young adult population, and in individuals involved in occupations requiring nocturnal shiftwork.[8] Less common causes of EDS are neurologic diseases inducing sleepiness: narcolepsy and idiopathic hypersomnolence. Daytime sleepiness is probably the most common side-effect of CNS active medications (Table 9.4). A major concern in such sleepy patients is the potential danger to self and others while working and/or driving motor vehicles.[31,32]

ALERTING MEDICATIONS

Medications that are used in somnolent patients to induce alertness include the amfetamines (dextroamfetamine (Dexedrine) and methylphenidate (Ritalin)) and pemoline (Cylert). The tendency of pemoline to cause acute hepatic failure has limited its usefulness. The amfetamines are considered to have high abuse potential and are Schedule II prescription drugs. Side-effects of these drugs include personality changes, tremor, hypertension (dextroamfetamine and methylphenidate), headaches, and gastrointestinal reflux.[9,32,33]

The newer alerting agent modafinil (Provigil) is pharmacologically distinct from the amfetamines and has much lower potential for abuse (Schedule IV). Modafinil is indicated for the treatment of narcolepsy, as well as the persistent sleepiness associated with obstructive sleep apnea in patients already being treated with CPAP. Modafinil is also indicated for the treatment of fatigue and daytime sleepiness in patients with shiftwork disorder.[34]

Table 9.3 Antidepressants: sedating agents in bold; insomnia-inducing agents in italics

Class[a]	Drug	Sleep-stage effects[b]	Indications
Tricyclic	**Trimipramine** **Nortriptyline** **Doxepin** **Amoxapine** **Amitryptyline** **Imipramine** **Amoxapine** **Protriptyline**[c] **Desipramine**	• Increased REMS latency • Decreased REMS (++), SWS latency, deep sleep, sleep latency	• Depression with insomnia • REMS and SWS suppression • Chronic pain • Fibromyalgia • Enuresis
Non-tricyclic sedating	**Maprotiline** **Mirtazapine**	• Increased REMS latency • Decreased SWS latency, REMS (++), sleep latency	• Depression • Depression with insomnia • REMS suppression
MAOI	**Phenelzine** **Tranylcypromine**	• Increased stage 4 • Decreased REMS latency, REMS (+++)	• Depression • REMS suppression
SSRIs	*Fluoxetine*[c] Paroxetine *Sertraline* Fluvoxamine Citalopram	• Increased REMS latency, sleep latency, stage 1 • Decreased REMS	• Depression • PTSD • OCD • Phobias • Cataplexy • Others
SNRI + NARI	Venlafaxine	• Increased REMS latency • Decreased sleep latency, REMS	• Depression
	Duloxetine	• Increased REMS, sleep latency	• Depression
DA/NERI	Bupropion	• Increased REMS latency, sleep latency	• Depression • Nicotine withdrawal
5-HT$_{1A}$ agonist	Buspirone	• Increased REMS latency • Decreased REMS	• Anxiety
Other	**Nefazodone**	• Increased REMS • Decreased sleep latency	• Depression • Depression with insomnia and anxiety

[a]MAOI, monoamine oxidase inhibitor; SSRI, selective serotonin reuptake inhibitor; SNRI, serotonin and norepinephrine reuptake inhibitor; DA/NERI, dopamine and norepinephrine reuptake inhibitor; 5-HT$_{1A}$, serotonin receptor type 1A.

[b]REMS, rapid eye movement sleep; SWS, slow-wave sleep; (+ ...) indicates higher levels of effect.

[c]Documented as a respiratory stimulant.

MEDICATION-INDUCED ALTERATIONS IN SLEEP STAGES AND SLEEP EEG

Polysomnographic recordings using electro-oculography (EOG), electromyography (EMG), and electroencephalography (EEG) can be used to divide sleep into stages. In some ways, sleep staging is an artificial construct designed for analysis of sleep based on the monitoring techniques that are currently available. However, research has revealed

Table 9.4   Medications reported in clinical trials and case reports to have sleepiness as a side-effect

Medication class[a]	Neurochemical basis for sleepiness[b]	Specific medications[c]
Antihistamines	Histamine receptor blockade	Azatadine [Optamine] Chlorpheniramine [Chlor-Trimeton] Dexbrompheniramine [Polaramine] Clemastine [Tavist] Cyproheptadine [Periactin] Diphenhydramine [Benadryl] Doxylamine [Unisom] Promethazine [Phenergan] Triprolidine [Actifed]
Antiparkinsonian agents	Dopamine receptor agonism	Benztropine [Cogentin] Biperiden [Akineton] Procyclidine [Kemadrin] Trihexiphendyl [Artane]
Antimuscarinic/antispasmotic	Varied effects	Atropine Belladona Dicyclomine [Bentyl] Glycopyrrolate [Robinul] Hyoscyamine Ipratropium bromide [Atrovent] Mepenzolate bromide [Cantil] Methscopolamine bromide [Pamine] Scopolamine
Skeletal muscle relaxants	Varied effects	Baclofen [Lioresal] Carisoprodol [Soma] Chlorzoxazone [Parafon forte] Cyclobenzaprine [Flexeril] Dantrolene [Dantrium] Metaxalone [Skelaxin] Methocarbamol [Robaxin] Orphenadrine [Norflex]
α-Adrenergic blocking agents	α_1-Adrenergic antagonism	Doxazosin [Cardura] Prazosin [Minipress] Terazosin [Hytrin]
β-Adrenergic blocking agents	β-Adrenergic antagonism	Acebutolol [Sectral] Atenolol [Tenormin] Betaxolol [Kerlone]

Continued...

Table 9.4 Continued...		
Medication class[a]	*Neurochemical basis for sleepiness*[b]	*Specific medications*[c]
		Bisoprolol [Zobeta]
		Carvedilol [Coreg]
		Esmolol [Brevibloc]
		Labetalol [Normodyne]
		Metoprolol [Lopressor]
		Nadolol [Corgard]
		Pindolol [Visken]
		Propranolol [Inderal]
		Sotalol [Betapace]
		Timolol [Blocadren]
Opiate agonists	Opioid receptor agonism (general CNS depression)	Codeine
		Fentanyl [Sublimaze]
		Hydrocodone
		Hydromorphone [Dilaudid]
		Levomethadyl [Orlamm]
		Levorphanol [Levo-Dromoran]
		Meperidine (pethidine) [Demerol]
		Methadone
		Morphine
		Opium
		Oxycodone
		Oxymorphone [Numorphan]
		Propoxyphene [Darvon]
		Sufentanil [Sufenta]
		Tramadol [Ultram]
Opiate partial agonists	Opioid receptor agonism (general CNS depression)	Buprenorphine [Buprenex]
		Butorphanol [Stadol]
		Nalbuphine [Stadol]
		Pentazocine [Talwin]
Anticonvulsants		
Barbiturates	GABA receptor agonism	Mephobarbital [Mebaral]
		Phenobarbital [Luminal]
		Primidone [Mysoline]
Benzodiazepines	GABA receptor agonism	Elonazepam [Klonopin]
Hydantoins	General effects?	Ethotoin [Peganone]
		Phenytoin [Dilantin]
		Fosphenytoin [Cerebyx]

Continued...

Table 9.4   Continued...

Medication class[a]	Neurochemical basis for sleepiness[b]	Specific medications[c]
Succinimides	General effects?	Ethosuximide [Zarontin] Methsuximide [Celontin]
Others	Varied effects, including GABA potentiation	Carbamazepine [Tegretol] Felbamate [Felbatol] Gabapentin [Neurontin] Lamotrigine [Lamictal] Levetiracetam [Keppra] Oxcarbazepine [Trileptal] Tigabine [Gabitril] Topiramate [Topamax] Valproic acid [Depakene] Zonisamide [Zonegran]
Antidepressants		
MAOIs	Norepinephrine, serotonin, and dopamine effects	Phenelzine [Nardil] Tranylcypromine [Parnate]
Tricyclics	Acetylcholine blockade; norepinephrine and serotonin uptake inhibition	Amitriptyline [Elavil] Clomipramine [Anafranil] Desipramine [Norpramin] Doxepin [Sinequan] Imipramine [Tofranil] Maprotiline [Ludiomil] Nortriptyline [Pamelor] Protriptyline [Vivactil] Trimipramine [Surmontil]
SSRIs	Serotonin uptake inhibition	Citalopram [Celexa] Escitalopram [Lexapro] Fluoxetine [Prozac] Fluvoxamine [Luvox] Paroxetine [Paxil] Sertraline [Zoloft]
Others	Serotonin, dopamine, and norepinephrine effects	Bupropion [Wellbutrin] Mirtazapine [Remeron] Nefazodone [Serazone] Trazadone [Deseryl] Venlafaxine [Effexor]
Antipsychotics	Dopamine receptor blockade; varied effects on histaminic, cholinergic and α-adrenergic receptors	Fluphenazine [Prolixin] Mesoridazine [Serentil] Perphenazine [Trilafon]

Continued...

Table 9.4 Continued...		
Medication class[a]	*Neurochemical basis for sleepiness*[b]	*Specific medications*[c]
		Prochlorperazine [Compazine]
		Thioridazine [Mellaril]
		Trifluperazine [Stelazine]
		Aripiprazole [Abilify]
		Clozapine [Clozaril]
		Haloperidol [Haldol]
		Loxapine [Loxitane]
		Molidone [Moban]
		Olanzapine [Zyprexa]
		Pimozide [Orap]
		Quetiapine [Seroquel]
		Risperidone [Risperdal]
		Thiothixene [Navane]
		Ziprasidone [Geodone]
Barbiturates	GABA receptor agonism	Amobarbital [Amytal]
		Butabarbital [Butisol]
		Mephobarbital [Mebaral]
		Pentobarbital [Nembutal]
		Phenobarbital [Luminal]
		Secobarbital [Seconal]
		Secobarbital/amobarbital [Tuinal]
Benzodiazepines	GABA receptor agonism	Alprazolam [Xanax]
		Chlordiazepoxide [Librium]
		Clorazepate [Tranxene]
		Diazepam [Valium]
		Estazolam [Prosom]
		Flurazepam [Dalmane]
		Lorazepam [Ativan]
		Midazolam [Versed]
		Oxazepam [Serax]
		Quazepam [Doral]
		Temazepam [Restoril]
		Triazolam [Halcion]
Anxiolytics; miscellaneous sedatives and hypnotics	GABA receptor agonism; varied effects	Buspirone [Buspar]
		Chloral hydrate
		Dexmedetomidine [Precedex]
		Droperidol [Inapsine]
		Hydroxyzine [Vistaril, Atarax]

Continued...

Table 9.4 Continued...		
Medication class[a]	Neurochemical basis for sleepiness[b]	Specific medications[c]
		Meprobamate [Equanil, Miltown] Promethazine [Phenergan] Zalepolon [Sonata] Zolpidem [Ambien] Eszopiclone [Estorra]
Antitussives	General?	Benzonatate [Tessalon] Dextromethorphan [Robitussin]
Antidiarrhea agents	Opioid, general?	Diphenoxylate [Lomotil] Loperamide [Imodium]
Antiemetics	Antihistamine and varied effects	Dimenhydrinate [Dramamine] Diphenidol [Vontrol] Meclizine [Antivert] Prochlorperazine [Compazine] Triethylperazine [Torecan] Trimethobenzamide [Tigan] Metoclopramide [Reglan]
Genitourinary smooth muscle relaxants	General?	Flavoxate [Urispas] Oxybutynin [Ditropan] Tolterodine [Detrol]

[a]MAOI, monoamine oxidase inhibitor; SSRI, selective serotonin reuptake inhibitor.

[b]CNS, central nervous system; GABA, γ-aminobutyric acid.

[c]Tradenames in square brackets.

that these sleep stages have physiologic and behavioral correlates that are clinically important.[8,27] Sleep-state alteration is frequently seen with the use of psychoactive medication. CNS-active medications often alter the occurrence, latency, and EEG characteristics of specific sleep/dream states, either with therapeutic intent or as side-effects. Even some non-pharmacologic therapies, such as oxygen, CPAP, and electroconvulsive therapy (ECT), can alter REM and deep sleep.[35] Medications that produce psychoactive effects alter the EEG. Typically, psychoactive medications alter background EEG frequencies and the occurrence, frequency, and latency of the various sleep stages (Tables 9.2 and 9.3).[36–38]

In general, drug-induced EEG changes are associated with characteristic behavioral effects. This relationship has been utilized to suggest therapeutic possibilities for medications producing characteristic EEG effects.[36,38]

SLEEP-STATE-SPECIFIC DIAGNOSES AND SYMPTOMS

Parasomnias are sleep disorders occurring during arousal, partial arousal, or sleep-state transition.[39] The arousal disorders are associated with arousals from deep sleep, usually during the first deep sleep episode of the night (typically 1–3 AM). Arousal disorders include sleep terrors, somnambulism (sleepwalking), and confusional arousals. REM sleep parasomnias include sleep paralysis, nightmare disorder, and REM behavior disorder. REM sleep alters many physiologic processes, and therefore it is not surprising that a variety of physical illnesses become symptomatic during REM sleep. Respiratory muscle atonia associated with REM sleep can result in increased sleep apnea, particularly in patients with chronic obstructive pulmonary disease (COPD). Reduced esophageal pressure, also characteristic of REM sleep, can result in symptomatic gastrointestinal reflux. Chronic diseases manifesting symptoms during REM sleep include angina, migraine, and cluster headache.[1] Nocturnal seizures, asthma, and panic attacks are more likely to occur in the non-REM (NREM) stages of sleep. The sleep manifestations of PTSD include stereotypic frightening dreams that occur either at sleep onset or during REM sleep. Such disordered dreaming can result in both sleep-onset and sleep-maintenance insomnia.[40]

MEDICATION EFFECTS ON SLEEP STAGES AND EEG

Medication-induced changes in sleep stages can lead to an increase in symptoms occurring during those specific sleep/dream states. For example, insomnia and nightmares are associated with the REM sleep rebound that occurs after discontinuation of REM-suppressive drugs (i.e., ethanol, barbiturates, and benzodiazepines). Medications such as lithium, opiates, and γ-hydroxybutyrate (GHB: sodium oxybate) that can cause an increase in deep sleep can induce arousal disorders such as somnambulism.[5,41]

The influence of psychoactive medications on sleep states has a positive side as well. For example, REM sleep-suppressive medications can be useful adjuncts in the treatment of REM sleep parasomnias and sleep-stage-specific symptoms. Both benzodiazepines and antidepressants can be used to decrease REM sleep. Similarly, the arousal disorders can be treated with medications affecting deep sleep (benzodiazepines and others) (Tables 9.2 and 9.3).[36,39,41] Clonazepam (Klonopin) is the medication most commonly utilized in the treatment of parasomnias, particularly in REM behavior disorder.

SLEEP-DIAGNOSIS-SPECIFIC MEDICATION EFFECTS

Respiratory effects

Most sedative medications depress respiratory drive with increasing dosage. Benzodiazepines, barbiturates, and opiates can exacerbate respiratory failure in patients with COPD, central sleep apnea, or restrictive lung disease. These medications can also negatively affect OSA, and may increase the potential for symptomatic sleep apnea in some population groups, such as patients being treated for chronic pain. The newer non-benzodiazepine hypnotics have demonstrated lower potential for respiratory depression. Methylprogesterone (Provera), protriptyline (Vivactyl), and fluoxetine (Prozac) have been documented to have respiratory stimulant effects that may be clinically useful in some patients.[15]

Enuresis

Enuresis, defined as persistent bedwetting more than twice a month past the age of 5 years, is present in 15% of 5-year-olds. Medication has been shown to be symptomatically useful. TCAs have been used for decades in this disorder, but there has been concern about cardiac effects and long-term safety in children. The current treatment of choice is desmopressin (DDAVP), which corrects the lack of cyclic antidiuretic hormone increase during sleep, typically seen in these patients. Symptoms can be controlled until neurophysiologic maturity occurs, with a resolution of nocturnal enuresis.[42]

Restless leg syndrome and periodic limb movement disorder

Symptoms of restless leg syndrome (RLS) include uncomfortable limb sensations at sleep onset, and motor restlessness relieved by exercise and exacerbated by relaxation. Periodic limb movement disorder (PLMD) is characterized by repetitive, stereotypic, limb movements occurring in 15–40 cycles in NREM sleep and often leading to recurrent arousals from sleep.[43] These associated disorders are quite common, occurring in up to 15% of the population, and increasing in frequency with age.[44] PLMD/RLS may develop during pregnancy and in patients with OSA, renal failure, or low serum ferritin levels, as well as in patients taking antidepressants (particularly SSRIs).[45]

Historically, both PLMD and RLS have been treated with benzodiazepines, particularly clonazepam (Klonopin).[39,46] Low dosages of dopamine precursors and dopamine receptor agonists at bedtime have been demonstrated to be efficacious in these disorders. Possible side-effects of these medications, which include carbidopa/levodopa (Sinemet), pergolide (Permax), pramipexole (Mirapex), ropinirole (Reguip), and selegiline (Eldepryl), are nausea, headache, tachyphylaxis, and augmentation of symptoms. The tendency of carbidopa/levodopa to induce tachyphylaxis and augmentation of symptoms of RLS/PLMD has limited its usefulness.[46,47] Requip has recently received FDA approval for treatment of restless leg syndrome.[48]

CIRCADIAN RHYTHM DISTURBANCE

A number of sleep disorders are linked to abnormally timed sleep–wake cycles. These include delayed and advanced sleep-phase syndromes (in which the sleep period is markedly later or earlier than what is socially accepted), jet lag, shiftwork, and certain sleep abnormalities associated with aging. Melatonin is the photoneuroendocrine transducer that conveys information controlling sleep–wake cycles and

circadian rhythms in the CNS. Low doses may be useful in treating these disorders.[49] Because it is marketed as a dietary supplement, there are minimal data on safety, side-effects, and drug interactions for this compound.[50] Ramelteon, a highly selective melatonin receptor agonist available by prescription has been shown to be useful in the treatment of circadian and chronic insomnia.[51] Jet lag and shiftwork disorders can also be effectively treated with bright-light therapy and the repetitive short-term use of sedative/hypnotics.[52]

CATAPLEXY

The primary symptoms of narcolepsy are daytime sleepiness and sleep attacks. A significant number of narcolepsy patients, however, also have hypnagogic hallucinations, sleep paralysis, and cataplexy – skeletal motor weakness associated with emotion when awake. For a subgroup of narcolepsy patients, cataplexy can be incapacitating. GHB (as sodium oxybate) has shown excellent efficacy in the treatment of cataplexy. Sodium oxybate, available in liquid form, is given as two doses in the first 2 hours of the night. This agent has a history of recreational misuse and has limited pharmacologic distribution; it is available as a class 3 agent for narcolepsy patients.[53]

CONCLUSIONS

Many medications disturb sleep or exacerbate the effect of chronic illnesses on sleep. Conversely, medications may be used therapeutically for specific sleep disorders. The effects of most sedative/hypnotic drugs on sedation and arousal is secondary to selective neurotransmitter effects rather than through non-specific CNS depression. The newer non-benzodiazepine sedative/hypnotic agents have lower addictive potential and toxicity than older agents and can be utilized on a long-term basis in patients with chronic insomnia. Benzodiazepines, antidepressants, and other agents are utilized for their sedative side-effects in anxious and insomniac patients. Drugs known to induce daytime sleepiness are associated with declines in daytime performance and increased rates of automobile accidents. One of the significant advances in sleep medicine has been the development and use of efficacious medications to treat sleep disorders – medications with minimal side-effects, low addictive potential, and limited toxicity in overdose.

REFERENCES

1. Reite ML, Nagel KE, Ruddy JR. The Evaluation and Management of Sleep Disorders. Washington, DC: American Psychiatric Press, 1990.
2. Thorpy MJ, ed. The International Classification of Sleep Disorders: Diagnosis and Coding Manual. Lawrence, KA: American Sleep Disorders Association and Allen Press, 1990.
3. Physicians Desk Reference, Thompson. Compton, New Jersey. 1990.
4. Buysse DJ. Drugs affecting sleep, sleepiness and performance. In: Monk TM, ed. Sleep, Sleepiness and Performance. Chichester, UK: Wiley, 1991: 4–31.
5. Pagel JF. Pharmachologic alterations of sleep and dream: a clinical framework for utilizing the electrophysiological and sleep stage effects of psychoactive medications. Hum Psychopharmacol 1996; 11: 217–23.
6. Richardson GS. Managing insomnia in the primary care setting: raising the issues. Sleep 2000; 23: S9–12.
7. Pivik RT. The several qualities of sleepiness: psychophysiological considerations. In: Monk TM, ed. Sleep, Sleepiness and Performance. Chichester, UK: Wiley, 1991: 3–38.
8. Kryger MH, Roth T, Dement WC. Principles and Practice of Sleep Medicine, 2nd edn. Philadelphia, PA: WB Saunders, 1994.
9. Wilens TE, Biederman J. The stimulants. Psychiatric Clin North Am 1992; 41: 191–222.
10. Mitler MM. Nonselective and selective benzodiazepine receptor agonists – Where are we today? Sleep 2000; 23(Suppl 1): S39–47.
11. Aldrich MS. Automobile accidents in patients with sleep disorders. Sleep 1989; 12: 487–94.
12. Ray WA, Griffen MR, Downey W. Benzodiazepines of long and short elimination half-life and the risk of hip fracture. JAMA 1989; 262: 3303–7.
13. Doghramji K. The need for flexibility in dosing hypnotic agents. Sleep 2000; 23(Suppl 1): S16–20.
14. Greenblatt DJ. Benzodiazepine hypnotics: sorting the pharmacodynamic facts. J Clin Psychiatry 1991; 52: 4–10.
15. George CFP. Perspectives in the management of insomnia in patients with chronic respiratory disorders. Sleep 2000; S1: S31–5.
16. Settle EC. Antidepressant drugs: disturbing and potentially dangerous adverse effects. J Clin Psychiatry 1998; 59(Suppl 16): 25–9.
17. Kessler RC, McGonagle KC, Zhao S. Epidemiology of psychiatric disorders. Arch Gen Psychiatry 1994; 51: 8–19.
18. Sateia MJ, Doghramji K, Hauri PJ, Morin CM. Evaluation of chronic insomnia. Sleep 2000; 23: 243–314.
19. Krystal A, Walsh J, Laska E, et al. Sustained efficacy of eszopiclone over 6 months of nightly treatment: results of randomized, double blind, placebo-controlled study in adults with chronic insomnia. Sleep 2003; 26: 793–9.
20. O'Hanlon JF, Ramaekers JG. Antihistamine effects on actual driving performance in a standard driving test: a summary of Dutch experience, 1989–94. Allergy 1995; 50: 234–42.
21. Pagel JF, Parnes BL. Medications for the treatment of sleep disorders: an overview. Primary Care Companion. J Clin Psychiatry 2001; 3: 118–25.
22. Weiler JM, Bloomfield JR, Woodworth GG, et al. Effects of fexofenadine, diphenhydramine, and alcohol on driving performance – a randomized, placebo controlled trial in the Iowa driving stimulator. Ann Intern Med 2000; 132: 354–63.
23. Ancoli-Israel S. Insomnia in the elderly: a review for the primary care practitioner. Sleep 2000; 23(Suppl 1): S23–30.
24. Vermeeren A, Danjou PE, O'Hanlon JF. Residual effects of evening and middle-of-the-night administration of zaleplon 10 and 20 mg on memory and actual driving performance. Hum Psychopharmacol Clin Exp 1998; 13: S98–107.
25. Stevenson C, Ernst E. Valerian for insomnia: a systemic review of randomized clinical trials. Sleep Med 2000; 1: 91–9.
26. Breslau N, Roth T, Rosenthal L, et al. Sleep disturbance and psychiatric disorder: a longitudinal epidemiological study of young adults. Biol Psychiatry 1996; 39: 411–18.
27. Ware JC, Brown FW, Moorad PJ, et al. Effects on sleep: a double blind study comparing trimimpramine

to imipramine in depressed insomniac patients. Sleep 1989; 12: 537–49.

28. Pagel JF. Disease, psychoactive medication, and sleep states. Primary Psychiatry 1996; 3: 47–51.

29. Rickles K, Schweizer E, Clary C, et al. Nefazodone and imipramine in major depression: a placebo controlled trial. Br J Psychiatry 1994; 164: 802–5.

30. Pagel JF, Zafralotfi S, Zammit G. How to prescribe a good night's sleep. Patient Care 1997; 2: 28, 81–94.

31. Volz HP, Sturm Y. Antidepressant drugs and psychomotor performance. Neuropsychobiology 1995; 31: 146–55.

32. Fry JM. Current issues in the diagnosis and management of narcolepsy. Neurology 1998; 50(2 Suppl 1): S1–48.

33. McClellan KJ, Spencer CM. Modafinil: a review of its pharmacology and clinical efficacy in the management of narcolepsy. CNS Drugs 1998; 9: 311–24.

34. Chervin RD. Sleepiness, fatigue, tiredness and lack of energy in obstructive sleep apnea. Chest 2000; 118: 372–9.

35. Hart LL, Middleton RK, Schott WJ. Drug treatment for sleep apnea. DICP Ann Pharmacother 1989; 23: 308–15.

36. Pagel JF. The treatment of insomnia. Am Fam Physician 1994; 49(6): 1417–22.

37. Mamdema JW, Danhof M. Electroencepalogram effect measures and relationships between pharmacokinetics and pharmachodynamics of centrally acting drugs. Clin Pharmacokinet 1992; 23: 191–215.

38. Itil TM. The discovery of psychotrophic drugs by computer-analyzed cerebral bioelectrical potentials (CEEG). Drug Dev Res 1981; 1: 373–407.

39. Schenck CH, Mahowald MW. Long-term, nightly benzodiazepine treatment of injurious parasomnias and other disorders of disrupted nocturnal sleep in 170 adults. Am J Med 1996; 100: 333–7.

40. Pagel JF. Nightmares and disorders of dreaming. Am Fam Physician 2000; 61: 2037–44.

41. Pagel JF, Heftner P. Drug induced nightmares – an etiology based review. Hum Psychopharmacol 2003; 18: 59–67.

42. Klauber GT. Clinical efficacy and safety of desmopressin in the treatment of nocturnal enuresis. J Pediatr 1989; 114: 719–22.

43. Walters AS. Toward a better definition of the restless leg syndrome. The International Restless Legs Syndrome Study Group. Mov Disord 1995; 10: 634–42.

44. Lavigne GJ, Montplaisir JY. Restless leg syndrome and sleep bruxism: prevalence and association among Canadians. Sleep 1994; 17: 739–43.

45. Boghen D, Lamothe L, Elie R, et al. The treatment of restless leg syndrome with clonazepam: a prospective controlled study. Can J Neurol Sci 1986; 13: 245–7.

46. Early CJ, Allen RP. Pergolide and carbidopa/levodopa treatment of the restless leg syndrome and periodic leg movements in sleep in a consecutive series of patients. Sleep 1996; 19: 801–10.

47. Ropinirole (Requip) for restless legs syndrome. Med Lett Drug Ther 2005; 47(1214): 62–4.

48. Stone BM, Turner C, Mills SL, Nicholson AN. Hypnotic activity of melatonin. Sleep 2000; 23: 663–70.

49. Arendt J, Middleton B, Stone B, Skene D. Complex effects of melatonin: evidence for photoperiodic responses in humans? Sleep 1999; 22: 625–36.

50. Erman M, Seiden D, Zammit G, Sainati S, Zhang J. An efficacy, safety, and dose-response study of Ramelton in patients with chronic primary insomnia. Sleep Med 2006; 7(1): 17–24.

51. Buxton OM, Copinschi G, Van Onderbergen A, et al. A benzodiazepine hypnotic facilitates adaptation of circadian rhythms and sleep–wake homeostasis to a eight hour delay shift simulating westward jet lag. Sleep 2000; 23: 915–28.

52. Mamelak M, Black J, Montplasier J, et al. A pilot study on the effects of oxybate on sleep architecture and daytime alertness in narcolepsy. Sleep 2004; 27: 1327–34.

10

Sleep and personality disorders

Samuel J Huber, C Robert Cloninger

INTRODUCTION – CHALLENGES AND LIMITATIONS

Contemporary research in sleep faces several significant methodologic and definitional challenges.[1] Although research criteria in insomnia and other sleep disorders have been developed, they have yet to be widely accepted. Also, longitudinal studies have not validated these criteria as identifying a discrete subset of pathology with clinical, prognostic, and etiologic correlates.[2]

Although difficulty with sleeping is a common concern throughout medicine, it remains difficult to distinguish between sleep as a symptom of another illness (e.g., depression) and sleep as a distinct category of function and dysfunction. As will be discussed below, a third possibility arises in the course of sleep research in psychosomatics, namely that sleep disturbance may be a predictive factor or vulnerability trait predicting future mental illness or its severity.

In the absence of validated criteria, attempts have been made to establish working definitions for sleep disorders, particularly insomnia.[2,3] Perhaps some of the variability of results can be accounted for by this heterogeneity of definition or the heterogeneity of the group identified for study. It is also important in this research to identify and acknowledge the impact of substance abuse and comorbid depressive illness on sleep and sleep architecture.[1,3]

Recent literature will be discussed below, with attention being paid to both sides of the sleep–personality relationship. A body of research exists that attends to the personality configurations of patients with sleep disorders, largely insomnia. A separate literature examines the sleep features of patients with personality disorders. We are unaware of attempts to unify the two. Sleep research in personality disorders to date has been limited by a focus on categorical diagnoses rather than specific personality traits or features of temperament and character. The role of sleep in the development of personality in childhood is not reviewed here, nor is the role of sleep in the exacerbation of personality diatheses.

PERSONALITY TRAITS IN PATIENTS WITH SLEEP DISORDERS

Difficulty with sleeping is a common complaint among adults, and is associated with significant utilization of healthcare resources in addition to being the source of significant psychosocial distress. Whether as part of a syndrome of illness or as a discrete primary disorder, insomnia is often comorbid with depression, personality disorders, and pulmonary, cardiovascular, or gastrointestinal disorders.[2] Given this high prevalence of comorbidity and general burden of illness and disability, sleep disorders have been a tempting subject of research to attempt to locate risk factors, vulnerability traits, or etiologic causes of insomnia and other sleep complaints. A number of general theories and hypotheses have been advanced to explain the development of insomnia and individual response to treatment.[3] These include a multifactorial approach that implicates high physiologic activation in addition to psychologic factors, particularly in perpetuating insomnia.[4,5] These factors may include anticipatory worry, anxiety, intrusive thoughts, or daytime personal problems. As reviewed below, some efforts have been made to investigate more systematically the role of personality and related factors in the development and persistence of sleep disorders, including insomnia, chronic fatigue, and sleep-disordered breathing.

Insomnia

A number of studies have sought to investigate a relationship between primary insomnia and psychologic or personality components with the intention of identifying either vulnerability factors for insomnia or hypothesizing a causal link. The Minnesota Multiphasic Personality Inventory (MMPI) is a research instrument that has been employed in the study of personality and related psychopathology for many years, and it has been a useful tool in the area of insomnia research. Several studies in the 1970s revealed pathologic deviations on MMPI scales, including Hypochondriasis, Hysteria, Depression, and Psychasthenia, leading to a characterization of patients with chronic insomnia as patients who tend to 'repress, inhibit and internalize stress and emotional conflicts'.[6]

Several studies have used the MMPI to study internalization of distress in insomnia.[4,7] Kales and Vgontas[7] also sought to link psychobehavioral factors to the development of persistent insomnia. Hauri and Fisher[8] reported more sensation-avoiding and guardedness among insomniacs versus dysthymic patients. In an examination of 74 insomniacs versus 26 good-sleeping controls, Levin et al[9] found elevated scores for insomniacs on the Hypochondriasis, Depression, Hysteria, Psychasthenia, and Psychopathic Deviate scales of the MMPI. Although none of the mean T-scores was clinically significant ($T>70$), 53% of poor-sleeping subjects had at least one scale in the $T>70$ range, the most common being Depression versus 16% of controls. This study did not assess for depression in poor-sleeping subjects.

In contrast to the homogeneous classification proposed in the 1970s and implicit in subsequent research, Edinger et al[6] noted substantial heterogeneity among insomniacs and hypothesized from the work of Kales and Vgontas[7] that this variance could be better explained through two separate subtypes of patients with insomnia. Edinger et al[6] applied a cluster analysis to the MMPI profiles of 100 nondepressed insomniacs and described approximately 90% of the variance in the sample, with significant differences in sleep history as well as response to treatment (Table 10.1). 'Type 1' insomniacs were more aroused and activated, less defended and had a greater history of childhood sleep problems than did 'type 2', with significantly lower scores on the Lying, Defensiveness, and Hypochondriasis scales, and higher Mania scores, although virtually none of these mean T-scales were in the pathologic range. Type 1 subjects also had a less robust response to treatment with a combination of sleep education, stimulus-control therapy, and progressive muscle relaxation. Type 2 patients had higher means on the Hysteria, Defensiveness, and Hypochondriasis scales, suggesting a more neurotic personality, as opposed to a more internalized type 1 personality. While these two subtypes may instead represent varying degrees

Table 10.1 Insomnia subtypes by MMPI, history and outcome variables

Type 1	Type 2
↑arousal	↓arousal/↑neuroticism
+childhood sleep problems	later onset
↓response to treatment	↑response to treatment
↑mania	↑hysteria
↑hypochondriasis	↑hypochondriasis
↓defensiveness	↑defensiveness

Adapted from: Edinger JD, Stout AL, Hoelscher TJ. *Psychosomatic Medicine* 1988; 50: 77–87 of severity of illness rather than underlying personality pathology or vulnerability, this finding also reiterates the idea that both physiologic arousal factors and psychologic response-to-stress factors play a role in insomnia.

In the contemporary setting, additional research tools have been developed to investigate components of personality, and these have been employed in the study of insomnia and other sleep disorders. The Temperament and Character Inventory (TCI) is a well-validated instrument based on the unified biosocial theory of personality developed by Cloninger and co-workers.[10,11] It is a true–false questionnaire that measures four dimensions of temperament – novelty-seeking (NS), harm avoidance (HA), reward dependence (RD), and persistence (P) – and three dimensions of character – self-directedness (SD), self-transcendence (ST), and cooperativeness (C).[12] There is evidence to suggest that these features have neurochemical correlates in brain and clinical correlates with regard to personality disorders as well as a differential response to treatment of depression and anxiety.[12–14] de Saint Hilaire et al[4] have used the TCI to investigate personality components in several sleep-related disorders. A study of 32 non-depressed patients with primary insomnia revealed significantly higher HA scores and lower SD scores in insomniacs versus normal controls. These were correlated with polysomnographic sleep variables related to insomnia. Sleep latency was positively correlated with HA. Harm avoidance and anticipatory worry (a subset of the HA scale) were negatively correlated with rapid eye movement (REM) latency. Insomniacs were higher

in all subscales of HA, including anticipatory worry, fear of uncertainty, shyness and fatigability. Patients and controls were not significantly different in the other aspects of temperament: reward dependence, novelty seeking or persistence (Table 10.2). Forty-three percent of the patients with high HA scores demonstrated a passive–aggressive profile (i.e., high on HA, NS, and RD), while 17% tended toward a passive–dependent personality type (i.e., high on HA and RD, and low on NS). Scores on the Hospital Anxiety and Depression Scale (HADS) were elevated for anxiety but not for depression. These findings are consistent with Fisher's hypothesis that insomnia may be related to sensation-avoiding behavior, which may be similar to TCI harm avoidance. In addition, they suggest that HA may be a vulnerability factor for insomnia. Furthermore, these findings are consistent with a previous finding that high HA and high RD combined with high persistence (P) are related to complaints of 'restless-sleep' on the Center for Epidemiologic Studies Depression Scale (CES-D).[15]

The de Saint Hilaire et al study raises anew the complication of considering insomnia or sleep disturbance as a symptom versus viewing insomnia as a discrete category of illness (Figure 10.1). Perlis et al[16] have suggested the commonsense notion that primary insomnia may be a prodromal symptom of affective illness, and anxiety or fatigue described by insomniacs may not be caused by their poor sleep. Harm avoidance has been correlated with serotonin 5-HT$_2$ receptor sensitivity, which is also thought to play a significant role in depression and anxiety – or at least in the treatment of these disorders with medications acting on serotonergic

Table 10.2	Temperament and character contributions to sleep-related disorders		
	Insomnia	*Sleep-disordered breathing*	*Chronic fatigue syndrome*
Harm avoidance	↑	–	↑
Reward dependence	±	–	↓
Persistence	±	–	±
Self-directedness	↓	–	

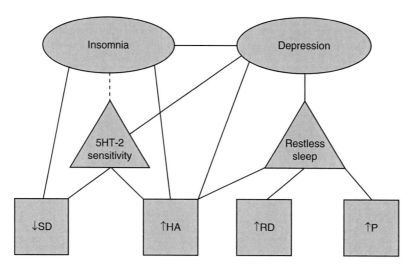

Figure 10.1   Summary of personality factors in insomnia and depression

neurons in the brain.[17] Both HA and serotonin are correlated with REM latency and non-REM (NREM) sleep, raising the hypothesis that serotonin is involved in insomnia and other sleep dysregulation.[4] It remains difficult to distinguish the role of HA and serotonin in depression from their role in sleep disorders or the possibility of HA as a vulnerability factor for depression, anxiety, or insomnia. Indeed, HA and SD may be vulnerability factors for depression via their impact on vulnerability for insomnia through a serotonin-mediated pathway. A definitive prospective trial to investigate vulnerability would follow non-depressed patients with insomnia with both high and low HA over time to assess for the development of depression or other affective illness. To our knowledge, this study has yet to be undertaken, but studies of siblings of depressives and controls do confirm high HA and low SD as vulnerability factors for major depression.[18]

Sleep-disordered breathing

Sleep-disordered breathing (SDB) is a general term used to describe a wide variety of sleep-related pulmonary conditions, including simple snoring, obstructive sleep apnea (OSA), sleep apnea syndrome (SAS), and other sequelae secondary to

nocturnal hypoxia. SDB often results in subjective complaints of fatigue and reduced alertness, and there has been recent academic interest in the development of concomitant or comorbid psychologic symptoms. Initial investigations suggested higher rates of personality and affective disorders in patients with SDB.[19,20] Associations have been suggested between SDB and hypochondriasis, conversion–hysteria, and possibly psychosis; however, recent studies have not identified apnea density or SDB as risk factors for personality disorders or affective illness.[20–22] Pillar and Lavie[23] studied psychologic sequelae in over 2000 patients with SDB, and failed to show a connection between the severity or existence of SAS and the development of depression or anxiety symptoms. In the same study, SAS was not associated with scores of somatization, obsession–compulsion, hostility, phobic anxiety, or paranoid ideation.

To further elucidate a possible connection between SDB and personality changes, Sforza et al[20] administered the TCI to 60 patients with reduced daytime alertness and snoring who presented to clinic for evaluation of possible OSA. Although there was a slight trend toward an increase in NS in patients with OSA, no relationship was found between apnea density and TCI variables (Table 10.2). The authors hypothesized that SDB and depression or personality disorders may not be causally related except by comorbid risk factors such as increased body mass index (BMI)/obesity, alcohol intake, and smoking. While these behaviors may be more likely in the setting of increased NS, it is more likely that NS is robustly related to the risk factors for OSA rather than being instrumental in the development of SDB. It is also possible that symptoms associated with SDB, including daytime sleepiness, reduced vigor and energy, or reduced lust for life, may be misinterpreted as symptoms of affective illness or personality disorder rather than primary sequelae of SDB.[20]

Chronic fatigue

Chronic fatigue syndrome (CFS) is a loosely defined constellation of symptoms without clear etiology, natural history, or consistent biologic marker. The central feature of the illness is persistent fatigue, which may or may not be related to a sleep disturbance. Diagnostic criteria have been developed by the US Centers for Disease Control and Prevention (CDC).[24] There are few systematic studies of the role of personality in fatiguing disorders. Furthermore, a consideration of fatigue suffers from the same methodologic difficulties as that of insomnia or poor sleep; that is, fatigue may be a symptom of affective illness or personality disorder or it may function as a discrete category of illness.

Christodoulou et al[25] hypothesized that a consideration of chronic fatigue from the standpoint of Cloninger's biosocial theory of personality would reveal common features of temperament or character associated with CFS. Based on previous observations that HA was elevated in patients with subjective chronic fatigue, Christodoulou et al[25] hypothesized that HA and P would also be elevated in patients with CFS defined by CDC criteria. The Tridimensional Personality Questionnaire (TPQ), a forerunner to the TCI, was administered to 38 patients with CFS as well as 40 patients with multiple sclerosis (MS) and 40 healthy controls. The study was controlled for depressive illness by clinical interview.

Both subjects with CFS and MS were found to have higher HA and lower RD than controls, with MS patients showing lower P than CFS subjects or controls (Table 10.2). Furthermore, Henderson and Tannock[26] found an increased incidence of personality disorders in 40 non-depressed CFS patients as assessed by structured clinical interview, with cluster C disorders being the most prominent. Notably, cluster B personality disorders were more prevalent in CFS patients with comorbid depression in the same study.

Examination of personality factors in chronic fatigue is complicated by a high level of overlap with somatization disorder, and in fact many of the diagnostic criteria for the two disorders are similar.[27,28] Patients with somatization disorder have been found to frequently meet criteria for a personality disorder, particularly the cluster B disorders, and the symptom profiles of patients with a cluster B disorder are often quite similar to those of patients with previously diagnosed somatization disorder.[29] As such, a specific link between chronic fatigue and a personality disorder is likely to be difficult to elucidate, independent of the risk for a personality disorder imparted by comorbid somatization.

SLEEP FEATURES IN PATIENTS WITH PERSONALITY DISORDERS

Human sleep can be characterized as having two main components: REM sleep and NREM sleep. The latter component is also referred to as slow-wave sleep, delta sleep, or deep sleep, and is sometimes divided into stages 1–4.[30] Polysomnography is a research tool used to identify these basic aspects of sleep architecture. In addition, observations may be made about the number of awakenings in an evening (sleep efficiency), time to onset of REM sleep (REM latency), and the amount of REM sleep (REM density). Additional variables have been identified for specialized analysis by some investigators through techniques such as spectral analysis (described, for example, by Philipsen et al[31]).

The current nosologic classification scheme of the 4th edition of the Diagnostic and Statistical Manual of Mental Disorders (DSM-IV) identifies several personality disorders among three clusters via behavioral criteria.[32] The most frequently studied of these disorders is borderline personality disorder (BPD) – due at least in part to features of the illness, including help-seeking and frequent psychosomatic complaints, that lend themselves well to study. While, overall, there is limited formal investigation of sleep characteristics of patients with personality disorders, the most investigated to date are BPD and antisocial personality disorder (ASP).

Borderline personality disorder

Careful investigation of fatigue, sleep features, and sleep architecture in patients with BPD can be complicated. Patients with BPD may report fatigue and other symptoms associated with major depressive disorder (MDD), and are often described as having comorbid depression. Efforts have been made on several fronts to examine the relation between BPD and MDD.[33] Sleep complaints are more frequent in BPD than in healthy controls.[34] There is a high prevalence of BPD among patients with somatization disorder, increasing the number of sleep complaints and somatoform complaints overall.[29] In general, BPD is associated with poor health-related lifestyle choices, risk factors for depression, and increased healthcare utilization.[35] Furthermore, rates of substance abuse, including alcoholism, are increased in patients with BPD, which may confound sleep study data.[36,37] Distinguishing a specific BPD-related signal in sleep studies from known confounding factors of MDD or subsyndromal depression has been a challenge in recent study design (Table 10.3).

To our knowledge, there have been approximately ten sleep-electroencephalography (EEG) studies in BPD.[31,38] The majority of these studies were not controlled for comorbid depressive illness, and those that acknowledged depression in research subjects did not often do so with standardized instruments.[39] The most common finding among

Table 10.3   Challenges and limitations in investigation of a personality disorders–sleep connection

- Sleep state misperception and interpretive behavior of personality disorders
- Decreased self-awareness of subjects
- Comorbid depression
- Comorbid substance abuse
- Comorbid somatization disorder
- DSM and behavioral criteria for personality disorder may result in inadequate or incomplete groupings

these studies was shortened REM latency, increased REM density, and overall disturbance of sleep continuity.[40–43] Similar findings have been reported in non-European and non-American populations, with similar methodologic shortcomings.[34]

More recently, several studies have controlled for comorbid depressive illness with mixed results. Akiskal et al[44] examined 24 non-depressed patients with BPD and found shortened REM latency in these patients versus non-BPD personality-disordered controls and healthy controls. This finding contributed to the hypothesis that affective disorders and BPD may have a common biologic origin or similar biologic pathways, or that at least a subset of BPD patients may be at elevated risk for affective illness.[44] Battaglia et al[45] examined ten never-depressed patients with BPD and correlated shortened REM latency with familial risk for depression in these patients. In a similar follow-up study, the same group found increased REM density in the first period of REM sleep to be related to risk for depressive illness in patients with BPD.[46] These authors have advanced these data to hypothesize a link between BPD and vulnerability for affective illness.

Current research has more effectively controlled for depressive illness and to some degree for alcohol usage. De la Fuente et al[47,48] were unable to differentiate between BPD, MDD, and normal controls on the basis of REM latency. Philipsen et al[31] studied conventional polysomnographic parameters as well as EEG spectral power analysis in 20 unmedicated, non-depressed female patients with BPD. No severe sleep problems were noted in the subjects versus healthy controls, but a significant discrepancy was noted between objective sleep measurements and subjective sleep quality. This raises the possibility that sleep disturbance in BPD may be more closely related to the psychologic correlates and interpretive behavior characteristic of BPD than to a primary neurobiologic mechanism. Indeed, complaints of subjectively poor sleep quality may be more consistent with the constellation of somatoform and psychoform symptoms seen in comorbid BPD and somatization disorder, with sleep-state misperception being part of a broader disturbance in self-awareness.

A second finding of the study by Philipsen et al[31] was that delta power in NREM sleep appears to be elevated in BPD. This is also consistent with findings in patients with antisocial personality disorder (ASP).[30,49] As will be discussed below, this similarity in NREM sleep between patients with BPD and ASP may be indicative of dysregulated impulse control and aggression, and lends itself to a serotonergic and dopaminergic hypothesis of impulse control, NREM sleep disturbance, and personality disorder.[31] It should be remembered that BPD and ASP, are clinically similar; patients with BPD are higher in HA than those with ASP, but are otherwise the same with regard to other aspects of personality.[50,51]

Overall, the most common sleep architecture change reported in polysomnographic evaluation of patients with BPD is shortened REM latency. This is an abnormality commonly seen in mood disorders.[39,52] It remains unclear whether these findings are confounded by comorbid depression, represent a vulnerability factor for comorbid depression, or predict response of BPD or sleep disturbance to antidepressant therapy.

Antisocial personality disorder and aggression

There is a limited yet significant body of research regarding sleep architecture and ASP. In a sleep-EEG study of 19 habitually violent and drug-free subjects with ASP, Lindberg et al[30] found an increase in slow-wave or deep sleep, with decreased sleep efficiency in the form of more frequent awakenings than controls. In contrast to other studies of psychiatric disorders, this appears to be the only instance of increased deep sleep among patients with psychopathology, although this finding may be consistent with observational findings in preadolescent boys with conduct disorder.[49] In a similar study, Lindberg et al[30] found that subjects with ASP (and by definition a history of conduct disorder) had a variable degree of impulsiveness that was correlated with variations in sleep architecture. More recently, this group found that in 14 habitually violent men with ASP, increases in amount and delta power of deep sleep correlated with a retrospective measure of childhood ADHD.[53] From these findings, Lindberg et al hypothesized a shared deficit related to sleep architecture among children with ADHD and adults who develop ASP. In addition, Philipsen et al[31] hypothesize a common pathway between ASP and BPD wherein impulse control and aggression are related to sleep architecture, perhaps through a serotonergic pathway with or without a dopaminergic component. While the $5-HT_{2c}$ receptor may play a role in slow-wave sleep regulation, and treatment with serotonergic medications may have some benefit in sleep regulation, it seems premature to declare a causal relationship.[54]

Complicating factors

As noted above, patients with personality disorders or pathologic disruptions of temperament and character have more somatic complaints overall, tend to utilize additional medical resources, and are prone to making poor health-related lifestyle choices.[35] In addition to their primary illness, these patients have elevated incidences of substance abuse and may be at elevated risk for MDD or other mood disorder.[12,51,55] The importance of acknowledging or controlling for depression in study designs has been discussed above. To our knowledge, limited efforts have been made at incorporating comorbid substance abuse, particularly alcoholism, into study design. Substance abuse may be a significant confounding factor in studies of personality disorders and sleep. On the other hand, 'self-medication' with alcohol or other drugs of abuse may initially develop in some patients as a response to a sleep disturbance. Furthermore, substance abuse may also impact the subjective experience or reporting of sleep quality, particularly in outpatient or ambulatory survey instruments.

Sleep features as a function of temperament and character

As explored above, there has been limited progress in investigation into the features of personality or personality disorders and sleep architecture or sleep disorders. This may be related in some part to the inherent difficulty in defining sleep as its own category of function and as separate from a symptom of depression or other mood syndrome. Another possibility is that the nosologic and phenomenologic schemes currently used in the clinical identification of personality disorders are inadequate or incomplete in a research setting, resulting in a heterogeneous population of research subjects. To date, sleep architecture, sleep disorders, or sleep quality have not been specific foci of research from investigators exploring Cloninger's unified biosocial theory of personality. However, some findings may add to the discussion of sleep and personality.

While it is reasonably well established that personality dimensions may predict scores on depression scales, this relationship has been further characterized by the finding that the qualitative experience of depressive symptoms is related to the personality structure of an individual.[15] In a study of personality and depressive symptoms, HA was related to total score on an inventory of depressive symptoms, including restless sleep. High RD combined with high P were also associated with restless sleep.[15] Both high HA and low SD have been established as risk factors for the development of depression.[18] Low SD is thought to be correlated with a significantly increased risk for personality disorder, and the combination of low SD and low C are thought to impart risk for mild personality disorder.[50,56]

By definition, P is an indicator of a tendency to persevere despite frustration or fatigue, although this dimension has not been specifically investigated with regard to sleep quality.

As noted above, HA and SD have been correlated with the development and persistence of sleep disturbance in the form of insomnia. These dimensions as measured by the TCI have also been associated with platelet $5-HT_2$ receptor sensitivity. While the impulsive personality disorders such as BPD and ASP are thought to be more related to high NS and low C, low SD also plays a role, and high HA is associated with comorbid depressive illness.[57] Although the findings reviewed above are individually limited, in total it is possible to suggest increased support for a serotonergic hypothesis of sleep, HA and SD, and vulnerability to comorbid depression. It is also possible that, as seen with MDD, the degree of HA or other personality dimensions may explain some of the variability in response to treatment of insomnia. Conversely, it is possible to surmise that alteration of sleep architecture may influence the severity of personality disturbance or offer a modality of therapy wherein SD, C, or impulsive behavior would be manipulated through changes in sleep.

SUMMARY

Progress, challenges, and limitations in investigation of a relationship between sleep and personality factors have largely followed those of its two component fields. Sleep research, in particular with regard to insomnia, is continually faced with the challenges of definition, validation, and confounding variables. Personality research is often limited by its measurement instruments and the heterogeneity of diagnostic schemes. Nevertheless, investigations from both sides of a sleep–personality research perspective have yielded interesting results, which have generated additional research questions and may also have clinical utility.

As reviewed above, there appears to be a relationship between HA, SD, serotonin, and vulnerability to both sleep disturbance and depression. Surprisingly, this relationship does not appear to extend to

SDB, while HA may yet play a role in CFS. HA and SD may influence not only the development of insomnia but also its perpetuation. It remains to be seen whether HA and serotonin represent only vulnerability factors for insomnia and depression, or whether they play an etiologic role as well.

While research regarding sleep components of personality disorders is complex and the recent iterations of more carefully controlled sleep-EEG studies have been largely equivocal with regard to REM latency, current evidence suggests an NREM sleep component to impulse-control-related personality disorders. These findings hold potential for therapeutic modalities involving modulation of sleep, impulsivity, and character components through pharmacologic intervention, self-awareness training, or alteration of sleep patterns.

REFERENCES

1. Zorumski CF. Chronic Insomnia: State of the Science. Grand Rounds Presentation, Washington University in St Louis, 20 September 2005.

2. National Institutes of Health. State-of-the-Science Conference Statement: Manifestations and Management of Chronic Insomnia in Adults. NIH: Bethesda, MD, 2005.

3. Silber MH. Chronic Insomnia. NEJM 2005; 353: 803–10.

4. de Saint Hilaire Z, Straub J, Pelissolo A. Temperament and character in primary insomnia. Eur Psychiatry 2005; 20: 188–92.

5. Shaver JLF, Johnston SK, Lentz MJ, Landis CA. Stress exposure, psychological distress, and physiological stress activation in midlife women with insomnia. Psychosomatic Med 2002; 64: 793–802.

6. Edinger JD, Stout AL, Hoelscher TJ. Cluster analysis of insomniacs' MMPI profiles: relation of subtypes to sleep history and treatment outcome. Psychosomatic Med 1988; 50: 77–87.

7. Kales A, Vgontas A. Predisposition to and development and persistence of chronic insomnia: importance of psychobehavioral factors. Arch Intern Med 1992; 152: 1570–2.

8. Hauri P, Fisher J. Persistent psychophysiologic insomnia. Sleep 1986; 9: 38–53.

9. Levin D, Bertelson AD, Lacks P. MMPI differences among mild and severe insomniacs and good sleepers. J Personality Assess 1984; 48: 126–9.

10. Cloninger CR, Svrakic DM, Przybeck TR. A psychobiological model of Temperament and Character Inventory (TCI). Arch Gen Psychiatry 1993; 50: 975–90.

11. Cloninger CR. A systematic method for clinical description and classification of personality variants. Arch Gen Psychiatry 1987; 44: 573–88.

12. Cloninger CR. Feeling Good: The Science of Well-being. Oxford: Oxford University Press, 2004.

13. Cloninger CR, Bayon C, Svrakic DM. Measurement of temperament and character in mood disorders: a model of fundamental mood states as personality types. J Affect Disord 1998; 51: 21–32.

14. Battaglia M, Przybeck TR, Bellodi L, Cloninger CR. Temperament dimensions explain the comorbidity of psychiatric disorders. Comprehensive Psychiatry 1996; 37: 292–8.

15. Grucza RA, Przybeck TR, Spitznagel EL, Cloninger CR. Personality and depressive symptoms: a multidimensional analysis. J Affect Disord 2003; 74: 123–30.

16. Perlis ML, Giles DE, Buysse DJ, et al. Which depressive symptoms are related to which sleep electroencephalographic variables? Biologic Psychiatry 1997; 42: 904–13.

17. Peirson AR, Heuchert JW, Thomala L, et al. Relationship between serotonin and the Temperament and Character Inventory. Psychiatric Res 1999; 89: 29–37.

18. Farmer A, Mahmood A, Redman K, et al. A sib-pair study of the Temperament and Character Inventory scales in major depression. Arch General Psychiatry 2003; 60: 490–6.

19. Kales A, Cadwell AB, Cadieux RJ. Severe obstructive sleep apnea – II: Associated psychopathology and psychosocial consequences. J Chronic Dis 1985; 38: 427–34.

20. Sforza E, de Saint Hilaire Z, Pelissolo A, Rochat T, Ibanez V. Personality, anxiety and mood traits in patients with sleep-related breathing disorders: effect of reduced daytime alertness. Sleep Med 2002; 3: 139–45.

21. Hudgel DW. Neuropsychiatric manifestation of obstructive sleep apnea. Int J Psychiatry Med 1989; 19: 11–22.

22. Beutler LE, Ware JC, Karacan I, Thornby JI. Differentiating psychological characteristics of patients with sleep apnea and narcolepsy. Sleep 1981; 4: 39–47.

23. Pillar G, Lavie P. Psychiatric symptoms in sleep apnea syndrome: effects of gender and respiratory disturbance index. Chest 1998; 114: 697–703.

24. Fukuda K, Straus SE, Hickie I, et al. The chronic fatigue syndrome: a comprehensive approach to its definition and study. Annals Intern Med 1994; 121: 953–9.

25. Christodoulou C, Deluca J, Johnson SK, et al. Examination of Cloninger's basic dimensions of personality

in fatiguing illness: chronic fatigue syndrome and multiple sclerosis. J Psychosomatic Res 1999; 47: 597–607.

26. Henderson M, Tannock C. Objective assessment of personality disorder in chronic fatigue syndrome. J Psychosomatic Res 2004; 56: 251–4.

27. Johnson SK, DeLuca J, Natelson BH. Assessing somatization disorder in the chronic fatigue syndrome. Psychosomatic Med 1996; 58: 50–7.

28. Price RK, North CS, Wessely S, Fraser VJ. Estimating the prevalence of chronic fatigue syndrome and associated symptoms in the community. Public Health Rep 1992; 107: 514–22.

29. Lenze EJ, Miller AR, Munir ZB, Pornnoppadol C, North CS. Psychiatric symptoms endorsed by somatization disorder patients in a psychiatric clinic. Ann Clin Psychiatry 1999; 11: 73–9.

30. Lindberg N, Tani P, Appelberg B, et al. Sleep among habitually violent offenders with antisocial personality disorder. Neuropsychobiology 2003; 47: 198–205.

31. Philipsen A, Feige B, Al-Shajlawi A, et al. Increased delta power and discrepancies in objective and subjective measurements in borderline personality disorder. J Psychiatric Res 2005; 39: 489–98.

32. American Psychiatric Association. Diagnostic and Statistical Manual of Mental Disorders, 4th edn (DSM-IV). Washington DC: APA 1994.

33. Koenigsberg HW, Anwunah I, New AS, et al. Relationship between depression and borderline personality disorder. Depression Anxiety 1999; 10: 158–67.

34. Asaad T, Okasha T, Okasha A. Sleep EEG findings in ICD-10 borderline personality disorder in Egypt. J Affect Disord 2002; 71: 11–18.

35. Frankenburg FR, Zanarini MC. The association between borderline personality disorder and chronic mental illnesses, poor health-related lifestyle choices and costly forms of health care utilization. J Clin Psychiatry 2004; 65: 1660–5.

36. Cloninger CR, Svrakic DM. Personality disorders. In: Sadock BJ, Sadock VA, eds. Comprehensive Textbook of Psychiatry. New York: Lippincott Williams & Wilkins, 2000: 1723–64.

37. Joyce PR, Mulder RT, Luty SE, et al. Borderline personality disorder in major depression: differential drug response and 6-month outcome. Compre Psychiatry 2003; 44: 35–43.

38. De la Fuente JM, Bobes J, Vizuete C, Mendlewicz J. Effects of carbamazepine on dexamethasone suppression and sleep electroencephalography in borderline personality disorder. Neuropsychobiology 2002; 45: 113–19.

39. Boutros NN, Torello M, McGlashan TH. Electrophysiological aberrations in borderline personality disorder: state of the evidence. J Neuropsychiatry Clin Neurosci 2003; 15: 145–54.

40. Bell J, Lycaki H, Jones D, Kelwala S, Sitaram N. Effect of preexisting borderline personality disorder on clinical and EEG sleep correlates of depression. Psychiatry Res 1983; 9: 115–23.

41. McNamara E, Reynolds III CF, Soloff PH, et al. EEG sleep evaluation of depression in borderline patients. Am J Psychiatry 1984; 141: 182–6.

42. Reynolds CF, Soloff PH, Kupfer DJ, et al. Depression in borderline patients: a prospective EEG sleep study. Psychiatry Res 1985; 14: 1–15.

43. Lahmeyer HW, Val E, Gaviria FM, et al. EEG sleep, lithium transport, dexamethasone suppression and monoamine oxidase activity in borderline personality disorder. Psychiatry Res 2002; 25: 19–30.

44. Akiskal HS, Yerevanian BI, Davis GC, King D, Lemmi H. The nosologic status of borderline personality: clinical and polysomnographic study. Am J Psychiatry 1985; 142: 192–8.

45. Battaglia M, Ferini-Strambi L, Smirne S, Bernardeschi L, Bellodi L. Ambulatory polysomnography of never-depressed borderline subjects: a high-risk approach to rapid eye movement latency. Biol Psychiatry 1993; 33: 326–34.

46. Battaglia M, Strambi LF, Bertella S, Bajo S, Bellodi L. First-cycle REM density in never-depressed subjects with borderline personality disorder. Biol Psychiatry 1999; 45: 1056–8.

47. De la Fuente JM, Bobes J, Vizuete C, Mendlewicz J. Sleep-EEG in borderline patients without concomitant major depression: a comparison with major depressives and normal control subjects. Psychiatry Res 2001; 105: 87–95.

48. De la Fuente JM, Bobes J, Morlan I, et al. Is the biological nature of depressive symptoms in borderline patients without concomitant Axis I pathology idiosyncratic? Sleep EEG comparison with recurrent brief major depression and control subjects. Psychiatry Res 2004; 129: 65–73.

49. Lindberg N, Tani P, Appelberg B, et al. Human impulse aggression: a sleep research perspective. J Psychiatric Res 2003; 37: 313–24.

50. Svrakic DM, Whitehead C, Przybeck TR, et al. Differential diagnosis of personality disorders by the seven factor model of temperament and character. Arch Gen Psychiatry 1993; 50: 991–9.

51. Cloninger CR. Antisocial personality disorder: a review. In: Maj M, Akiskal HS, Mezzich JE, Okasha A, eds.

Personality Disorders: Evidence and Experience in Psychiatry. Chichester, UK: Wiley, 2005: 125–9.

52. Benson KL, King R, Gordon D. Sleep patterns in borderline personality disorder. J Affect Disord 1990; 18: 267–73.

53. Lindberg N, Tani P, Porkka-Heiskanen T, et al. ADHD and sleep in homicidal men with antisocial personality disorder. Neuropsychobiology 2004; 50: 41–7.

54. Sharpley AL, Elliott JM, Attenburrow MJ, Cowen PJ. Slow wave sleep in humans: role of 5-HT$_{2A}$ and 5-HT$_{2C}$ receptors. Neuropharmacology 1994; 33: 467–71.

55. Cloninger CR. A unified biosocial theory of personality and its role in development of anxiety states. Psychiatric Dev 1986; 3: 167–226.

56. Cloninger CR, Svrakic DM. Differentiating normal and abnormal personality by the seven-factor personality model. In: Strack S, Lorr M, eds. Differentiating Normal and Abnormal Personality. New York: Springer-Verlag, 1994; 40–64.

57. Cloninger CR. A practical way to diagnose personality disorder: a proposal. J Personality Disord 2000; 14: 99–108.

11

A review of dreaming by psychiatric patients: An update

Milton Kramer, Zvjezdan Nuhic

INTRODUCTION

There has long been an assumption that there is an intimate relationship between dreams and mental disorders. Epigrammatic statements that 'the madman is a waking dreamer',[1] that 'dreams [are] a brief madness and madness a long dream',[2] that if we 'let the dreamer walk about and act like a person awake …, we [would] have the clinical picture of dementia praecox [schizophrenia]',[3] and that if 'we could find out about dreams, we would find out about insanity'[4] reflect the conviction about the close relationship between dreams and profound emotional disturbance. This view enlivened efforts to study dreaming to gain insights into the problems of the mentally ill.

In the literature review that introduces *The Interpretation of Dreams*, Freud[5] has a section on 'The relations between dreams and mental diseases'. He points out that when he 'speaks of the relationship of dreams to mental disorders [he has] three things in mind: (1) etiological and clinical connections, as when a dream represents a psychotic state, or introduces it, or is left over from it; (2) modifications to which dream-life is subject in cases of mental disease; and (3) intrinsic connections between dreams and psychosis, analogies pointing to their being essentially akin.'

The published work on dreams and psychopathologic state touches on all three areas of Freud's concern.[6] There are reports of psychotic states appearing to begin with a dream or a series of dreams, and there is certainly a literature, which continues to pursue analogies between dreams and psychosis. However, the vast majority of the work that has been done on dreams and psychopathologic states devotes itself to the 'modifications to which dream life is subject in cases of mental disease' and will be the focus of this report. Freud was of the opinion that as we better understand dreams, it will enhance our understanding of psychosis. Hartmann[7] is of a similar opinion.

There is a potential confusion between a psychopathology of dreams and dreams in a psychopathologic state. The former refers to alternations in the dreaming process that may be seen as abnormal, whereas the latter refers to the dreams that are the concomitants of a mental disorder. A dream that awakens the dreamer in a terrified state, generally with accompanying frightening dream content, a nightmare, would be a psychopathologic dream.[7] A dream report from a patient suffering from schizophrenia would be a dream from a person in a psychopathologic state. The dream may or may not be unique, either pathonomonically or statistically, to that state. Strangers occurring more frequently in the dreams of schizophrenics than in normals or depressed individuals is a statistical change in dream content in a psychopathologic condition.[8]

A psychologic examination of the dream is a study of the manifest content of the dream. Jones[9] pointed out that a psychology of dreams must rest on a study of the elements of which it is composed, the manifest dream images. Even Freud[10] pointed out '… that in some cases the façade of the dream directly reveals the dream's actual nucleus'. However, his almost exclusive focus on the latent dream content and his dismissal of the reported manifest dream retarded the study of dream reports. Calvin Hall[11] in the modern era has presented quantitative methods to assess dream content and has encouraged a scientific approach to the examination of the dream.

The study of the dream is an undertaking fraught with many difficulties. The dream experience cannot be directly observed, and its study is still dependent on the dream report. The dream is experienced during one state, sleep, and reported during another state, wakefulness. The problems of examining verbal reports of inner experiences are compounded by the change in state necessary to obtain the dream report. The study of lucid dreaming[12] opens the possibility of examining the dream experience while it is occurring, but the work so far on lucid dreaming has been more directed at demonstrating its occurrence than utilizing it as a method for studying the dream experience.

The verbal nature of the dream report needs to be addressed. Does the form of the dream obtained in the dream report reflect the dream as experienced or is it a result of the verbal style of the dreamer? An appropriate report of a waking experience becomes a necessary control if the study of the form of the dream is undertaken. For example, is the 'apparently' non-linear description of an experience the same for a subject in describing a waking experience as in describing a dream experience? If it is, then the finding of non-linearity cannot be considered a property of the dream experience, but rather it is an aspect of the dreamer's verbal style.

There are those who see the dream as an ineffable experience whose essence is destroyed by scientific study, by quantification.[13] The present survey is of quantitative reports. Quantification does not have to damage the essence of the dream experience.

There are significant methodologic issues that influence the dream content found in dream reports. These issues relate to the collection and measurement of the dream report.[14] They apply generally to dreams obtained either from night-time awakenings or from morning reports. There are seven collection factors that influence dream content: (1) the place in which the dream is experienced and collected; (2) the method of awakening the dreamer; (3) the context of the interpersonal situation in which the dream report is given; (4) the style of the collection interview; (5) the time of night and stage of sleep from which the sleeper is awakened; (6) the method of recording the dream report; and (7) the type of subject from whom the dream is collected. In addition, there are five problems that are related to the quantification of dream content that need to be considered: (1) the verbal nature of the dream report; (2) the definition of the scoreable protocol; (3) the effect of dream length on the type of measurement made; (4) the methods of quantifying dream content; and (5) the validity and reliability of the measurement. These factors need to be considered in studying the reports of dreams both separately and in interaction, as they affect the results obtained.

Interest in the dream has been kept alive by the depth psychologists[15] and by the 'man in the street',[16] while the scientific study of the dream has been significantly stimulated by the amount of the dream experience that can be recovered relatively close to the time of occurrence in rapid eye movement (REM) sleep,[17,18] and this has opened the possibility for manipulative (experimental) studies of dreaming.

In 1953, Ramsey[19] published a review of studies of dreaming. These were all from the pre-REM literature. Overall, he cited some 121 articles and books, of which 20 at most were studies of the dreams of six patient groups. The amount of information available from 20 publications would be woefully inadequate to characterize the dreams of psychopathologic groups. Ramsey concluded that the research was scientifically inadequate. Very few of the studies were so designed and reported that they could be replicated to validate their findings. He found that the dream studies were weak in not adequately (1) describing the population under study, i.e., their gender, age, intelligence, health, economic status, and education; (2) limiting the group of subjects under study; (3) using control groups; (4) defining more adequately the characteristics of the dreams; (5) treating the data statistically; and (6) controlling for interviewer bias.

The literature dealing with the nature of the relationship between dreaming and mental illness has been reviewed on several occasions,[20–24] with the last detailed review, covering the literature up to 1975, having been published in 1979.[23] That review focused on 75 reports in 71 articles in six patient groups, namely schizophrenia, depression, disturbing dreams, alcoholism, chronic brain syndrome, and mental retardation. Seventy-one articles were covered, four of which referred to more than one diagnostic group of interest. The scientific adequacy of the publications covered in that review was quite problematic, but a picture of dream content in some psychopathologic states began to emerge.

Since that review, only one other review article on dream content in psychiatric conditions has appeared.[25] The report was an extension of the previous work[23] and used as its database relevant studies and cases reports found in *Psychological Abstracts* from 1977 through 1990. It was of interest in that many of the findings of the previous review[23] were supported and some additional groups were examined. Unfortunately, as only 35 articles were cited, covering nine diagnostic groups, the scope of the review was limited. Meanwhile, a review of sleep physiology in psychiatric disorders has been published by Benca.[26]

METHOD

For the present report, an extensive title search of the English language periodical literature on dreams was undertaken. The basic source of bibliographic

Table 11.1 Extent of periodical literature search for dreams in psychiatric disorders

	Number of citations	
	1975[23]	2005
Citations found	2503	5484
Citations requested	1410	496[a]
Citations obtained	1359	493
Citations unavailable	51	3
Citations reviewed	71[b]	94[c]
Citations not reviewed	17	0

[a]Limited to Schizophrenia, Depression, Post-Traumatic Stress Disorder, Eating Disorders, Organic Brain Disorders, and Alcoholism and Drug Abuse
[b]Two articles had three studies each
[c]Two articles had three studies each and one had two studies

information was Medline (1966–2005). Dream was used as a descriptor to generate a basic 5484-item list (Table 11.1). This list was then searched for the six psychopathologic categories of interest, namely schizophrenia, depression, post-traumatic stress disorder (PTSD), eating disorders, organic brain disorder, and alcoholism and drug abuse. Some 496 articles published since 1976 were selected.

Of those 496 articles, 493 were obtained and examined. Ninety-four articles with dream content were included in the review. In the case of PTSD, all the appropriate articles available from 1966 on were reviewed. Two of the publications had three studies each and one had two studies. Each study was reviewed as a separate article, giving a total of 98 studies (Table 11.2).

The studies utilized for this review were categorized along 53 parameters covering the areas of (1) the type, nature, and site of the studies; (2) the description of the patient sample; (3) the description of the control sample; (4) the method of dream content collection; (5) the method of scoring the dream content; (6) the nature of the statistical analysis; and (7) the dream content results obtained. The review of the various parameters established only the presence or absence of the

Table 11.2 Psychiatric disorder studies with dream content reported

	Number of studies		
	1975[23]	2005	Refs (2005)
Schizophrenia	30	8	35–42
Depression	14	20[a]	45–65
Post-traumatic stress disorder (PTSD)	17[b]	46[a]	66–129
Eating disorders	0	11	130–140
Organic brain disorder	5	6	141–146
Alcoholism and drug abuse	5	7	149–155
Total	71	98	

[a]References 55 and 67 each included three studies
[b]Included nightmares and anxiety dreams

category, not its adequacy, with the exception of the statistical category.

RESULTS

The current update (1976–2005) yielded 94 articles covering 98 studies in six psychiatric conditions of concern (Table 11.2). There were 8 articles about schizophrenia, 18 articles with 20 studies about depression, 44 articles with 46 studies about PTSD, 11 articles on eating disorders, 6 articles on organic brain disorder, and 7 articles on alcoholism and drug abuse. In the earlier review, there had been 30 studies on schizophrenia, 14 on depression, 17 on disturbing dreams (PTSD and nightmares), 5 on organic brain disorder, and 5 on alcoholism. The findings from the 98 studies are presented under six content headings and are compared with the findings from the earlier review.[23]

Type, nature, and site of studies (Table 11.3)

In the current update (1976–2005), 67% of the reports on the six conditions are of studies. This is encouraging, as single case reports are less likely to

Table 11.3 Type, nature, and site of studies

	Percentage of studies	
	1975[23]	2005
Type of report		
Study	77	67
Case report	23	33
Nature of report		
Descriptive	37	69
Separate groups	51	27
Repeated measures	12	4
Site of data collection		
Sleep laboratory	32	27
Non-laboratory	68	73
Subject–control in separate groups		
Sick–sick	53	46
Sick–well	29	29
Both	18	25

provide leads about fundamental aspects of the dream life of a particular patient group. Interestingly, there is a 10% increase in case reports compared with our 1975 review, which showed 23% case reports and 77% studies. The increase in the number of case reports may reflect an interest in trying to capture some aspect of the reported dream life of a patient group that has not been adequately described in the literature[22] – for example the effects of physical illness, medication, or residence.

The trend toward increased description is underlined in that currently 69% of the reports were descriptive in nature, compared with 37% reported earlier. Comparison of the target patient group to another (control) group has fallen from 51% to 27%, while following an aspect of the manifest dream content across time or condition change (ill-to-well or vice versa) has declined from 12% to 4%.

It appears that the concern voiced by Ramsey[19] in reviewing the pre-REM era of dream studies, and in the earlier review,[23] about the neglect of appropriate research designs to build a scientifically sound literature about dream studies remains an issue to this day.

The sleep laboratory has not become an increased source for collecting dream reports, as only 27% of current studies and 32% in the earlier review were in the dream laboratory. This may reflect the fact that researchers are not convinced of the value of waking subjects at night to collect a larger, more complete sample of dreams, or that those interested in dream content do not have such a facility available, and therefore base their work instead on reports of spontaneously recalled dreams from home studies. We know that the site in which the dream is experienced and collected influences the content.[14]

It is heartening to see that the value of comparing the index group with another ill group or with both an ill and a well (normal) group has been maintained. In both reviews, 71% of studies had at least a sick–sick comparison.

It is unfortunate that available designs have not been systematically applied. It had been suggested, based on the earlier review,[23] that a content or theme generated from a descriptive report, case study, or literature review be appropriately compared in a separate group study with an ill and well (normal) group and then be studied in a repeated measure design to establish if the finding was limited to the illness (state) or was linked to a predisposition to the condition (trait). Our knowledge of the dream life of psychopathologic groups will remain limited without more systematic study.

Adequacy of description of patient sample (Table 11.4)

Sample size

The overall sample sizes for both sleep laboratory and non-laboratory studies appear to be adequate. The mean laboratory sample size has almost doubled from 12 to 22, comparing the earlier review with the current one. The mean number of subjects in the non-laboratory studies, although still adequate, has decreased from 246 to 97.

Patient selection

Greater attention has been paid to describing the basis for selecting patients in the various reports. In 56% of the studies, the selection basis is provided, whereas in earlier studies, only 31% provided this information. This information is essential to understand the nature of the group studied, as well as providing the minimal information needed for replication.

Basis of diagnosis

There is a slight increase from 45% to 48% in providing the basis for the diagnosis. Without this information, no judgment can be made about whether the classification of the patient was made on reasonable and reproducible grounds. Was the patient classified as schizophrenic because he was delusional or because he met some criteria such as those in DSM-IV?[27]

Specificity of diagnosis

The problem of categorizing the patient as to 'subtype' has been considerably less well attended to in the current than in the earlier review. Only 23% of studies provided the operational basis for subtyping of the patient (e.g., major depressive disorder or

Table 11.4   Description of patient sample

	Patient sample size			
	Total		Original	
	1975[23]	2005	1975[23]	2005
Number of studies				
Laboratory	24	27	17	22
Non-laboratory	51	71	46	69
Total number of subjects				
Laboratory	297	594	234	496
Non-laboratory	12 528	6693	5966	5034
Mean number of subjects per study				
Laboratory	12	22	14	22
Non-laboratory	246	97	130	73

	Percentage of studies			
	1975[23]		2005	
	Yes	No	Yes	No
A. Basis of selection	31	69	56	44
B. Basis of diagnosis	45	55	48	52
C. Specificity of diagnosis	48	52	23	77
D. Drugs or physical treatment	24	76	36	64
E. Demography:				
1. Sex	85	15	88	12
2. Age	69	31	67	33
3. Race	27	73	26	74
4. Education	29	71	22	78
5. Marital status	29	71	30	70
6. Socioeconomic class	25	75	12	88
F. General health	5	95	29	71
G. Original sample	81	19	89	11
H. Site of patient residence:				
1. In hospital	57		28	
2. Out of hospital	28		62	
3. Both	11		10	
4. Not given	4		0	

dysthymia), while 48% included this information in the earlier review.[23]

Drugs or physical treatment

In slightly over one-third of the patient studies (36%), mention is made of the treatment status of the patient. This is up from the 24% in the earlier review. In neither case is this adequate, as we have reason to believe that medication and physical treatments can effect the psychology of dreaming as well as the physiology of sleep.[22] The problem is that if one obtains a positive finding in a study, one would not know whether to attribute it to the psychopathologic state, the treatment, or an interaction between the two.

Demography

There is an awareness in both the current and previous[23] reviews that the gender and age of subjects are parameters that do indeed influence the content of the dreams. Gender is reported in 88% of the current studies and age is reported in 67%, compared with 85% and 69%, respectively, in the earlier review.[23] The other demographic variables – race, education, marital status, and social class – are reported less often (12% vs 30%), and, indeed, they have less influence on dream content.[28]

General health

There has been a significant increase in reporting the general health status of the patient population: from 5% in the previous review[23] to 29% of studies in the current review. The physical health status of a patient group is a potentially confounding variable, as it may either independently or in interaction affect the dream report content.[22]

Original sample

In 89% of studies, the sample used was an original one. This is slightly larger than the 81% of studies in the earlier review.[23]

Site of patient residence

There has been a major shift in dream studies of patients with psychopathology from studying those in the hospital (57%) to those out of the hospital (62%). This may reflect the current practice of treating patients outside the hospital. Setting impacts the contents of the dream[29] and is universally reported (96% in the 1975 review and 100% in the present review).

Adequacy of description of control sample (separate group studies) (Table 11.5)

The descriptions of the control group in the 27 separate group studies are more complete than those found for all of the other studies and are significantly improved over those reported in the earlier review.[23] To illustrate, 56% of the current overall sample reported the basis for selecting their target group. Thirty-seven percent of the separate group studies reported the basis for selection of the control sample in the earlier review,[23] while in the current review, 83% of the studies provided the basis for selecting the control sample. For 15 descriptors (A through I in Table 11.5), the studies in the current review presented more complete data for 8 (A, B, C, D, E-1, E-3, F, G) of 12 parameters compared with what was reported in the previous review.[23]

Method of dream content collection (Table 11.6)

The major interest in dream content studies, whether of psychopathologic or normal individuals, is what is contained in the dream report. How the report is obtained, scored or categorized, counted, and statistically analyzed is basic to establishing what the subject is dreaming about.

The nature and extent of the sampling of the dream life of a psychopathologic population is reflected in the number of nights (in laboratory studies) or days (in non-laboratory studies) of dream collection that were attempted, the number of dreams collected, and the percentage of dream recall achieved. The sampling process in the current review reflects less attention to the number of days or nights

Table 11.5   Description of control sample (separate groups only)

	Patient sample size			
	Total		Original	
	1975[23]	2005	1975[23]	2005
Number of studies				
Laboratory	10	10	8	9
Non-laboratory	28	17	23	17
Total number of subjects				
Laboratory	166	167	143	127
Non-laboratory	1843	1007	1703	1007
Mean number of subjects per study				
Laboratory	17	17	18	14
Non-laboratory	66	72	74	72

	Percentage of studies			
	1975[23]		2005	
	Yes	No	Yes	No
A. Basis of selection	37	63	83	17
B. Basis of diagnosis	26	74	71	29
C. Specificity of diagnosis	24	76	50	50
D. Drugs or physical treatment	5	76	54	46
E. Demography:				
1. Sex	76	24	92	8
2. Age	68	32	62	38
3. Race	18	82	25	75
4. Education	33	67	21	79
5. Marital status	24	76	12	88
6. Socioeconomic class	26	74	12	88
F. General health	11	89	33	67
G. Original sample	80	20	88	12
H. Site of patient residence:				
1. In hospital	42		25	
2. Out of hospital	34		75	
3. Both	24		0	

Table 11.6	Dream content collection variables				
		Percentage of studies			
		1975[23]		2005	
		Yes	No	Yes	No
A.	Number of days or nights	52	48	38	62
B.	Number of dreams	57	43	58	42
C.	Percent dream recall	35	65	22	78
D.	Who collected dreams	67	33	46	54
E.	When dreams collected	55	45	51	49
F.	Mode of awakening[a]	38	62	22	78
G.	Protocol for obtaining dreams	15	85	19	81
H.	Mode of recording dreams	87	13	27	73
I.	Associations obtained	37	63	34	66

[a]Only applicable to laboratory studies

of collection or to the percentage recall than in the earlier studies. The number of days or nights was reported in 52% of the previous studies, versus 38% in the current studies, while the percentage dream recall was reported in 35% versus 22%.

The interpersonal setting[30] and the mode of dream inquiry[13] may influence the nature of any content obtained. In the previous review, 67% of the articles reported who and 55% reported when the dreams were collected, compared with 46% and 51%, respectively, in the current review. There has been a decrease in reporting both variables – more significantly in who collected the dream – indicating a failure to appreciate the effect of the interpersonal situations on what is reported.

Although known to influence content, the mode of awakening[31] the subject in laboratory studies remains infrequently reported at 22%. The protection against interviewer bias provided by a fixed protocol for obtaining a dream report also remains low at 19%. The mode of recording the report and whether associations are obtained is reported in one-third or less of the current reports.

Unfortunately, the major methodologic problems in dream collection studies remain unchanged. The basic sampling procedures are often not reported. The failure in 81% of studies to use a fixed protocol to protect against interviewer bias is of great concern. Moreover, the low rate of reporting the mode of awakening in laboratory studies (22%) also contributes to the problems in characterizing the dream life of patient groups. The neglect of these crucial parameters contributes to our difficulties in assessing the adequacy of a study, in comparing the results from one study to another, and in being able to resolve discrepancies between studies.

Method of scoring dream content (Table 11.7)

Little or no attention was paid in the articles under review to reporting on protocol preparation (6%), on whether the raters were 'blind' (18%), or on the reliability of the scorers (11%). In 33% of the studies, only one rater did the rating, The type of

Table 11.7 Dream content scoring variables

	Percentage of studies			
	1975[23]		2005	
	Yes	No	Yes	No
A. Protocol preparation	28	72	6	94
B. 'Blind' raters	28	72	18	82
C. Reliability reported	27	73	11	89
D. Number of scorers used:				
1.		68		33
2.		27		6
3.		5		0
4. Not given		0		61
E. Type of scale:				
1. Item		20[a]		32
2. Thematic		77[a]		6
3. Not given		3[a]		62
F. Scale source:				
1. Standard		22[a]		18
2. Ad hoc		78[a]		20
3. Not given		0[a]		62

[a]Modified

scale and source of the scale was given in only 38% of the studies. These issues were reported at a lower frequency than in the earlier review, where they were also given inadequate attention. The failure to use more than one 'blind' rater whose reliability has been established and checked periodically attributes a remarkable faith in the objectivity and consistency of human performance.

The limited use of standard rating scales (18% currently and 22% in the previous review) underlines a core problem in the field of dream research. Failure to describe the basic elements in the manifest dream report with a standard device, and then to build special or inferential scoring from these identifiable parameters, severely limits the development of a body of knowledge in which one study builds on another and in which any given study is potentially relatable to another.[32]

Nature of statistical analysis (Table 11.8)

The percentage of studies in which any statistical analysis was reported is only 33% currently, compared with 41% in the previous survey.[23] In the 30 studies reporting statistical results, the number of tests was reported in almost all studies (90%), the statistic was by and large appropriate to the design and the data (80%), and the comparisons were generally preplanned (77%).

The content of the dream in psychopathologic states can be developed only from studies with acceptable statistical treatment of the data collected.

Table 11.8   Nature of the statistical analysis

	Percentage of studies			
	1975[23]		2005	
	Yes	No	Yes	No
A. Are statistical tests reported?	41	59	33	67
B. Are the number of tests reported?[a]	81	19	90	10
C. Are the statistics appropriate?[a]				
1. To the design?	81	19	80	20
2. To the data?	55	45	80	20
D. What is the nature of the comparison?[a]				
1. Preplanned	48		77	
2. Post hoc	52		23	
E. Significant results[a]	81		73	

[a]These studies reported statistical tests

DREAM CONTENT RESULTS

This limits the core data pool to 30 of the 90 studies. The non-statistical articles, either case reports or studies, provide leads for further more systematic study. However, only a small group of studies remains to characterize a large area of interest.

In 1976, Frosch[6] wrote a critical review entitled 'The psychoanalytic contributions to the relationship between dreams and psychosis', which provided some partial answers to Freud's questions about the relationship. Frosch concluded that (1) 'although there are many apparent similarities between dreams and psychosis, they do differ in some basic respects; certainly in so far as the factors are concerned which play a role in their production', (2) 'there is no consensus as to whether the manifest dream was of itself a meaningful guide to the presence of psychosis … [some] felt it was the latent content that was most telling [while others] seemed to feel that there might be features about the manifest form and content which could be of

significance, indicating the presence of a psychosis. It [was] felt by some investigators that the patient's attitude toward the dream, difficulties in differentiating the dream from reality, and the persistence of dream like states invading the waking life (that) may offer clues to the possibly psychotic nature of dreams', and (3) '[in regard] to whether there are dreams which presage psychosis, there was some suggestive evidence that this was the case'.

Schizophrenia

Schizophrenics are less interested in their dreams and their dreams are more primitive (i.e., less complex, more direct, and more sexual, anxious, and hostile), and showed evidence of their thought disorder in being more bizarre and implausible.[23] In a mixed patient population, which included schizophrenics, Lesse[33] reported that mounting anxiety could increase or decrease dream reporting. With increasing anxiety, motion and affect in the manifest dream are increased. And, a decrease in affect in the manifest dream is the first change seen during successful phenothiazine therapy.

Strangers were the most frequent dream characters in schizoprenics. Hallucinations and dream content were relatable, and the degree of paranoia (awake and in dreaming) was similar, contrary to Freud's[34] compensatory view of waking and dreaming in paranoia. An updated literature review yielded only eight articles on dream content in schizophrenic states,[35–42] – a surprisingly small number that added little to our understanding.

Lobotomized schizophrenics[43] had a lower dream recall rate in the laboratory (10.4%) than non-schizophrenics (46.7%), but both were lower than in another study.[44]

Depression

Depressed patients were found to dream as frequently as non-depressed, but the dreams were shorter and had a paucity of traumatic or depressive content even after depression had lifted.[23] Family members were more frequent in their dreams. When hostility was present, it could be directed at or away from the dreamer – while in schizophrenia, it was directed at the dreamer. Depressed patients had in their dreams more friendly and fewer aggressive interactions than schizophrenics, but more failure and misfortune. With clinical improvement, hostility decreased, while intimacy, motility, and heterosexuality increased.

The view that begins to emerge more clearly from the updated review[32,45–65] is that in depression there is a decrease in the frequency[47,49–52,55,64,65] and length[51,52,55,56,64] of the dream reports. Their dreams are often commonplace, but at times have content characteristics[45,50,52,57] of high interest. There is an increase in dreams of death themes in depressed suicidal patients and in bipolars before becoming manic.[45,52] There may also be an increase in family roles in the dreams of the depressed.[46,51,55]

Masochism in the dreams of the depressed appears more clearly in women than in men, and is more likely a trait than a state characteristic.[32,53,54,57–59] It is evident that a past focus is not universal in the dreams of the depressed, nor is it unique to the depressed state.[49–53,56,58] Affects such as anxiety and hostility are not prominent in the dreams of the depressed.[45,53,57,61] The content of their dreams may have prognostic significance for the response of the depressed patient to treatment or the spontaneous outcome of the depression.[49,54]

A most striking implication of these findings about dreaming in the depressed is that the affective state of the dreamer covaries with the content of the dream.[45,46,48,50,55–57] Changes in dreams across the night may contribute to the dreamer's coping capacity,[56,57,60,63,65] as has been suggested by Kramer.[62] Changes in dream content across the night alter the affective condition of the dreamer and contribute to the adaptive state of the dreamer the next day. Mood-regulation processes may have an implication for the treatment of depression. Untreated depressed subjects reporting more negative dreams at the beginning of the night than at the end of the night are more likely to be in remission after 1 year.[63] In contrast, a failure to self-regulate mood is associated with a suicidal tendency.[65]

Post-traumatic stress disorder

A widespread interest in PTSD has developed since the Vietnam war, including the dreams of such patients.[66–129] PTSD was only included in the official nomenclature of the American Psychiatric Association in 1980, although it had been described in the psychiatric literature for over 100 years.[66,81,89]

In a review article, Ross et al[68] attempt to demonstrate that sleep disturbance is the hallmark of PTSD. They based their hypothesis upon the mentation difference between REM and non-REM (NREM) sleep. They characterized the dreams of PTSD patients as vivid, affect-laden, disturbing, outside the realm of current waking experience (although representative of an earlier life experience), repetitive, stereotyped, and easy to recall. They proposed that the dream disturbance is relatively specific for the disorder[69,112] and that PTSD may fundamentally be a disorder of the REM sleep mechanism. However, as the nightmare in REM sleep occurs early in the night, when there is less REM and is associated with gross body movements, they acknowledged that abnormal non-REM sleep mechanisms may also be involved, and speculated that the neural circuitry involved in PTSD may be similar to that in accentuated startle behavior.[68] Ross et al[70] took exception to Reynold's[69] suggestion that the dream in PTSD is the same as that occurring in traumatized depressives, and pointed out that the dreams of traumatized depressives are not dreamlike and do not incorporate the trauma.[56,107] According to Ross et al[68] the dream in PTSD is repetitive and, more importantly, stereotyped.

In contrast, Kramer[71] viewed the disturbing dream as the hallmark of PTSD rather than the sleep disturbance. Green et al[72] have suggested that the unique aspect of PTSD is indeed the intrusive symptoms, including intrusive images and recurrent dreams and nightmares. They pointed out that not all dreams are direct recapitulations of the trauma. For them, these intrusive images may be the hallmark of PTSD. The view of Green et al[72] was based on the suggestion by Brett and Ostroff,[73] who pointed out that there has been a neglect of post-traumatic imagery, which they postulated to be the core of PTSD. They lamented the lack of research into the range, content, and patterning of the imagery.[102] Interestingly, Fisher et al[74,105] pointed out that trauma sufferers may have disturbing arousals that can come out of both REM and NREM (stages 4 and 2) sleep. This view was confirmed by Schlosburg and Benjamin,[75] Kramer and Kinney,[76] and Dagan et al.[124] Questions arise whether the sleep disturbance in PTSD involves more than REM sleep mechanisms and whether the imagery and dreams, reported by PTSD patients are stereotyped and REM-bound,[94] as Ross et al[68] postulate.

There has been a relative lack of attention with regard to the range, content, and patterning of the nightmares in PTSD. It was found that there can be different types of nightmares,[78,84,85,88] that themes may be unrelated to the trauma[67,90,128] (with one study finding a strong association between recalled dream content and a war experience[127]), and that the traumatic dream can change across time.[100,101,103,111,115] The traumatic nightmare is seen to reflect classical Freudian dreamwork mechanisms[77,79,80,84–86] and is not a meaningless reenactment of the trauma.

An adequate characterization of the phenomenology of the disturbing dream in PTSD remains to be done.[96,97,110] The dream experience is disturbing, but this may be more a reaction to the dream than the dream itself.[120] The affect-laden nature of the disturbing dream cannot be confirmed, and expectations may influence the perception of what the dream should be like in PTSD.[129] The content of the disturbing dream may be outside the realm of current waking experience, but it is linked to earlier childhood experiences,[77,79,80,85–87,99,109,116] and can be reactivated later in life.[82–84,88,91–93] The vividness of the dream has not been adequately addressed. The dream in PTSD is not easily recalled. Patients with active PTSD have a lower dream recall rate[67,104,106] than normals, but higher than that of well-adjusted former PTSD patients.[113]

A consensus has begun to emerge from the PTSD dream literature, suggesting that the hallmark of PTSD is a disturbance in psychologic dreaming and possibly of NREM sleep early in the night.[95] Disturbed dreaming covaries with combat exposure[117] and the experience of torture,[118] – not with the complaint of a sleep disturbance. The disturbing dream tends to occur early during sleep,[108] as do increases in movement,[67,119] spontaneous awakenings,[120,121] autonomic discharge,[122] elevated arousal threshold,[123–125] and a heightened startle response.[125,126] The disturbing dream is not sleep-stage-bound, and may emerge out of REM or NREM sleep.[74–76] Stereotypical dream content is not the sine qua non of the dream in PTSD. Failure or avoidance of dream recall may be an adaptational strategy in PTSD.[113,114]

Eating disorders

Anorexics and bulimics[130–140] both report dreams, and such dreams may be useful in therapy. For eating disorder patients, the rate of dream recall is low on self-report questionnaires, but normal in the sleep laboratory. Dreaming of food is high in eating disorder patients – higher in bulimics then anorexics.

Aggressive dreams are less common in eating disorder patients then normals.

Brain damage

The previous review[23] found five articles on brain-damaged patients. These studies reported that there was a decrease in dream reporting with age and dementia. More recent studies[141–148] of brain-injured patients have reported the value of dream exploration in psychotherapy. A questionnaire study of aged individuals found no relationship between dream report frequency and the degree of brain atrophy on computed tomography scan. Repetitive visual imagery in brain-damaged patients was not REM-bound. Focal brain damage studies suggest the anatomic substrate for dream formation. The dream content of right-hemispherectomized patients was similar to the content of the control subjects, which suggests that the left hemisphere plays a critical role in dream generation.[146]

Alcoholism and drug abuse

In the previous review,[23] the dreams of alcoholics could be distinguished from those of non-alcoholics. The alcoholic had more oral references in his dreams, was more often the object of aggression, and had fewer sexual interactions. Those detoxifying alcoholics who dreamed about drinking maintained sobriety for a longer period. The implication of dreaming about drinking or drug use as a predictor of abstinence remains unclear.[149–155] However, it raises the possibility that what one dreams about may have adaptive significance. Drug dreams in patients with cocaine dependence and bipolar disorder are similar to those in patients with pure substance dependence.[155]

CONCLUSIONS

It is apparent that the mysteries of psychosis have not been revealed through the study of dreams. The paucity of studies in some conditions and the relative lack of scientific rigor throughout continue to plague the study of dreams in psychiatric conditions. However, in some areas, such as depression and PTSD, we do know more about dreaming than we did previously.

Detailed phenomenologic descriptions are needed of the dream experience in normals and in the various psychiatric illnesses, in and out of the laboratory, utilizing quantitative techniques to capture various aspects of the experience. These results can then be compared statistically in between-group and repeated-measure experiments, as was recommended in the previous review.[23] Further, study of the dream construction process, of the dream as a dependent measure, applying the manipulations suggested by Tart[156] and the analytic techniques described by Kramer et al,[157] Montangero,[158] and Cipolli,[159] would enhance our understanding of the cognitive process in dreaming.

The most intriguing insight that emerges from this review is that what one does or does not dream about may contribute to the waking adaptational process.[57,62,113,114,152,153,160] Manipulating the dream by controlled incorporation of characters or events into the dream[161] and assessing the daytime consequences would treat the dream as an independent variable and contribute to our understanding of the functional significance of dreaming.

ACKNOWLEDGMENTS

The assistance of Mike Douglas, Valerie Ratchford, and Linda Kittrell, the library staff at Bethesda Oak Hospital, Cincinnati, Ohio, is gratefully acknowledged, as well as the support of Lydia Friedman, James Verlander, and the library staff of the Maimonides Medical Center, Brooklyn, New York.

REFERENCES

1. Kant I. Quoted in Freud S. The Interpretation of Dreams. Volumes IV and V of the Standard Edition. London: Hogarth Press, 1953: 90.

2. Schopenhauer A. Quoted in Freud S. The Interpretation of Dreams. Volumes IV and V of the Standard Edition. London: Hogarth Press, 1953: 90.

3. Jung C. The Psychology of Dementia Praecox. London: Princeton University Press, 1960: 86.

4. Jackson J. In: Taylor J, ed. Selected Writings of John Hughlings Jackson, Volume 2. New York: Basic Books, 1958: 45.

5. Freud S. The Interpretation of Dreams. Volumes IV and V of the Standard Edition. London: Hogarth Press, 1953.

6. Frosch J. Psychoanalytic contributions to the relationship between dreams and psychosis – a critical survey. Int J Psychoanal Psychother 1976; 5: 39–63.

7. Hartmann E. The Nightmare: The Psychology and Biology of Terrifying Dreams. London: Harper and Row, 1981.

8. Kramer M, Baldridge B, Whitman R, et al. An exploration of the manifest dream in schizophrenia and depressed patients. Dis Nerv Syst 1969; 30: 126–36.

9. Jones R. Dream interpretation and the psychology of dreaming. J Am Psychoanal Assoc 1965; 13: 304–19.

10. Freud S. On Dreams. Volume V of the Standard Edition. London: Hogarth Press, 1958: 667.

11. Hall C, Van de Castle R. The Content Analysis of Dreams. New York: Appleton, 1966.

12. LaBerge S, Rheingold H. Exploring the World of Lucid Dreaming. New York: Ballentine, 1990.

13. Boss M. The Analysis of Dreams. New York: Philosophical Library, 1958.

14. Kramer M, Winget C, Roth T. Problems in the definition of the REM dream. In: Levin P, Koella W, eds. Sleep, 1974. Basel: S Karger, 1975.

15. Kramer M, ed. Dream Psychology and the New Biology of Dreaming. Springfield, IL: Charles C Thomas, 1969.

16. Weiss H. Oneirocritica Americana. Bull NY Public Library 1944; 48: 519–41.

17. Aserinsky E, Kleitman N. Regularly occurring periods of eye motility and concomitant phenomena during sleep. Science 1953; 118: 273–4.

18. Aserinsky E, Kleitman N. Two types of ocular motility in sleep. J Appl Physiol 1955; 8: 1–10.

19. Ramsey G. Studies of dreaming. Psychol Bull 1953; 50: 432–55.

20. Kramer M. Manifest dream content in psychopathological states. In: Kramer M, ed. Dream Psychology and the New Biology of Dreaming. Springfield, IL: Charles C Thomas, 1969: 377–96.

21. Kramer M. Manifest dream content in normal and psychopathological states. Arch Gen Psychiatry 1970; 22: 149–59.

22. Kramer M, Roth T. Dreams in psychopathological groups: a critical review. In: Williams R, Karacan I, eds. Sleep Disorders: Diagnosis and Treatment. New York: Wiley, 1978: 323–49.

23. Kramer M, Roth T. Dreams in psychopathology. In: Wolman B, ed. Handbook of Dreams: Research, Theories and Applications. New York: Van Norstrand Reinhold, 1979: 361–87.

24. Kramer M. Dream content in psychiatric conditions: an overview of sleep laboratory studies. In: Perris C, Struwe G, Jansson B, eds. Biological Psychiatry 1981. New York: Elsevier/North-Holland, 1981: 306–9.

25. Mellen R, Duffey T, Craig S. Manifest content in the dreams of clinical population. J Mental Health Counseling 1993; 15: 170–83.

26. Benca R. Sleep in psychiatric disorders. Neurol Clin 1996; 14: 739–64.

27. American Psychiatric Association. Diagnostic and Statistical Manual of Mental Disorders, 4th edn (DSM-IV). Washington, DC: American Psychiatric Association Press, 1994.

28. Kramer M, Winget C, Whitman R. A city dreams: a survey approach to normative dream content. Am J Psychiatry 1971; 127: 1350–6.

29. Piccione P, Thomas S, Roth T, Kramer M. Incorporation of the laboratory situation in dreams. Sleep Res 1976; 5: 120 (abst).

30. Whitman R, Kramer M, Baldridge B. Which dream does the patient tell? Arch Gen Psychiatry 1963; 8: 277–82.

31. Goodenough D, Lewis H, Shapiro A, et al. Dream reporting following abrupt and gradual awakenings from different types of sleep. J Pers Soc Psychol 1965; 2: 170–9.

32. Clark J, Trinder J, Kramer M, et al. An approach to the content analysis of dream content scales. Sleep Res 1972; 1: 118 (abst).

33. Lesse S. Psychiatric symptoms in relationship to the intensity of anxiety. Psychother Psychosom 1974; 23: 94–102.

34. Freud S. Some Neurotic Mechanisms in Jealousy, Paranoia and Homosexuality. Volume XVIII of the Standard Edition. London: Hogarth Press, 1955.

35. Ushijima S. On recovery from the post psychotic collapse in schizophrenia. Jpn J Psychiat Neurol 1988; 42: 199–207.

36. Deutsch H. A case that throws light on the mechanism of regression in schizophrenia. Psychoanal Rev 1985; 72: 1–8.

37. Meloy J. Thought organization and primary process in the parents of schizophrenics. Br J Med Psychol 1984; 57: 279–81.

38. Wilmer H. Dream seminar for chronic schizophrenic patients. Psychiatry 1982; 45: 351–60.

39. Ohira K, Kato N, Namura I, et al. A psychopathology of schizophrenic dreaming: a feeling of passivity. Sleep Res 1979; 8: 170 (abst).

40. Van de Castle R. Manifest content of schizophrenic dreams. Sleep Res 1974; 3: 126 (abst).

41. Hadjez J, Stein D, Gabbay U, et al. Dream content of schizophrenic, nonschizophrenic mentally ill, and community control adolescents. Adolescence 2003; 38: 331–42.

42. Stompe T, Ritter K, Ortwein-Swoboda G, et al. Anxiety and hostility in the manifest dreams of schizophrenic patients. J Nerv Ment Dis 2003; 191: 806–12.

43. Jus A, Jus K, Villeneuve A, et al. Studies on dream recall in chronic schizophrenic patients after prefrontal lobotomy. Biol Psychiat 1973; 6: 275–93.

44. Solms M. The Neuropsychology of Dreams: A Clinico-Anatomical Study. Mahwah, NJ: Lawrence Erlbaum Associates, 1997.

45. Beauchemin K, Hays P. Prevailing mood, mood changes and dreams in bipolar disorder. J Affect Disord 1995; 35: 41–9.

46. Brenman E. Separation: a clinical problem. Int J Psychoanal 1982; 63: 303–10.

47. Mathew R, Largen J, Cleghorn J. Biological symptoms of depression. Psychosom Med 1979; 41: 439–43.

48. Levitan H. The relationship between mania and the memory of pain: a hypothesis. Bull Menninger Clin 1977; 41: 145–61.

49. Greenberg R, Pearlman C, Blacher R, et al. Depression: variability of intrapsychic and sleep parameters. J Am Acad Psychoanal 1990; 18: 233–46.

50. Beauchemin K, Hays P. Dreaming away depression: the role of REM sleep and dreaming in affective disorders. J Affect Disord 1996; 41: 125–33.

51. Barrett D, Loeffler M. Comparision of dream content of depressed versus non-depressed dreamers. Psychol Rep 1992; 70: 403–6.

52. Firth S, Blouin J, Natarajan C, et al. A comparison of the manifest content in dreams of suicidal, depressed and violent patients. Can J Psychiatry 1986; 31: 48–51.

53. Dow B, Kelsoe J, Gillen J. Sleep and dreams in Vietnam PTSD and depression. Biol Psychiatry 1996; 39: 42–50.

54. Cartwright R, Wood E. The contribution of dream masochism to the sex ratio difference in major depression. Psychiat Res 1993; 46: 165–73.

55. Riemann D, Low H, Schredl M, et al. Investigations of morning and laboratory dream recall and content in depressive patients during baseline conditions and under antidepressive treatment with trimipramine. Psychiat J Univ Ottawa 1990; 15: 93–9.

56. Cartwright R, Lloyd S, Knight S, et al. Broken dreams. A study of the effects of divorce and depression on dream content. Psychiatry 1984; 47: 251–9.

57. Trenholme I, Cartwright R, Greenberg G. Dream dimension differences during a life change. Psychiatry Res 1984; 12: 35–45.

58. Hauri P. Dreams of patients remitted from reactive depression. J Abn Psychol 1976; 85: 1–10.

59. Beck A. Depression: Clinical, Experimental and Theoretical Aspects. New York: Harper and Row, 1967.

60. Cartwright R. Dreams that work: the relation of dream incorporation to adaptation to stressful events. Dreaming 1991; 1: 3–9.

61. Strauch I, Meier B. In Search of Dreams: Results of Experimental Dream Research. Albany, NY: State University of New York Press, 1966: 234.

62. Kramer M. The selective mood regulatory function of dreaming: an update and revision. In: Moffitt A, Kramer M, Hofmann R, eds. The Functions of Dreaming. Albany, NY: State University of New York Press, 1993: 139–95.

63. Cartwright R, Young AM, Mercer P, et al. Role of REM sleep and dream variables in the prediction of remission from depression. Psychiatry Res 1998; 80: 249–55.

64. Armitage R, Rochlen A, Fitch T, et al. Dream recall and major depression: a preliminary report. Dreaming 1995; 5: 189–97.

65. Agargun YM, Cartwright R. REM sleep, dream variables and suicidality in depressed patients. Psychiatry Res 2003; 119: 33–9.

66. Erichson J. On Concussion of the Spine. New York: Bermingham, 1882. Cited In: Modlin H. Is there an Assault Syndrome? Bull Am Acad Psychiatry Law 1985; 13: 139–45.

67. Mellman T, Kulick-Bell R, Ashlock L, et al. Sleep events among veterans with combat-related post traumatic stress disorder. Am J Psychiatry 1995; 152: 110–15.

68. Ross R, Ball W, Sullivan K, et al. Sleep disturbances as the hallmark of post traumatic stress disorder. Am J Psychiatry 1989; 146: 697–707.

69. Reynold C. Sleep disturbance in post traumatic stress disorder: pathogenic or epiphenomenal? Am J Psychiatry 1989; 146: 695–6.

70. Ross R, Ball W, Sullivan K, et al. Sleep disturbance in post traumatic stress disorder. Am J Psychiatry 1990; 147: 374.

71. Kramer M. Dream disturbances. Psychiat Ann 1979; 9: 366–76.

72. Green B, Lindy J, Grace M. Post traumatic stress disorder: toward DSM IV. J Nerv Ment Dis 1985; 173: 406–11.

73. Brett E, Ostroff R. Imagery and post traumatic stress disorder: an overview. Am J Psychiatry 1985; 142: 417–24.

74. Fisher C, Kahn E, Edwards A, et al. A physiological study of nightmares and night terrors. J Nerv Ment Dis 1973; 2: 275–98.

75. Schlosberg A, Benjamin M. Sleep patterns in three acute combat fatigue cases. J Clin Psychiatry 1978; 39: 546–9.

76. Kramer M, Kinney L. Sleep patterns in trauma victims with disturbed dreaming. Psychiat J Univ Ottawa 1988; 13: 12–16.

77. Lansky M. Nightmares of a hospitalized rape victim. Bull Menninger Clin 1995; 59: 4–14.

78. Straker G. Integrating African and Western healing practices in South Africa. Am J Psychother 1994; 48: 455–67.

79. Lansky M. The transformation of affect in post traumatic nightmares. Bull Menninger Clin 1991; 55: 470–90.

80. Silvan-Adams A, Silvan M. 'A Dream is the fullfillment of a wish': traumatic dream, repetition compulsion and the Pleasure Principle. Int J Psychoanal 1990; 71: 513–22.

81. Modlin H. Is there an Assault Syndrome? Bull Am Acad Psychiatry Law 1985; 13: 139–45.

82. Van Dyke C, Zilberg N, McKinnon J. Post traumatic stress disorder: a thirty year delay in a World War II veteran. Am J Psychiatry 1985; 142: 1070–3.

83. Wells B, Chu C, Johnson R, et al. Buspirone in the treatment of post traumatic stress disorder. Pharmacotherapy 1991; 11: 340–3.

84. Siegel L. Holocaust survivors in Hasidic and Ultra-Orthodox Jewish populations. J Contemp Psychother 1980; 11: 5–31.

85. Dowling S. Dreams and dreaming in relation to trauma in childhood. Int J Psychoanal 1983; 63: 157–66.

86. de Saussure J. Dreams and dreaming in relation to trauma in childhood. Int J Psychoanal 1982; 63: 167–75.

87. Puk G. Treating traumatic memories: a case report on the eye movement desensitization procedure. J Behav Ther Exp Psychiatry 1991; 22: 149–51.

88. Schreuder J. Post traumatic re-experiencing in older people: working through or covering up? Am J Psychother 1996; 50: 231–42.

89. Helzer J, Robins L, McEvoy M. Post traumatic stress disorder in the general population: findings of the Epidemiologic Catchment Area Survey. N Engl J Med 1987; 317: 1630–4.

90. Watson I. Post traumatic stress disorder in Australian prisoners of the Japanese: a clinical study. Aust NZ J Psychiatry 1993; 27: 20–9.

91. Kuch K, Cox B. Symptoms of PTSD in 124 survivors of the Holocaust. Am J Psychiatry 1992; 149: 337–40.

92. Mollica R, Wyshak G, Lavelle J. The psychosocial impact of the war trauma and torture on Southeast Asian refugees. Am J Psychiatry 1987; 144: 1567–72.

93. Goldstein G, VanKammen W, Shelly C, et al. Survivors of imprisonment in the Pacific Theater during World War II. Am J Psychiatry 1987; 144: 1210–13.

94. Burstein A. Dream disturbances and flashbacks. J Clin Psychiatry 1984; 45: 46.

95. Woodward S, Arsenault E, Bliwise D, et al. The temporal distribution of combat nightmares in Vietnam combat veterans. Sleep Res 1991; 20: 152 (abst).

96. Woodward S, Arsenault E, Bliwise D, et al. Physical symptoms accompanying dream reports in combat veterans. Sleep Res 1991; 20: 153 (abst).

97. Horowitz M, Wilner N, Kaltreider N, et al. Signs and symptoms of post traumatic stress disorder. Arch Gen Psychiatry 1980; 37: 85–92.

98. Wilkinson C. Aftermath of a disaster: the collapse of the Hyatt Regency Hotel Skywalks. Am J Psychiatry 1983; 140: 1134–9.

99. Terr L. Children of Chowchilla. In: Solnit A, Eissler R, Freud A, Kris M, Neubauer P, eds. The Psychoanalytic Study of the Child. New Haven, CT: Yale University Press, 1979: 547–623.

100. Titchener J, Kapp F. Family and character change at Buffalo Creek. Am J Psychiatry 1976; 133: 295–9.

101. Brockway S. Group treatment of combat nightmares in post-traumatic stress disorder. J Contemp Psychother 1987; 17: 270–84.

102. Kramer M, Schoen L, Kinney L. Nightmares in Vietnam veterans. J Am Acad Psychoanal 1987; 15: 67–81.

103. Kinzie J, Sack R, Riley C. The polysomnographic effects of clonidine on sleep disorders in post traumatic stress disorder: a pilot study with Cambodian patients. J Nerv Ment Dis 1994; 182: 585–7.

104. Hefez A, Metz L, Lavie P. Long-term effects of extreme situational stress on sleep and dreaming. Am J Psychiatry 1987; 144: 344–7.

105. Fisher C, Byrne J, Edwards A, et al. A physiological study of nightmares. J Am Psychoanal Assoc 1970; 18: 747–82.

106. Dagan Y, Lavie P. Subjective and objective characteristics of sleep and dreaming in war related PTSD patients: lack of relationships. Sleep Res 1991; 20A: 270 (abst).

107. Deekin M, Bridenbaugh R. Depression and nightmares among Vietnam veterans in a military psychiatry outpatient clinic. Mil Med 1987; 152: 590–1.

108. van der Kolk B, Blitz R, Burr W, et al. Nightmares and trauma: a comparison of nightmares after combat with lifelong nightmares in veterans. Am J Psychiatry 1984; 14: 187–90.

109. Terr L. Life attitudes, dreams and psychic trauma in a group of 'normal' children. J Am Acad Child Psychiatry 1983; 22: 221–30.

110. Defazio V, Rustn S, Diamond A. Symptom development in Vietnam Era veterans. Am J Orthopsychiatry 1975; 45: 158–63.

111. Archibald H, Long D, Miller C, et al. Gross stress reaction in combat: a 15 year followup. Am J Psychiatry 1962; 119: 317–22.

112. Ross R, Ball W, Dinges D, et al. Rapid eye movement sleep disturbance in post traumatic stress disorder. Biol Psychiatry 1994; 35: 195–202.

113. Lavie P, Kaminer H. Dreams that poison sleep: dreaming in Holocaust survivors. Dreaming 1991; 1: 11–21.

114. Kramer M, Schoen L, Kinney L. The dream experience in dream-disturbed Vietnam veterans. In: van der Kolk B, ed. Post Traumatic Stress Disorders: Psychological and Biologic Sequelae. Washington, DC: American Psychiatric Association Press, 1984: 81–95.

115. Kellett S, Beail N. The treatment of chronic posttraumatic nightmares using psychodynamic–interpersonal psychotherapy: a single case study. Br J Med Psychol 1997; 70: 35–49.

116. Terr L. Chowchilla revisited: the effects of psychic trauma four years after a school-bus kidnapping. Am J Psychiatry 1983; 140: 1543–50.

117. Neylan T, Marmar C, Metzler M, et al. Sleep disturbances in the Vietnam Generation: findings from a nationally representative sample of male veterans. Am J Psychiatry 1998; 155: 929–33.

118. Shrestha N, Sharma B, Van Ommeren M, et al. Impact of torture on refugees within the Development World: symptomatology among Bhutanese refugees in Nepal. JAMA 1998; 280: 443–8.

119. Lavie P, Hertz G. Increased sleep motility and respiration rates in combat neurotic patients. Biol Psychiatry 1979; 14: 983–7.

120. Kramer M, Schoen L, Kinney L. Psychological and behavioral features of disturbed dreamers. Psychiat J Univ Ottawa 1984; 9: 102–6.

121. Schoen L, Kramer M, Kinney L. Arousal patterns in non-REM dream disturbed veterans. Sleep Res 1983; 12: 315 (abst).

122. Wilmer H. The healing nightmare: war dreams of Vietnam veterans. In: Barrett D, ed. Trauma and Dreams. Cambridge, MA: Harvard University Press, 1996: 92.

123. Schoen L, Kramer M, Kinney L. Auditory thresholds in the dream disturbed. Sleep Res 1984; 13: 102 (abst).

124. Dagan Y, Lavie P, Bleich A. Elevated awakening threshold in sleep stage 3–4 in war related posttraumatic stress disorder. Biol Psychiatry 1991; 30: 618–22.

125. Kramer M, Kinney L. Vigilance and avoidance during sleep in U.S. Vietnam War veterans with post traumatic stress disorder. J Nerv Mental Dis 2003; 191: 1–3.

126. Kinney L, Schoen L, Kramer M. Responsivity of night terror patients in sleep. Sleep Res 1983; 12: 193 (abst).

127. Schreuder BJ, van Egmond M, Klein WC, et al. Daily reports of posttraumatic nightmares and anxiety dreams in Dutch war victims. J Anxiety Disord 1998; 12: 511–24.

128. Esposito K, Benitez A, Barza L, et al. Evaluation of dream content in combat-related PTSD. J Trauma Stress 1999; 12: 681–7.

129. Taub J, Kramer M, Arand D, et al. Nightmare dreams and nightmare confabulations. Compr Psychiatry 1978; 19: 285–91.

130. Jackson C, Tabin J, Russell J, et al. Themes of death: Helmut Thoma's 'Anorexia Nervosa' (1967) – A Research Note. Int J Eat Disord 1993; 14: 433–7.

131. Jackson C, Beumont P, Thornton C, et al. Dreams of death: Von Weizsacker's dreams in so-called endogenic anorexia – A Research Note. Int J Eat Disord 1993; 13: 329–32.

132. Wilson C. Dream interpretation. In: Wilson C, ed. Fear of Being Fat: The Treatment of Anorexia Nervosa and Bulimia. New York: Jason Aronson, 1983: 245–54.

133. Wilson C. The fear of being fat and anorexia nervosa. Int J Psychoanal Psychother 1982/83; 9: 233–55.

134. Wells L. Anorexia nervosa: an illness of young adults. Psychiat Q 1980; 52: 270–82.

135. Sprince M. Early psychic disturbances in anorexic and bulimic patients as reflected in the psychoanalytic process. J Child Psychother 1984; 10: 199–215.

136. Levitan H. Implications of certain dreams reported by patients in a bulimic phase of anorexia nervosa. Can J Psychiatry 1981; 26: 228–31.

137. Hudson J, Bruch H, DeTrinis J, et al. Content analysis of dreams of anorexia nervosa patients. Sleep Res 1978; 7: 176 (abst).

138. Brink S, Allan J. Dreams of anorexic and bulimic women: a research study. J Anal Psychol 1992; 37: 275–97.

139. Frayn D. The incidence and significance of perceptual qualities in the reported dreams of patients with anorexia nervosa. Can J Psychiatry 1991; 36: 517–20.

140. Dippel B, Lauer C, Riemann D, et al. Psychother Psychosom 1987; 48: 165–9.

141. Stern B, Stern J. On the use of dreams as a means of diagnosis of brain injured patients. Scand J Rehab Med Suppl 1985; 12: 44–6.

142. Stern M, Stern B. Psychotherapy in cases of brain damage: a possible mission. Brain Injury 1990; 4: 297–304.

143. Benyakar M, Tadir M, Groswasser Z, et al. Dreams in head-injured patients. Brain Injury 1988; 2: 351–6.

144. Nathan R, Rose-Itkoff C, Lord G. Dreams, first memories and brain atrophy in the elderly. Hillside J Clin Psychiatry 1981; 3: 139–48.

145. Askenasy J, Gruskiewicz J, Braun J, et al. Repetitive visual images in severe war head injuries. Resuscitation 1986; 13: 191–201.

146. McCormik L, Nielsen M, Ptito M, et al. REM sleep dream mentation in right hemispherectomized patients. Neuropsychologia 1997; 35: 695–701.

147. Turner J, Graffam J. Deceased loved ones in the dreams of mentally retarded adults. Am J Ment Retard 1987; 92: 282–9.

148. Voelm C, Kossor M, Duran E. Dream work with the mentally retarded. Psychiat J Univ Ottawa 1988; 13: 85–90.

149. Cernovsky Z. MMPI and nightmares in male alcoholics. Percept Mot Skills 1985; 61: 841–2.

150. Cernovsky Z. MMPI and nightmare reports in women addicted to alcohol and other drugs. Percept Mot Skills 1986; 62: 717–18.

151. Fiss H. Dream content and response to withdrawal from alcohol. Sleep Res 1980; 9: 152 (abst).

152. Christo G, Franex C. Addicts' drug related dreams: their frequency and relationship to six-month outcomes. Substance Use Misuse 1996; 31: 1–15.

153. Denizen N. Alcoholic dreams. Alc Treat Q 1988; 5: 133–9.

154. Reid SD, Simeon DT. Progression of dreams of crack cocaine abusers as a predictor of treatment outcome: a preliminary report. J Nerv Ment Dis 2001; 189: 854–7.

155. Yee T, Perantie DC, Dhanani N, et al. Drug dreams in outpatients with bipolar disorder and cocaine dependance. J Nerv Ment Dis 2004; 192: 238–42.

156. Tart C. From spontaneous event to lucidity: a review of attempts to consciously control nocturnal dreaming. In: Wolman B, ed. Handbook of Dreams: Research, Theories and Applications. New York: Van Nostrand Reinhold, 1979: 226–68.

157. Kramer M, Whitman R, Baldridge B, et al. Patterns of dreaming: the interrelationship of the dreams of a night. J Nerv Ment Dis 1964; 139: 426–39.

158. Montangero J. Dream, problem solving and creativity. In: Corrado C, Foulkes D, eds. Dreaming as Cognition. New York: Harvester–Wheatsheaf, 1993: 93–113.

159. Cipolli C. The narrative structure of dreams: linguistic tools of analysis. In: Horne J, ed. Sleep 90. Bochum: Pontenagel Press, 1990: 281–4.

160. Koulack D. To Catch a Dream: Exploration of Dreaming. Albany, NY: State University of New York Press, 1991.

161. Kramer M, Kinney L, Scharf M. Dream incorporation and dream function. In: Koella W. Sleep 1982. Basel: S Karger, 1983: 369–71.

12

Sleep and headache disorders

Jeanetta C Rains, David M Biondi, Donald B Penzien, J Steven Poceta

INTRODUCTION

The association between sleep and headache disorders was recognized well over a century ago. Early observations described the influence of sleep in both provoking and relieving headaches.[1,2] For example, in 1871, Wright[1] in his headache textbook observed that, among other headache triggers, 'The causes that predispose to the occurrence of sick headache [include] insufficient sleep' (p 32) and 'waking from a deep sleep' (p 94). Wright also identified headache as a likely consequence of obstructive sleep apnea or obesity hypoventilation syndrome in his description of the 'predisposition to suffer from headaches' related to 'The habit of the body, age of the patient, with insufficient exercise, over-indulgence in sleep' (pp 71–72). Such early clinical observations foretold later research concerning sleep-related headache precipitants and headache secondary to sleep-disordered breathing.

Systematic research into sleep-related headache has lagged far behind clinical and anecdotal observations. It has only been within the last quarter-century that an empirical literature has emerged, chiefly comprising descriptive studies, parallel group comparisons, and single-group treatment outcome studies. Unfortunately, widely varying research methods, measures, and samples have yielded some inconsistencies in outcome and interpretation across studies. Reviewers agree that the specific nature, magnitude and underlying mechanisms of the relationship are not well defined.[3–12]

Paiva et al[7] proposed several hypothetical associations to account for the relationships between sleep and headache; Dodick et al[4] succinctly summarized these potential relationships (Table 12.1). Headache may be a cause as well as a consequence of sleep disorder or disturbance, and both may occur secondary to underlying medical illness or other pathologic conditions.

It is likely that the sources of sleep-related headache are multifactorial, and cases supporting each association may be found. The collective literature as discussed in this chapter reveals specific headache patterns potentially indicative of sleep disorders, suggests common anatomic structures and neurochemical processes involved in sleep and headache, and suggests the value of sleep regulation as a key component of head pain management for a substantial portion of headache sufferers.

Table 12.1 Potential relationship between headache and sleep[a]

- Headache is a symptom of a primary sleep disturbance
- Sleep disturbance is a symptom of a primary headache disorder
- Sleep disturbance and headache are symptoms of an unrelated medical disorder
- Sleep disturbance and headache are both manifestations of a similar underlying pathogenesis

[a]Reproduced from Dodick DW, et al. Headache 2003; 43: 282–92[4]

This chapter reviews the diagnosis and classification of sleep-related headache, the prevalence of the disorders, headache diagnosis-specific sleep parameters identified in research, potential physiologic mechanisms, and treatment implications, and discusses the limitations of existing research.

DIAGNOSIS AND CLASSIFICATION

International Classification of Headache Disorders, 2nd edition (ICHD-II)

The International Headache Society's ICHD-II[13] nosology includes two specific diagnoses for sleep-related headaches – 'Sleep apnea headache' and 'Hypnic headache' – and lists sleep disturbance among symptoms of anxiety disorders that may be associated with headache. Sleep apnea headache

(ICHD-II Code 10.1.3: Table 12.2) is coded as a subclassification of '10.1 Headache attributed to hypoxia or hypercapnia' under the major code heading '10. Headache attributed to disorders of homeostasis'. Although the category 'sleep apnea headache' was included in the original ICHD, the label was listed without diagnostic criteria. To our knowledge, these newly published diagnostic criteria have not been empirically validated and have rarely been applied in studies of sleep apnea headache. Although it appears that they may not have employed a strict application of the ICHD-II diagnostic criteria for sleep apnea headache diagnosis, Alberti et al[14] described a small sample of apneic patients with awakening headache, of whom only 7 of 19 patients fulfilled ICHD-II criterion A for sleep apnea headache (pressing quality, bilateral location, resolution ⩽30 minutes, and no

---

Table 12.2   ICHD-II diagnostic criteria for sleep apnea headache[a]

10.1.3 Sleep apnea headache

A. Recurrent headache with at least one of the following characteristics and fulfilling criteria C and D:
   1. Occurs on >15 days per month
   2. Bilateral, pressing quality and not accompanied by nausea, photophobia or phonophobia
   3. Each headache resolves within 30 minutes
B. Sleep apnea (respiratory disturbance index ⩾ 5) demonstrated by overnight polysomnography
C. Headache is present upon awakening
D. Headache ceases within 72 hours, and does not recur, after effective treatment of sleep apnea

4.5 Hypnic headache

Attacks of dull headache that always awaken the patient from sleep.

A. Dull headache fulfilling criteria B–D
B. Develops only during sleep and awakens patient
C. At least two of the following characteristics:
   1. Occurs >15 times per month
   2. Lasts ⩾15 minutes after waking
   3. First occurs after age of 50 years
D. No autonomic symptoms and no more than one of nausea, photophobia, or phonophobia
E. Not attributed to another disorder

[a]Reproduced from International Headache Society. Cephalalgia 2004; 24(Suppl 1): 1–151

accompanying symptoms). The remaining patients met criteria for migraine ($n = 1$), frequent episodic ($n = 8$), or chronic ($n = 3$) tension-type headache. Headache reportedly resolved in under 1 hour in only 26% of cases with headache on awakening, while meeting criterion A, #3 requires that headaches resolve within 30 minutes. Whether headaches resolved with treatment of sleep apnea (which is necessary to fulfill criterion D) was not reported as part of the study.

In the ICHD-II, 'Hypnic Headache' (ICHD-II Code 4.5: Table 12.2) is coded under the category of '4. Other primary headaches'. Hypnic headache occurs only during sleep and awakens the patient, is not associated with autonomic symptoms, and involves no more than one of the following: nausea, photophobia, or phonophobia. Hypnic headache diagnosis requires two of the following features: occurs at least 15 times per month; lasts more than 15 minutes (but usually less than 180); headache onset after age 50. This diagnosis was not included in the original ICHD, and although a series of case reports of patients meeting ICHD-II criteria for hypnic headache have now been published, the new criteria have yet to be empirically validated.

International Classification of Sleep Disorders, 2nd edition (ICSD-II)

The American Academy of Sleep Medicine's ICSD-II[15] categorizes 'Sleep-related headaches' among 'Sleep disorder associated with conditions classifiable elsewhere'. This denotes a small list of specific medical conditions that are not considered primary sleep disorders but are frequently a reason for referral to sleep specialists or encountered in the differential diagnosis of sleep disorders. The criteria for sleep-related headaches state: 'The patient complains of headache during sleep or upon awakening from sleep', and would include a variety of primary headache diagnoses such as migraine, cluster, chronic paroxysmal hemicrania, and hypnic headache, as well as headache associated with other medical and sleep disorders. Within ICSD-II, headache is also listed among associated

symptoms for sleep-related bruxism and physical symptoms occurring in response to sleep loss with insomnia. 'Morning headache' is listed among symptoms for sleep-related hypoventilation or hypoxemic syndromes and obstructive sleep apnea (pediatric).

'Exploding head syndrome' is classified under parasomnias by ICSD-II. Criteria for this diagnosis include waking from sleep or the wake–sleep transition with a sense of noise or explosion that is usually frightening to the patient, and is notable for the absence of pain. The syndrome is not included in ICHD-II headache diagnoses, but, despite the absence of pain, it is often described among rare or short-lived headache disorders, and may present to headache or sleep specialists.[16,17]

Comparing and contrasting ICHD-II and ICSD-II

The respective diagnostic nosologies for headache and sleep disorders both recognize and offer at least some provision for classification of sleep-related headaches. Both ICHD-II and ICSD-II recognize a potential association between headache and sleep-related breathing disorders. The terminology 'morning headache' (also known as awakening headache and nocturnal headache) is commonly employed in the sleep literature to refer to any headache temporally related to sleep, but it is a rarely found nomenclature in headache journals and other literature. Morning headache is not well defined with respect to headache features other than timing of the headache – this represents a challenge in equating headache diagnoses across the sleep and headache literatures. Future research and clinical management would benefit from further study and refinement of diagnostic provisions for this presentation of headache. ICSD-II accounts for the potential that primary headaches can be temporally related to sleep; under a categorization of 'sleep disorders associated with conditions classifiable elsewhere', ICSD-II would presumably lead the diagnostician to headache nosologies for specific headache diagnoses. Greater diagnostic precision is needed to better understand the association of sleep and various headaches in research and to direct clinicians to appropriate treatments in clinical practice.

PREVALENCE

Headache patient populations

A high prevalence of sleep disorders and sleep-related complaints has been observed in studies of headache patients. This evidence is derived from descriptive studies (with and without comparison groups as controls), and (although rarely) studies utilizing polysomnography to assess sleep. The largest clinical study published to date reported the prevalence of sleep complaints obtained from 1283 migraineurs presenting for headache treatment.[18] Within this migraine population, sleep disturbance and oversleeping were recognized as headache precipitants (i.e., headache triggers) by 50% and 37% of patients, respectively, while 85% reported sleeping as a means to relieve headache. Many patients reported difficulty initiating sleep (53%) and maintaining sleep (61%), at least occasionally. Morning headaches were reported by 71% of migraineurs. Although insomnia was not systematically assessed, chronically shortened sleep patterns similar to those characteristics of insomnia were observed in 38% of migraineurs (sleeping on average 6 hours or less per night). Shortened sleep patterns were associated with more frequent and more severe migraine.

In a clinical sample of 289 headache patients, Maizels and Burchette[19] observed a high prevalence of insomnia (60%) and fatigue (73%), and observed insomnia to be more common among patients with chronic versus episodic headache. Paiva et al[20] described sleep-related headache in 28 of 50 consecutive headache patients, with the large majority of patients reporting difficulty initiating (82.1%) and maintaining sleep (92.9%). The average nightly sleep duration for the entire sample was only 5.6 hours.

Relative to an age- and gender-matched comparison group (less than one headache per month), Spierings et al[21] found that headache patients presenting for specialty treatment slept significantly shorter durations (6.7 hours vs 7.0 hours), reported more difficulty initiating sleep (31.4 minutes vs 21.1 minutes), and took longer to fall back asleep after awakenings during the night (28.5 minutes vs 14.6 minutes). The study also observed that, as a group, only women with headache experienced fatigue of greater intensity than gender-matched controls, whereas men with headache reported more difficulty initiating sleep and falling back asleep after awakenings than controls. Although much less is known about pediatric than adult sleep-related headache, one study observed a significantly higher prevalence of insomnia, narcolepsy, and excessive daytime sleepiness among children with headache in a pediatric neurology clinic than in age- and sex-matched non-headache controls within the clinic.[22] Contradicting previous literature, however, Luc et al[22] did not observe a higher prevalence of sleep apnea, restlessness, and parasomnias among pediatric headache sufferers.

Paiva et al[7] reported results of polysomnography from 25 headache clinic patients complaining of morning headache. Sleep disorders were diagnosed in 13 of 25 patients, including obstructive sleep apnea (OSA), periodic limb movements and fibrositis. Paiva et al[23] extended this line of research and reported that 17% of headache clinic patients (49 of 288 patients) reported that headaches were sleep-related in at least 75% of headache episodes. Polysomnography revealed the presence of a primary sleep disorder (OSA, periodic limb movements, fibrositis, or psychophysiologic insomnia) in 53% of the 49 patients with sleep-related headache, in contrast with only 9% of the total sample. With the exception of the cases with periodic limb movements ($n = 8$), treatment of the primary sleep disorder resolved headache.

Collectively, these clinical studies of headache patients suggest that sleep complaints are common in this population. Although the full spectrum of sleep complaints has not generally been assessed, these studies tend to emphasize and report a high prevalence of insomnia among headache sufferers.

Sleep-disordered patient populations

This review identified only a single published study that examined the prevalence of headache in sleep-disordered patients representing the full range of sleep disorders. Goder et al[24] examined morning headaches in 432 sleep clinic patients who underwent polysomnography and 30 healthy controls. Polysomnographic recordings from nights before morning headache were compared with nights without subsequent headache. Patients with sleep disorders reported significantly more headaches than healthy controls (34% vs 7%). The study specifically examined the occurrence of tension-type headache the morning after polysomnographic recordings. Patients with migraine and other headaches that occurred during the night were not included, because the authors wished to exclude the direct adverse influence of pain on sleep architecture. Twenty-five percent (108/432) of sleep-disordered patients reported morning tension-type headache within 30 minutes of waking, compared with only 3% of controls. Any headache versus the specific description of 'morning headache after polysomnography', respectively, occurred in 27% versus 22% of patients with sleep breathing disorders, 28% versus 26% of patients with insomnia, 22% versus 19% of patients with restless legs, 50% versus 38% of patients with hypersomnia, 22% versus 15% of patients with parasomnias, and finally 46% versus 16% of patients with other sleep disorders. The occurrence of morning headache in the sleep laboratory was associated with decreases in total sleep time, sleep efficiency, and amount of rapid eye movement (REM) sleep and with an increase in the wake time during the preceding night, leading the authors to conclude that morning headaches in patients with sleep disorders might be associated with particular disturbances of the preceding night's sleep.

Headache has not commonly been described among sleep-disordered patients except specifically in relation to sleep-disordered breathing. Headache (not otherwise specified) in relation to OSA has been examined in a number of studies, with the occurrence of headache within this population varying widely from 15% to 60%.[25–28] Morning headache, although common among sleep disorders, appears most strongly associated with sleep apnea. Headache of any diurnal pattern was reported by 49% of apneics and 48% of insomniacs in the sleep clinic patient population, while 'morning headaches' were significantly more common among apneics (74%) than among insomniacs (40%).[14]

Epidemiologic studies

Several epidemiologic studies assessing sleep in relation to headache were identified. Ohayon[29] reported the findings of a European study of 18 980 telephone interviews estimating the prevalence of 'chronic morning headache' to be 7.6% (with chronic morning headache characterized as occurring 'daily', 'often', or 'sometimes'). Prevalence rates were higher in women than in men (8.4% vs 6.7%). More individuals with morning headache than individuals without headache reported sleep complaints; specific complaints included insomnia (odds ratio, OR, 2.1), circadian rhythm disorder (OR 1.97), loud snoring (OR 1.42), sleep-related breathing disorder (OR 1.51), nightmares (OR 1.39), and other dyssomnia (OR 2.30). Odds ratios were greater for all sleep disorders except insomnia, when the data were reanalyzed in a model that only used information obtained from individuals with 'daily' morning headache. Significant comorbidities were identified between headache and major depression alone (OR 2.70), anxiety alone (OR 1.98), and the combination of both 'depression and anxiety disorders' (OR 3.51). Not surprisingly, heavy alcohol use was also associated with morning headache (OR 1.83). In contrast, morning headaches were not associated with caffeine use, as those who did not drink coffee exhibited greater morning headache than those who drank at least one cup per day; this argues against the hypothesis that morning headache was attributable to caffeine withdrawal among this large sample.

In a large cross-sectional epidemiologic study of headache disorders, Rasmussen[30] examined the prevalence of sleep complaints among persons with migraine and tension-type headache relative to the general population. Sleep complaints were more common among tension-type than migraine headache sufferers and the population at large. Non-refreshing sleep was associated with migraine for both males and females, and with tension-type headache among females. Snoring was associated with migraine in women only. Onset of headache usually occurred during sleep or upon awakening for 24% of migraineurs and 12% of tension headache, with morning headache occurring more commonly among individuals having migraine than tension headache.

In establishing the diagnosis of sleep-disordered breathing, snoring is considered a *sensitive* though not *specific* indicator for sleep apnea in epidemiologic research. A large cross-sectional study of Danish middle-aged and elderly males identified a strong statistical relationship between snoring and non-specific headache (i.e., having any form of headache).[31,32] Considering both females and males, a Swedish study combining epidemiologic and sleep clinic data reported that headache occurred more commonly among patients with heavy snoring and sleep apnea than among the general population.[33] Morning headache, in particular, was reported by 18% of snorers and apneics versus only 5% of controls. In a case–control epidemiologic survey conducted within the USA, Scher et al[34] compared the prevalence of snoring in a group of chronic daily headache sufferers ($n = 206$) with a group of episodic headache sufferers ($n = 507$). Habitual snoring was more common among chronic daily than among episodic headache sufferers (24% vs 14%, respectively), leading the authors to speculate that sleep disorders may provide a target for intervention for some patients with chronic daily headache. Conversely, in Australia, Olson et al[35] found that morning headaches were not related to apneics (based on questionnaire and respiratory home monitoring) compared with snorers (OR 0.2) or non-snorers (OR 0.1).

These data are correlative in nature and do not address causality. However, the findings are consistent with a hypothesis that headache, particularly morning headache and chronic headache, is a potential consequence of sleep-disordered breathing or of another related and covarying function.

MEASUREMENT OF SLEEP

Polysomnography

The gold standard of objective sleep measurement is polysomnography, with its full overnight assessment of multiple physiologic parameters, including sleep, breathing, cardiac, movement, etc.[36] Testing is usually attended, laboratory-based, under continuous visual surveillance via closed-circuit television, and videotaped. Daytime sleepiness under similar controls is quantified by the Multiple Sleep Latency Test (MSLT), while the ability to remain awake may be assessed with the Maintenance of Wakefulness Test (MWT).[37] All are well-validated objective measures of sleep and wakefulness under standardized conditions with available normative data for a variety of sleep-disordered populations and normal controls. Typically, polysomnography is necessary to document the extent and severity of sleep-disordered breathing and parasomnias. Movement disorders such as restless legs syndrome and periodic limb movement disorder sometimes require polysomnography to ascertain impact on sleep and to guide therapy. Narcolepsy is typically diagnosed after polysomnography and MSLT. MWT is most often used to formally assess alertness after treatment of a sleep disorder that may impair alertness. When headache is evaluated in relation to sleep, polysomnography can indicate the timing, specific sleep stage, and antecedent events of the headache. Limited-channel EEG cassette recordings may be used to assess sleep parameters only.[38]

Actigraphy

This activity monitor or motion detector has been used to infer sleep and waking states based on activity level.[39] The patient wears a small wristwatch-like recording device that records and stores activity data, which are later downloaded for evaluation. Sleep is inferred by extended periods of inactivity so that approximate sleep time can be determined for patients who are relatively inactive during sleep and maintain a normal activity level while awake. Actigraphy may be a cost-effective tool for validating self-report diary data and measuring the timing and duration of sleep in circadian rhythm disorders and insomnia over days or weeks. Statistical correlations for actigraphy with 1 night of polysomnography varied by the sleep variable of interest, such as time in bed ($r = 0.99$), total sleep time ($r = 0.68$), sleep onset ($r = 0.87$), wake after sleep onset ($r = 0.69$), total wake time ($r = 0.74$), and sleep efficiency ($r = 0.67$).[40] Actigraphy has been employed in migraine research,[41,42] although rarely.

Questionnaires

A wide variety of questionnaires are available to assess sleep disorders, sleep quality, daytime sleepiness, sleep-related psychosocial functioning, impairment, and quality of life. Questionnaires vary in level of psychometric development, and are reviewed elsewhere.[43,44] Interestingly, validated questionnaires have rarely been utilized in studies of sleep-related headaches.

Sleep diary

Paper and pencil and electronic sleep diaries are probably the most commonly used systematic self-report tools for sleep assessment. With once-a-day monitoring, subjective estimates can be obtained over time in the regularity, duration, and quality of sleep. Typical findings of general interest are latency to sleep onset, number and duration of nocturnal awakenings, total sleep time relative to time in bed (i.e., sleep efficiency), sleep quality ratings, daytime sleepiness and alertness, and napping. Monitoring can also include other specific variables that are potentially related to sleep, such as headache (combined headache/sleep diary). Interestingly, sleep diaries are seldom employed in headache research, although headache diaries are commonly used and familiar tools for headache research.

HEADACHE DIAGNOSIS – SPECIFIC REVIEW

Migraine

Migraine, to some degree, has been examined in relation to sleep stage, circadian patterns, and sleep-related precipitants. Early studies using polysomnography associated migraine (and cluster headache) with REM sleep.[45,46] Dexter[47] later examined polysomnography in five patients with migraine reporting sleep as a precipitant of headache. An association was found between migraine and REM sleep as well as slow-wave sleep (sleep stages 3 and 4, delta sleep). More recently, using 4-channel EEG recordings, Drake et al[38] observed minimal sleep disturbance between patients with episodic migraine between attacks, with only modestly increased REM latencies and proportions. In contrast, they observed patients with tension headaches had significant sleep disturbances (i.e., reduced sleep time and sleep efficiency, decreased sleep latency but frequent awakenings, increased nocturnal movements, and marked reduction in slow-wave sleep) without change in REM sleep or latency. Patients with chronic headache with mixed features of migraine and tension headache likewise had significant sleep disturbance (i.e., reduced sleep time, increased awakenings, and diminished slow-wave sleep), but with REM sleep that was decreased in amount and reduced in latency. Drake et al[38] speculated that the chronic forms of headache may be worsened by chronically poor sleep. It is unclear why they chose not to speculate about the converse (i.e., that chronically poor sleep may be a consequence of chronic headache).

A prospective longitudinal study examined migraine chronobiology over a 3-year period in 1698 migraineurs (3582 migraine attacks).[48] Nearly half of all migraine attacks occurred between the hours of 4 AM and 9 AM. Interestingly, this period of time would typically encompass the later stages of the sleep cycle, where the longest and most dense REM sleep would normally dominate, and the early waking hours of the day. Migraine has been observed to have a greater than expected prevalence in some individuals having specific sleep disorders. Narcolepsy, a disorder of REM sleep, has been linked to migraine.[49,50] In a study of 100 confirmed narcoleptics, the prevalence of migraine was two- to fourfold greater in narcoleptics than would be expected based on migraine prevalence in the general population.

Headache may be precipitated, or 'triggered', by dysregulation of sleep patterns. Among patients with migraine (and tension-type headache), changes in sleep patterns (e.g., sleep disturbance, sleep loss, and oversleeping) are routinely listed among the most commonly observed precipitants of headache.[18–20,51–56] A polysomnographic study demonstrated that sleep on nights preceding migraine attacks was characterized by findings of decreased cortical activation during sleep (i.e., fewer arousals, decreased REM density, decreased beta power in slow-wave sleep, and decreased alpha in the first REM period).[57] A study of pediatric migraine using actigraphy found decreased motor activity on nights preceding migraine relative to controls and nights not followed by migraine.[41]

In addition to acting as a potential precipitant to headache, sleep has been demonstrated to be a palliative treatment for migraine headache. Migraine attacks are often relieved by overnight sleep or a daytime nap,[18,47,57,58] particularly in children.[59,60]

Tension-type headache

Relative to migraine, tension-type headache has only been rarely assessed with respect to sleep. In the EEG study by Drake et al[38] referred to above, the investigators examined the recordings of patients with episodic and chronic tension headache as well as migraine. Notably, subjects with tension headache did not exhibit the changes in REM sleep or latency that were noted in migraineurs, but did exhibit reduced sleep time and sleep efficiency, decreased sleep latency, frequent awakenings, increased nocturnal movements, and marked reduction in slow-wave sleep.

Similar to a pattern that is well established in migraine, sleep dysregulation may precipitate tension headache. Houle et al[55] observed in a time-series fashion that both short (<6 hours) and long sleep periods (>8.5 hours) were associated with more occurrences of tension headache. Other studies have similarly related sleep disturbance to tension headache.[20,21,56,61]

Cluster headache

Cluster headache has an estimated prevalence of less than 1% of the population.[62] Seventy-five percent of cluster headache episodes were found to occur between the hours of 9 PM and 10 AM.[63] Cluster headache has been specifically associated with REM sleep and sleep-disordered breathing. A study of 37 cluster headache patients who underwent polysomnography identified an 8.4-fold increase in the incidence of obstructive sleep apnea relative to age and gender-matched controls (58% vs 14%, respectively) and this risk increased over 24-fold among patients with a body mass index (BMI) >25.[64] Another uncontrolled study of 31 cluster headache patients who underwent polysomnography observed OSA in 80% (25/31).[65] A marked increase in the incidence of sleep-disordered breathing had been noted in earlier research,[66,67] and treatment of sleep apnea had been observed to improve cluster headache control.[66,68] Cluster headache attacks that have occurred during polysomnographic recordings have been linked to REM sleep, at least in cases of episodic cluster,[47] although perhaps not for patients having the chronic form[69] of cluster headache. Available evidence indicates a marked increased incidence of sleep-disordered breathing among cluster patients,[66,67] and that treatment of the apnea can improve this form of headache.[66,68]

Chronic paroxysmal hemicrania

Chronic paroxysmal hemicrania (CPH)[13] is a variant of cluster headache, but with female preponderance, more frequent headache attacks, and attacks of shorter duration. CPH is characterized by disproportionately nocturnal attacks.[70] Like cluster headache, CPH can have predictable nocturnal patterns and has been associated with REM sleep; because of this pattern, it is sometimes referred to as an 'REM-locked' headache disorder.[71,72]

Hypnic headache

This form of headache is relatively rare and is, by definition, confined to sleep. Its true prevalence in the population is not known, but it is estimated to occur in only 0.07–0.1% of patients seen in a specialty headache clinic setting.[73,74] Hypnic headaches tend to occur in the middle or later portion of the night, with patients being abruptly awakened with pain. A meta-analysis pooled data from the 71 cases of hypnic headache found published in medical literature.[74] The average duration of hypnic headache was 67 ± 44 minutes (range 15–180 minutes), and the frequency of attacks was 1.2 ± 0.9 per 24 hours. The majority (77%) reported the onset of headache between 120 and 480 minutes after sleep onset. Polysomnography was available for seven of the published cases. There were only four occurrences of headache during polysomnography; among these four cases, three episodes emerged from REM sleep and one from slow-wave sleep. Manni et al[75] observed polysomnography in 10 hypnic headache sufferers; for the five patients (6 headache episodes) in whom headache occurred during polysomnography, two episodes occurred in REM and four in non-REM (NREM) sleep stages (two during stage 2 and two during stage 3 headache). A few cases have reported an association between hypnic

headaches and sleep disorders such as decreased sleep efficiency, restless legs, snoring, and sleep apnea.[74]

Morning headache

Although not a formal diagnosis, morning headache is probably the most common form of headache studied in relation to sleep and usually in relation to sleep-disordered breathing. As noted above, between 15% and 60% of sleep apneics report morning headaches.[7,14,23,25–28,67,76,77] The pathogenic basis of morning headache was initially presumed to be a consequence of abnormal respiration (e.g., hypoxemia or hypercapnia). This hypothesis would be supported by polysomnographic research yielding a dose–response relationship between the severity of sleep apnea (e.g., number of apneic events and severity of nocturnal oxygen desaturation) and severity of morning headache;[14,28] resolution or improvement in headache following treatment of sleep apnea with non-invasive positive pressure ventilation treatment or surgical modification of the upper airway to improve breathing;[23,27,66,68,78,79] and a higher incidence of morning headache in apneics than in similarly sleep-disturbed insomniacs.[14]

Although evidence associating headache with sleep-disordered breathing via respiratory dysfunction appears compelling, contradicting studies dispute this hypothesis.[80–82] In some cases, morning headache was observed to be more common among patients with non-respiratory sleep disorders such as periodic limb movements.[26] A study evaluated 432 patients with various sleep disorders by using data obtained from two nights of polysomnography, and compared these results with data obtained from 30 healthy controls.[83] Individuals with sleep apnea exhibited a higher occurrence of morning headache than did controls. However, patients with sleep disorders other than apnea had higher occurrence of morning headache, and the apneics with headache in this study generally had milder headache conditions. Analysis of the sleep parameters for nights associated with morning

Table 12.3 Potential mechanisms for morning headache in sleep-disordered breathing

- Hypoxemia and hypercapnic vasodilatation
- Autonomic surges and blood pressure dysregulation associated with resuscitative arousals
- Sleep dysregulation (sleep fragmentation, sleep-stage alteration, sleep deprivation) from resuscitative arousals
- Increased intracranial pressure during apneas
- Daytime sleepiness and fatigue
- Changes in head and neck position, with altered muscle tension and afferent activity

headache compared with nights not associated with morning headache indicated that morning headache was directly associated with decreased total sleep time, lower sleep efficiency, and lower amounts of REM.

In summary, although clinical observations and a meager body of clinical research have established a relationship between sleep-disordered breathing and headache, the pathophysiologic mechanisms of this relationship are still generally unknown. It is not clear if the pathogenic basis of this association is related to a *specific* respiratory mechanism, a *nonspecific* consequence of the sleep disorder (i.e., autonomic arousal, sleep dysregulation/deprivation, intracranial cerebrospinal fluid pressure changes, or cervical/cranial muscle tension), or a complex combination of these factors (Table 12.3).

Exploding head syndrome

Considered rare and benign[84] and probably a sleep rather than a headache disorder, exploding head syndrome has been seldom studied. In one study of nine patients with a history of the syndrome using polysomnographic recordings, five patients reported the sensation of 'explosions' during the recording period, and in each case the EEG demonstrated that the patients were awake and relaxed. Two attacks were characterized by EEG arousals, while no EEG changes were observed in

the remaining three. No epileptiform activity was recorded in any case.[85]

MECHANISMS

The convergence of sleep and headache disorders is generally believed to have its basis in neuro-anatomic connections and neurophysiologic mechanisms, involving especially the hypothalamus, serotonin, and perhaps melatonin.[4] Wakefulness depends principally on the functioning of the reticular activating system in the brainstem, maintained by influences of cortical neurotransmitters such as norepinephrine (noradrenaline), dopamine, and acetylcholine. NREM sleep is primarily controlled by influences from the basal forebrain, with NREM sleep functions maintained by γ-aminobutyric acid (GABA) from basal forebrain neurons. REM sleep-generating processes have been localized within the dorsolateral pontine tegmentum. REM sleep is initiated by release of acetylcholine, which activates pontine neurons. Serotonin is abundant in the dorsal raphe nuclei and has a well-established but incompletely delineated role in acute migraine. The trigeminal nucleus caudalis in the pons and midbrain has been considered to be a potential 'migraine generator' by some researchers, since there appears to be activation of vascular structures supplied by this nucleus during migraine attacks.[86,87] However, many migraine symptoms, especially those associated with prodrome and aura, are more likely to be the result of hypothalamic or cerebral cortical activity, and include clinical features such as yawning, hunger, cravings, fatigue, mood changes, and sensory and visual distortions. The hypothalamus, which is the location of the suprachiasmatic nuclei, has extensive connections, some of which include connections to the limbic system, pineal gland (a source of neuronal melatonin), and brainstem nuclei involved in autonomic efferent control (nucleus tractus solitarius), sleep stage and motor control (locus ceruleus), and pain modulation (periaquaductal gray matter). The hypothalamus has exhibited specific activation during cluster headache attacks.[88] Melatonin is well established as a factor in circadian rhythmicity, and might have therapeutic efficacy in cluster headache.[89,90] Further study of headache syndromes that exhibit chronobiologic patterns, such as cluster headache, have the most potential to provide a clearer understanding of the anatomic and physiologic links between headache and sleep.

CLINICAL IMPLICATIONS

While there are no empirically established algorithms to guide clinical practice, there are now at least a few empirically supported tenets. The review provided in this chapter suggests the following:

- Morning headache is a particular although non-specific indicator for sleep disorders.

- The identification and management of a primary sleep disorder in the presence of headache may improve or resolve the headache (headache secondary to primary sleep disorder).

- Headache patients exhibit a high incidence of sleep disturbance, which might trigger or exacerbate headache.

- Headache may improve with regulation of sleep.

- Sleep efficiency might improve with effective headache control.

For headache practitioners, several sources[3,7,8,11] have emphasized the merits of a thorough clinical interview examining the headache pattern and history in relation to the sleep/wake cycle. When headache frequently occurs during or after sleep onset or upon awakening, it is prudent to screen for presence of significant sleep disorder or disturbance. The identification of obstructive sleep apnea or other sleep-related breathing abnormalities is particularly important because of the potential for headache to improve with treatment of the apnea[23,27,28,66,68,78,79] as well as to avert the significant morbidity and mortality associated with sleep apnea.[91] Clinical symptoms[92] and risk factors[93,94] for OSA are presented in Table 12.4. An overweight headache sufferer, such as those with a BMI ≥ 25, awakening with headache should particularly be questioned about snoring and other symptoms of sleep apnea.[64] Adding to the conundrum are observations that obesity might also be a risk factor for the transformation of episodic headache to chronic headache forms, thereby creating a potentially adverse influence on sleep efficiency and a vicious cycle of headache and sleep disturbance.[95]

Table 12.4   Obstructive sleep apnea: signs and symptoms

Clinical symptoms	Risk factors
• Habitual snoring	• Obesity (increased body mass index, neck, chest, waist, hips)
• Wake gasping	• Male gender (male preponderance less in elderly)
• Witnessed apnea	• Age (positive correlation)
• Morning headache	• Family history
• Hypersomnia or insomnia	• Craniofacial morphology and oral anatomy
• Night sweats	• Neuromuscular disorders
• Nocturia	• Substances (e.g., tobacco, alcohol, sedatives)

The probable presence of OSA, hypersomnia, and other sleep disorders warrants referrals for polysomnographic confirmation of the diagnosis and initiation of appropriate treatment. Identification and management of primary sleep disorders can be crucial not only for optimal head pain management but also for managing the often substantial medical consequences of the sleep disorders themselves. Reevaluation of the headache 1 month following the initiation of treatment for the sleep disorders is recommended. Notably, morning headache related to sleep apnea might present as tension-type, migraine, cluster, or other non-specific headaches.[14]

Sleep disturbances may trigger or exacerbate headache, and therefore identification of sleep-related triggers may facilitate management of primary headache disorders.[18–21,51–53,55,56] Headache triggers are probably most accurately identified by prospective self-monitoring, because patients are often unaware of behavioral and psychosocial precipitants. Headache diaries can be highly informative for patients and clinicians to identify previously unrecognized headache patterns and precipitants. Figure 12.1 shows a headache diary structured to identify sleep patterns and disturbance as well as a wide range of other common headache triggers (see the Appendix for patient instructions). The diary yields information concerning regularity of the sleep/wake cycle, disorders of sleep onset and maintenance, total sleep time and efficiency, napping, etc. Sleep disturbance can be treated with behavioral sleep management and pharmacologic therapy, with outcomes being monitored in the headache diary over time. Sleep patterns may impact the choice of prophylactic headache treatments, with more sedating agents being preferred in cases of insomnia and more alerting or neutral agents for hypersomnolent headache patients.[3,8,11] Behavioral and psychosocial factors that can trigger or exacerbate both headache and sleep disorders (e.g., stress, caffeine use, and lifestyle) also warrant careful assessment, and may prove important targets for treatment for patients with sleep-related headaches.

LIMITATIONS OF THE RESEARCH LITERATURE

The evidence base concerning sleep and headache is characterized by significant methodologic limitations that probably account, at least in part, for inconsistent results identified in the literature described above. These limitations are wide-ranging and encompass such concerns as lack of standard criteria to determine headache and sleep disorder diagnoses, inappropriate research design, inadequate sampling methods, lack of objective outcome measures, and inconsistencies in data reporting. Historically, the nosologies to diagnose sleep-related headaches have provided little guidance. Although improved over earlier versions, even the revised editions of ICHD-II and ICSD-II have not been empirically validated and continue to be imprecise in their provisions for sleep-related headache and not particularly consistent with each other. Many studies have reported no formal headache diagnosis so as to allow a comparison of symptoms and outcomes across studies. The popular terminology 'morning headache' likely includes many different forms of headache with varying pathophysiologies, and introduces substantial variance into the research equation.

Research methods have varied widely across studies, and sampling methods and study populations are often not well described. Earlier studies, in particular, employed very small and selected diagnostic groups rather than larger unselected samples of headache patients or the general population. A small number of subjects might be unavoidable in some circumstances because of the rarity of certain disorders (e.g., hypnic headache and chronic paroxysmal hemicrania). However, it is a more common circumstance that a clinical study was designed to employ samples of convenience, which are unlikely to adequately represent the population and phenomenon of interest. Many studies report single-group outcomes, and few have employed rigorous controls.

Many of the available studies have relied on unsystematically collected and subjective data.

DAILY HEADACHE SELF-MONITORING FORM

NAME:

SOCIAL SECURITY NUMBER:

PATIENT ID NUMBER:

DIRECTIONS: Four times each day, please rate your headache intensity, disability level, and stress using the rating scales below. Mark the times that you were sleeping and eating by coloring (or putting x) in the boxes. You may indicate ½ hour increments by coloring ½ of a box (or use slash). Also, record body temperature, whether menstruating, and rating of sleep amount and sleep quality.

HEADACHE INTENSITY

10 EXTREMELY PAINFUL....My headache is so painful that I can't do anything
9
8 VERY PAINFUL............My headache makes concentration difficult, but i can perform demanding tasks.
7
6 PAINFUL....................My headache is painful, but i can continue what i am doing.
5
4 MILDLY PAINFUL...........I can ignore my headache most of the time.
3
2 SLIGHTLY PAINFUL.......I only notice my headache when I focus my attention on it.
1
0 NO HEADACHE

DISABILITY

10 COMPLETELY IMPAIRED (Bedrest)
9
8 SEVERELY IMPAIRED
7
6 MODERATELY IMPAIRED
5
4 MILDLY IMPAIRED
3
2 MINIMALLY IMPAIRED
1
0 NO IMPAIRMENT

STRESS

10 EXTREMELY
9
8 VERY
7
6 MODERATELY
5
4 MILDLY
3
2 SLIGHTLY
1
0 NO STRESS

SLEEP AMOUNT

10 TOO MUCH
9
8
7
6
5 PERFECT
4
3
2
1
0 TOO LITTLE

SLEEP QUALITY

10 EXCELLENT
9
8 VERY GOOD
7
6 GOOD
5
4 FAIR
3
2 POOR
1
0 VERY POOR

WEEKLY MEDICATION LIST (AND AMOUNT):

	12a	1a	2a	3a	4a	5a	6a	7a	8a	9a	10a	11a	12p	1p	2p	3p	4p	5p	6p	7p	8p	9p	10p	11p
MONDAY DATE:																								
HEADACHE:																								
DISABILITY:																								
STRESS:																								
SLEEP:																								
MEAL/SNACK:																								

TEMP

MENSES Y - N

SLEEP AMOUNT

SLEEP QUALITY

COMMENTS:

MEDICATION (AND AMOUNT):

Figure 12.1 Headache diary: daily headache monitoring in relation to precipitants – sleep, stress, meals, menstruation (reproduced from Rhudy JL, Penzien DB, Rains JC. Self-Management Training Program for Chronic Headache: Therapist Manual, 2006, with permission from the authors)

The studies that did use objective polysomno-graphic data to quantify measures of sleep have tended to include small numbers of subjects. In other studies that did include a larger number of subjects, the polysomnographic data were often collected for other clinical purposes and not specif-ically in a study that was prospectively designed to evaluate the associations of sleep and headache. No doubt, this limitation is an unfortunate con-sequence of the substantial costs and labor involved in conducting polysomnography. While there are cost-competitive tools available, such as actigraphy and EEG cassette recordings, these have rarely been employed. Even very low-cost tools, such as standardized questionnaires and dia-ries, have been rarely utilized in this field of study. Finally, reporting of results, as in many areas of research, has been highly variable. A research base with commonly inconsistent diagnoses, low statis-tical power, skewed populations, multiple sources of variance, limited controls, and often lacking objective measurement and inconsistent reporting, is likely to yield the contradictory outcomes and interpretations observed in the review provided by this chapter.

CONCLUSIONS

The association between headache and sleep has been long recognized in the medical literature, but is still not well understood. Although few clini-cians would dispute the substantial comorbidity of headache and sleep disorders, the nature, extent, and causes of this comorbidity are debated. The empirical literature has yielded inconsistencies and, in some cases, highly divergent outcomes, no doubt due in part to methodologic limitations among studies comprising the evidence base (e.g., imprecise diagnoses, small numbers of subjects, varied sampling methods, lack of objective sleep measures, other non-standardized measures, and inconsistent reporting). It is highly probable that the pathogenic sources of sleep-related headache

are multifactorial and stem from the involvement of common neuroanatomic structures and neuro-physiologic processes. With rapid scientific advan-ces and the growth in knowledge regarding the complex interrelationships of functional ana-tomic, neurologic, and molecular processes occur-ring over the last decade, there is great promise that future research specifically designed to exam-ine and better understand the associations of headache and sleep disorders is close at hand. Regardless, there are now at least a few empirically supported tenets to guide clinicians in identifying headache that is a consequence of primary sleep disorders, identifying sleep variables that may impact headache threshold, and thereby provi-ding a means by which to improve headache management.

REFERENCES

1. Wright H. Headaches: Their Causes and Their Cures. Philadelphia, PA: Lindsay & Blakiston, 1871.
2. Liveing E. On Megrim, Sick-Headache, and Some Allied Disorders: A Contribution to the Pathology of Nervous Storms. London: Churchill, 1873.
3. Biondi DM. Headaches and their relationship to sleep. Dent Clin North Am 2001; 45: 685–700.
4. Dodick DW, Eross EJ, Parish JM. Clinical, anato-mical, and physiologic relationship between sleep and headache. Headache 2003; 43: 282–92.
5. Jennum P, Jensen R. Sleep and headache. Sleep Med Rev 2002; 6: 471–9.
6. Moldofsky H. Sleep and pain. Sleep Med Rev 2001; 5: 385–96.
7. Paiva T, Batista A, Martins P, Martins A. The rela-tionship between headaches and sleep disturbances. Headache 1995; 35: 590–6.
8. Poceta JS. Sleep-related headache. Curr Treat Options Neurol 2002; 4: 121–8.
9. Poceta JS. Sleep-related headache syndromes. Curr Pain Headache Rep 2003; 7: 281–7.
10. Rains JC, Penzien DB. Chronic headache and sleep dis-turbance. Curr Pain Headache Rep 2002; 6: 498–504.
11. Rains JC, Poceta JS. Sleep-related headache syn-dromes. In: Avidan AY, ed. Seminars in Neurology, Vol 25. New York: Thieme, 2005; 69–80.

12. Sahota PK, Dexter JD. Sleep and headache syndromes: a clinical review. Headache 1990; 30: 80–4.

13. International Headache Society. International Classification of Headache Disorders, Second Edition. Cephalalgia 2004; 24(Suppl 1): 1–151.

14. Alberti A, Mazzotta G, Gallinella E, Sarchielli P. Headache characteristics in obstructive sleep apnea and insomnia. Acta Neurol Scand 2005; 111: 309–16.

15. American Academy of Sleep Medicine. International Classification of Sleep Disorders, 2nd edn: Diagnostic and Coding Manual. Westchester, IL: American Academy of Sleep Medicine, 2005.

16. Rozen TD. Short-lasting headaches syndromes and treatment options. Curr Pain Headache Rep 2004; 8: 268–73.

17. Casucci G, d'Onofrio F, Torelli P. Rare primary headaches: clinical insights. Neurol Sci 2004; 25: S77–83.

18. Kelman L, Rains JC. Headache and sleep: examination of sleep patterns and complaints in a large clinical sample of migraineurs. Headache 2005; 45: 904–10.

19. Maizels M, Burchette R. Somatic symptoms in headache patients: the influence of headache diagnosis, frequency, and comorbidity. Headache 2004; 44: 983–93.

20. Paiva T, Esperanca P, Martins I, Batista A, Martins P. Sleep disorders in headache patients. Headache Q 1992; 3: 438–42.

21. Spierings EL, van Hoof MJ. Fatigue and sleep in chronic headache sufferers: an age- and sex-controlled questionnaire study. Headache 1997; 37: 549–52.

22. Luc ME, Gupta A, Brinberg JM, Reddick D, Kohrman MH. Characterization of symptoms of sleep disorders in children with headache. Pediatr Neurol 2006; 34: 7–12.

23. Paiva T, Farinha A, Martins A, Batista A, Guilleminault C. Chronic headaches and sleep disorders. Arch Intern Med 1997; 157: 1701–5.

24. Goder R, Friege L, Fritzer G, et al. Morning headaches in patients with sleep disorders: a systematic polysomnographic study. Sleep Med 2003; 4: 385–91.

25. Guilleminault C, Eldridge FL, Tilkian A, Simmons FB, Dement WC. Sleep apnea due to upper airway obstruction: a review of 25 cases. Arch Intern Med 1977; 137: 296–300.

26. Aldrich MS, Chauncey JB. Are morning headaches part of obstructive sleep apnea syndrome? Arch Intern Med 1990; 150: 1265–7.

27. Poceta JS, Dalessio DJ. Identification and treatment of sleep apnea in patients with chronic headache. Headache 1995; 35: 586–9.

28. Loh NK, Dinner DS, Foldvary N, Skobieranda F, Yew WW. Do patients with obstructive sleep apnea wake up with headaches? Arch Intern Med 1999; 159: 1765–8.

29. Ohayon MM. Prevalence and risk factors of morning headaches in the general population. Arch Intern Med 2004; 164: 97–102.

30. Rasmussen BK. Migraine and tension-type headache in the general population: precipitating factors, female hormones, sleep pattern and relation to lifestyle. Pain 1993; 53: 65–72.

31. Jennum P, Hein HO, Suadicani P, Gyntelberg F. Headache and cognitive dysfunctions in snorers. A cross-sectional study of 3323 men aged 54 to 74 years: the Copenhagen Male Study. Arch Neurol 1994; 51: 937–42.

32. Jennum P, Sjol A. Self-assessed cognitive function in snorers and sleep apneics. An epidemiological study of 1,504 females and males aged 30–60 years: the Dan–MONICA II Study. Eur Neurol 1994; 34: 204–8.

33. Ulfberg J, Carter N, Talback M, Edling C. Headache, snoring and sleep apnoea. J Neurol 1996; 243: 621–5.

34. Scher AI, Lipton RB, Stewart WF. Habitual snoring as a risk factor for chronic daily headache. Neurology 2003; 60: 1366–8.

35. Olson LG, King MT, Hensley MJ, Saunders NA. A community study of snoring and sleep-disordered breathing. Symptoms. Am J Respir Crit Care Med 1995; 152: 707–10.

36. Kushida CA, Littner MR, Morgenthaler T, et al. Practice parameters for the indications for polysomnography and related procedures: an update for 2005. Sleep 2005; 28: 499–521.

37. Littner MR, Kushida C, Wise M, et al. Standards of Practice Committee of the American Academy of Sleep Medicine. Practice parameters for clinical use of the multiple sleep latency test and the maintenance of wakefulness test. Sleep 2005; 28: 113–21.

38. Drake ME Jr, Pakalnis A, Andrews JM, Bogner JE. Nocturnal sleep recording with cassette EEG in chronic headaches. Headache 1990; 30: 600–3.

39. Saadeh A, Hauri PJ, Kripke DF, Lavie P. The role of actigraphy in the evaluation of sleep disorders. Sleep 1995; 18: 288–302.

40. Edinger JD, Means MK, Stechuchak KM, Olsen MK. A pilot study of inexpensive sleep-assessment devices. Behav Sleep Med 2004; 2: 41–9.

41. Bruni O, Russo PM, Violani C, Guidetti V. Sleep and migraine: an actigraphic study. Cephalalgia 2004; 24: 134–9.

42. Capuano A, Vollono C, Rubino M, et al. Hypnic headache: actigraphic and polysomnographic study of a case. Cephalalgia 2005; 25: 466–9.

43. Devine EB, Hakim Z, Green J. A systematic review of patient-reported outcome instruments measuring sleep dysfunction in adults. Pharmacoeconomics 2005; 23: 889–912.

44. Moule DE, Hall M, Pilkonis PA, Buysse DJ. Self-report measures of insomnia in adults: rationales, choices, and needs. Sleep Med Rev 2004; 8: 177–98.

45. Dexter JD, Weitzman ED. The relationship of nocturnal headaches to sleep stage patterns. Neurology 1970; 20: 513–18.

46. Hsu LK, Crisp AH, Kalucy RS, et al. Early morning migraine. Nocturnal plasma levels of catecholamines, tryptophan, glucose, and free fatty acids and sleep encephalographs. Lancet 1977; i: 447–51.

47. Dexter JD. The relationship between stage III + IV + REM sleep and arousals with migraine. Headache 1979; 19: 364–9.

48. Fox AW, Davis RL. Migraine chronobiology. Headache 1998; 38: 436–41.

49. Dahmen N, Kasten M, Wieczorek S, et al. Increased frequency of migraine in narcoleptic patients: a confirmatory study. Cephalalgia 2003; 23: 14–19.

50. Dahmen N, Querings K, Grun B, Bierbrauer J. Increased frequency of migraine in narcoleptic patients. Neurology 1999; 52: 1291–3.

51. Blau JN. Sleep deprivation headache. Cephalalgia 1990; 10: 157–60.

52. Inamorato E, Minatti-Hannuch SN, Zukerman E. The role of sleep in migraine attacks. Arq Neuropsiquiatr 1993; 51: 429–32.

53. Turner LC, Molgaard CA, Gardner CH, Rothrock JF, Stang PE. Migraine trigger factors in non-clinical Mexican–American population in San Diego county: implications for etiology. Cephalalgia 1995; 15: 523–30.

54. Spierings EL, Ranke AH, Honkoop PC. Precipitating and aggravating factors of migraine versus tension-type headache. Headache 2001; 41: 554–8.

55. Houle TT, Rains JC, Penzien DB, Lauzon JJ, Mosley TH. Biobehavioral precipitants of headache: time-series analysis of stress and sleep on headache activity. Headache 2004; 44: 533–4.

56. Boardman HF, Thomas E, Millson DS, Croft PR. Psychological, sleep, lifestyle, and comorbid associations with headache. Headache 2005; 45: 657–69.

57. Goder R, Fritzer G, Kapsokalyvas A, et al. Polysomnographic findings in nights preceding a migraine attack. Cephalalgia 2001; 21: 31–7.

58. Bag B, Karabulut N. Pain-relieving factors in migraine and tension-type headache. Int J Clin Pract 2005; 59: 760–3.

59. Rossi LN. Headache in childhood. Childs Nerv Syst 1989; 5: 129–34.

60. Parrino L, Pietrini V, Spaggiari MC, Terzano MG. Acute confusional migraine attacks resolved by sleep: lack of significant abnormalities in post-ictal polyomnograms. Cephalalgia 1986; 6: 95–100.

61. Holroyd KA, Stensland M, Lipchik GL, et al. Psychosocial correlates and impact of chronic tension-type headaches. Headache 2000; 40: 3–16.

62. Finkel AG. Epidemiology of cluster headache. Curr Pain Headache Rep 2003; 7: 144–9.

63. Russell D. Cluster headache: severity and temporal profiles of attacks and patient activity prior to and during attacks. Cephalalgia 1981; 1: 209–16.

64. Nobre ME, Leal AJ, Filho PM. Investigation into sleep disturbance of patients suffering from cluster headache. Cephalalgia 2005; 25: 488–92.

65. Graff-Radford SB, Newman A. Obstructive sleep apnea and cluster headache. Headache 2004; 44: 607–10.

66. Chervin RD, Zallek SN, Lin X, et al. Sleep disordered breathing in patients with cluster headache. Neurology 2000; 54: 2302–6.

67. Kudrow L, McGinty DJ, Phillips ER, Stevenson M. Sleep apnea in cluster headache. Cephalalgia 1984; 4: 33–8.

68. Buckle P, Kerr P, Kryger M. Nocturnal cluster headache associated with sleep apnea. A case report. Sleep 1993; 16: 487–9.

69. Pfaffenrath V, Pollmann W, Ruther E, Lund R, Hajak G. Onset of nocturnal attacks of chronic cluster headache in relation to sleep stages. Acta Neurol Scand 1986; 73: 403–7.

70. Russell D. Chronic paroxysmal hemicrania: severity, duration and time of occurrence of attacks. Cephalalgia 1984; 4: 53–6.

71. Kayed K, Sjaastad O. Nocturnal and early morning headaches. Ann Clin Res 1985; 17: 243–6.

72. Newman LC, Goadsby PJ. Unusual primary headache disorders. In: Silberstein LR, Palessio DJ, eds. Wolff's Headache and other Head Pain. New York: Oxford University Press, 2001; 310–24.

73. Dodick DW, Mosek AC, Campbell JK. The hypnic ('alarm clock') headache syndrome. Cephalalgia 1998; 18: 152–6.

74. Evers S, Goadsby PJ. Hypnic headache: clinical features, pathophysiology, and treatment. Neurology 2003; 60: 905–9.

75. Manni R, Sances G, Terzaghi M, Ghiotto N, Nappi G. Hypnic headache: PSG evidence of both REM- and NREM-related attacks. Neurology 2004; 62: 1411–13.

76. Biber MP. Nocturnal neck movements and sleep apnea in headache. Headache 1988; 28: 673–4.

77. Boutros NN. Headache in sleep apnea. Tex Med 1989; 85: 34–5.

78. Kiely JL, Murphy M, McNicholas WT. Subjective efficacy of nasal CPAP therapy in obstructive sleep apnoea syndrome: a prospective controlled study. Eur Respir J 1999; 13: 1086–90.

79. Davis JA, Fine ED, Maniglia AJ. Uvulopalatopharyngoplasty for obstructive sleep apnea in adults: clinical correlation with polysomnographic results. Ear Nose Throat J 1993; 72: 63–6.

80. Sand T, Hagen K, Schrader H. Sleep apnea and chronic headache. Cephalalgia 2003; 23: 90–5.

81. Greenough GP, Nowell PD, Sateia MJ. Headache complaints in relation to nocturnal oxygen saturation among patients with sleep apnea syndrome. Sleep Med 2002; 3: 361–4.

82. Idiman F, Oztura I, Baklan B, Ozturk V, Kursad F, Pakoz B. Headache in sleep apnea syndrome. Headache 2004; 44: 603–6.

83. Goder R, Friege L, Fritzer G, et al. Morning headaches in patients with sleep disorders: a systematic polysomnographic study. Sleep Med 2003; 4: 385–91.

84. Pearce JM. Clinical features of the exploding head syndrome. J Neurol Neurosurg Psychiatry 1989; 52: 907–10.

85. Sachs C, Svanborg E. The exploding head syndrome: polysomnographic recordings and therapeutic suggestions. Sleep 1991; 14: 263–6.

86. Welch KM. Contemporary concepts of migraine pathogenesis. Neurology 2003; 61(8 Suppl 4): S2–8.

87. Bartsch T, Goadsby PJ. The trigeminocervical complex and migraine: current concepts and synthesis. Curr Pain Headache Rep 2003; 7: 371–6.

88. Goadsby PJ, May A. PET demonstration of hypothalamic activation in cluster headache. Neurology 1999; 52: 1522.

89. Gagnier JJ. The therapeutic potential of melatonin in migraines and other headache types. Altern Med Rev 2001; 6: 383–9.

90. Nagtegaal JE, Smits MG, Swart AC, Kerkhof GA, van der Meer YG. Melatonin-responsive headache in delayed sleep phase syndrome: preliminary observations. Headache 1998; 38: 303–7.

91. Systematic Review of the Literature Regarding the Diagnosis of Sleep Apnea. Summary, Evidence Report/ Technology Assessment: Number 1, December 1998. Agency for Health Care Policy and Research, Rockville, MD. http://www.ahrq.gov/clinic/epcsums/apneasum.htm.

92. Tishler PV, Larkin EK, Schluchter MD, Redline S. Incidence of sleep-disordered breathing in an urban adult population: the relative importance of risk factors in the development of sleep-disordered breathing. JAMA 2003; 289: 2230–7.

93. Young T, Shahar E, Nieto FJ, et al. Sleep Heart Health Study Research Group. Predictors of sleep-disordered breathing in community-dwelling adults: the Sleep Heart Health Study. Arch Intern Med 2002; 162: 893–900.

94. Cakirer B, Hans MG, Graham G, et al. The relationship between craniofacial morphology and obstructive sleep apnea in whites and in African–Americans. Am J Respir Crit Care Med 2001; 163: 947–50.

95. Scher AI, Stewart WF, Ricci JA, Lipton RB. Factors associated with the onset and remission of chronic daily headache in a population-based study. Pain 2003; 106: 81–9.

APPENDIX*

Instructions for Daily Headache Self-Monitoring Form

Self-Management Training Program for Chronic Headache

These forms are designed to help you keep a careful record of your: daily headache intensity levels, stress, disability, medication use, meal pattern, sleep (pattern, quality, amount), basal temperature (women only), and menses (women only). Each page contains seven grids – one for each day of the week. You may want to fold the sheet so you can carry it with you in your pocket or purse. Each grid has several spaces running horizontally that correspond with times of the day (12 AM to 11 PM) for each day of the week. These boxes will be used to keep track of headache intensity, disability, stress, sleep, and meals. On top of the page are rating scales for headache intensity, disability, stress, sleep amount, and sleep quality. There is a large box at the top of the front page for listing medications that you take weekly. There are also boxes for keeping track of daily medications that are not used regularly. And finally, there is space available for making daily comments on any day of the week.

We would like you to rate each day's headache intensity, disability, and stress at least *four* times each day. Most people find it easiest to make ratings at the same times each day. People also find it helpful to pair the act of recording with some other daily event to help them remember to record. For example, you might record (1) at breakfast or when you first get up, (2) at lunch time or when you hear noon church bells, (3) at supper time or when you first get home from work or school, and (4) at bedtime or when your favorite evening TV show begins. If you should happen to forget to make a recording at your usual time, please fill in the grid just as soon as you remember. In addition, whenever you take medication for a headache, please indicate the amount and type of medication in the space provided for that day.

Each time you update the grid put the ratings in the boxes that correspond to the time of day that you are rating. For example, if you are making ratings for 6 AM Monday, then indicate the level of your headache, disability, and stress in the boxes of the column for 6 AM Monday. Put the number in the box that best describes how you are feeling at that time. For headache intensity you will put a number from 0 (*NO HEADACHE*) to 10 (*EXTREMELY PAINFUL HEADACHE*), for disability level you will put a number from 0 (*NO IMPAIRMENT*) to 10 (*COMPLETELY IMPAIRED*), and for stress you will put a number from 0 (*NO STRESS*) to 10 (*EXTREMELY STRESSED*). Don't be overly concerned with the exact rating level you select; your first impression is probably the best estimate. If you have a day with no headache, please be sure to complete the grid anyway. To indicate your sleeping pattern, you will place an 'X' in the boxes that correspond with times that you were asleep. If you slept for only half of the hour, then place a '/' in the box. For indicating meals and snacks, place an 'X' in the hourly boxes that correspond with times of the day that you ate a meal or a snack.

Also, once a day you will rate your sleep amount and your sleep quality in the single boxes to the right of each day's grid. When you rate your sleep amount, you will place the number corresponding to how much you think you slept from 0 (*TOO LITTLE*) to 10 (*TOO MUCH*). When you make this rating, we want you to tell us what you feel about your sleep amount, not how much experts tell you you should have. For example, some people might sleep 8 hours, but still feel like it was too little. On the other hand, other people might sleep 8 hours and think it was too much. Additionally, you will rate your sleep

*Reproduced from Rhudy JL, Penzien DB, Rains JC. Self-Management Training Program for Chronic Headache: Therapist Manual, 2006, with permission of the authors.

quality by placing the number corresponding to your experience ranging from 0 (*VERY POOR*) to 10 (*EXCELLENT*).

EXAMPLE FORM

[The following notes refer to an example form not shown in this book.] You can see that on Monday, Marcy reported NO HEADACHE (intensity 0) at 6:00 AM when she got up. At noon, she had a SLIGHTLY PAINFUL (intensity 2) headache, by supper time (6:00 PM) she reported a PAINFUL (intensity 6) headache, and just before bed (10:30 PM) it had decreased to SLIGHTLY PAINFUL (intensity 2). Her level of disability was the same throughout the day, MINIMALLY IMPAIRED (2) at 6:00 AM, 12:00 PM, 6:00 PM, and 10:30 PM. But, Marcy has a stressful job, so her stress level decreased after she came home from work. It started out as VERY STRESSED (8) when she awoke (9:00 AM) and remained high at noon. Her stressed dropped by supper (6:00 PM) to SLIGHTLY (2) and she experienced NO STRESS (0) as she went to sleep (10:30 PM).

To indicate that she awoke at 6:00 AM, she marked an 'X' in the boxes corresponding to 12AM, 1AM, 2AM, 3AM, 4AM, and 5AM. She took a 30 min nap at 7:30 PM, so she put a '/' mark in the sleep box corresponding to 7:00 PM. She fell asleep at 10:30, so she put a '/' mark in the sleep box for 10:00 PM, and an 'X' in the sleep box corresponding to 11 PM. She ate breakfast at 7:00 AM, lunch at 12:00 PM, a snack at 3:00 PM, and supper at 6:00 PM. Therefore, she placed 'X's in the meal/snack boxes for 7 AM, 12 PM, 3 PM, and 6 PM.

Upon waking, Marcy took her body temperature and found that it was 98.6°, so she indicated this in the box marked 'TEMP'. Since she was not menstruating on Monday, she circled the 'N'. Marcy also made a subjective rating of her sleep amount by putting a 3 in that box, indicating it was somewhat too little. She thought the sleep that she did get was FAIR, so she placed a '4' in the box for 'SLEEP QUALITY'.

Marcy took 2 aspirin and 1 butalbital (50 mg) for her headache on Monday. She also noted in the comments box that her nap seemed to help reduce her headache intensity.

When filling out each grid, please be sure to write your name and the dates of the week on each page. If you have any questions about these recording procedures, feel free to call and ask for advice.

13

Sleep and infection

Linda A Toth, Ming Ding, Rita A Trammell

SLEEP AND HEALTH

Sleepiness and sleep quality broadly influence measures of general health, particularly impacting perceptions about energy and fatigue. Obtaining adequate amounts of sleep is generally viewed as important for promoting clear thinking and feelings of general well-being and for reducing accidents and related injuries. For example, studies of medical interns and residents indicate that fatigue related to loss of sleep increases numbers of motor vehicle accidents and medical errors and could decrease the quality of patient care.[1,2] In another study, healthy young adults exposed to one night of sleep loss had slower and more variable reaction times, more errors of commission and omission, and impaired error correction.[3] Such studies indicate that in these general ways, sleep promotes performance.

Some epidemiologic studies of human populations support a relationship between unusually short night-time sleep durations and decreased life expectancy, although others do not.[4–10] In *Drosophila*, a point mutation in the *Shaker* gene results in a short-sleep phenotype and reduced lifespan.[11] This finding indicates that even a single gene can profoundly affect both sleep and survival. Sleep may be as important as proper nutrition for general health and well-being and has been called 'nutrition for the brain'.[12] Adequate amounts of sleep may promote resistance to infectious disease, and sleep loss

may temporarily impair immune responses and increase susceptibility to infection.[13,14]

DOES SLEEP INFLUENCE THE IMMUNE RESPONSE?

The immune system functions at both local and systemic levels to generate complex coordinated and highly regulated host defense responses that affect the entire organism. Sleep, like an immune response, is characterized by a complex and highly regulated alteration of endocrine and autonomic and central nervous system (CNS) processes. The complexity, multifaceted nature, and systemic scope of these two physiologic processes suggest the likelihood of interactions. Thus, physiologic differences between the states of sleep and wakefulness could differentially modulate immune responses.[15] For example, early nocturnal sleep, which is dominated by slow-wave sleep (SWS), is associated with a shift in the Th1/Th2 cytokine balance toward increased Th1 activity, with an increase in the ratio of interferon-γ to interleukin-4 (IFN-γ to IL-4)-producing T helper cells; in contrast, during late nocturnal sleep, in which rapid eye movement sleep (REMS) is dominant, the Th1/Th2 balance shifts toward Th2 dominance.[16] However, an important issue in the evaluation of sleep-related alterations in immune function is the determination of whether small but statistically significant changes in immune indices reflect biologic or clinical significance.[17,18]

Some data suggest that sleep patterns reflect the progression of disease processes, the prognosis, or the clinical outcome. For example, in rabbits inoculated with *E. coli*, *S. aureus* or *C. albicans*, a prolonged phase of enhanced sleep after microbial challenge is associated with a more favorable prognosis and less severe clinical signs than in a short period of enhanced sleep.[19,20] Rabbits that eventually die exhibit significantly less sleep than rabbits that survive the infection, whereas animals with the greatest increases in SWS have the lowest mortality rates.[20] Associations between absent or diminished sleep, reduced electroencephalogram (EEG) amplitude, and imminent death also occur in aged mice prior to spontaneous death,[21] in mice with fatal experimental rabies infections,[22,23] and in rats that die subsequent to chronic sleep deprivation and septicemia.[24–26] The total amount of sleep and the EEG amplitude during sleep also gradually decline in rabbits that are chronically infected with trypanosomes.[27] These observations suggest a prognostic value for sleep during infectious disease, but also imply that sleep may promote recuperation, potentially via facilitation of immune efficacy.

DOES SLEEP LOSS INFLUENCE THE IMMUNE RESPONSE?

The impact of sleep loss on immune competence is difficult to assess experimentally. Because stress influences the immune response, effects caused by loss of sleep must be differentiated from those associated with non-specific stress generated by the procedure used to induce sleep loss. Some approaches to inducing sleep loss in animals elicit relatively few of the classic physiologic signs of non-specific stress (e.g. the so-called disk-over-water method),[28] whereas others (e.g. the 'flower pot' method of causing REMs deprivation) cause responses traditionally thought to reflect stress (e.g., elevated catecholamines or glucocorticoids).[29,30] Increased catecholamines or glucocorticoids are generally not present in humans undergoing sleep deprivation,[31–35] perhaps because humans can voluntarily choose to go without sleep. However, the sleep loss that humans experience as a 'normal' facet of life may frequently be associated with stressful situations that necessitate or otherwise contribute to loss of sleep (e.g., examinations, bereavement, shift work, or depression).

Several human studies have quantified various measures of immune function after varying periods of partial or total sleep deprivation. These studies typically use small numbers of subjects and vary substantially in terms of the parameters measured, the environment of the subjects, the degree of sleep loss, and other factors. Some studies report that sleep deprivation alters particular immune parameters,[31,33,35,36] whereas others do not find significant changes.[18,37] For example, in studies evaluating natural killer (NK) cell numbers or activity, some groups report increases in sleep-deprived subjects,[31] whereas others report decreases.[33,38] Some studies report altered responses to antigens or mitogens.[31,33,35,36] For example, volunteers who underwent influenza vaccination in association with chronic partial sleep restriction generated less than half the antibody titer of participants who were permitted normal sleep.[39] Similarly, one group reported that mice that were immunized against influenza virus in association with sleep deprivation failed to clear the virus from the lung upon subsequent challenge, whereas rested mice completely cleared the virus, but others have failed to replicate this finding.[40] A comparison of immune function in persons with chronic insomnia or good sleep implies that chronic insomnia is associated with lower numbers of cells in various lymphocyte subpopulations and perhaps with an associated impairment of cellular immune competence.[41] Monocytes collected from persons who have undergone sleep loss show greater ability to produce tumor necrosis factor α (TNF-α) and IL-1β[42] when stimulated with endotoxin.[44] Sleep loss also leads to enhanced nocturnal plasma IL-1-like and IL-2-like activity.[33] An increased infection rate has been reported in some studies of sleep-deprived subjects,[43] but not in others.[31]

Most reports evaluating the impact of sleep loss on the immune system have studied animals or people that are overtly healthy and that are not experiencing a substantive immunologic challenge coincident with sleep loss. However, fragmented sleep, non-restorative sleep, and inadequate amounts of sleep could severely impact elderly or patient populations despite few significant adverse immune consequences in young, healthy individuals. Furthermore, stress- or illness-induced activation of the glucocorticoid system could act synergistically with sleep loss to impair host defense responses such as antibody production or microbial clearance.[44] For example, chronic stress that is associated with sleep loss impairs immune responses to influenza vaccination in elderly humans.[45] Sleep disruption can be profound in hospitalized patients and nursing home residents.[46,47] For example, SWS occupies less than 1% of the night during the 5–8 days after open-heart surgery.[46,48] A better understanding of such interactions could have important health implications for hospitalized patients and nursing home residents, who commonly experience severe disruptions in normal patterns of sleep.

The contention that sleep loss impairs immune competence is most strongly supported by observations that chronic sleep deprivation of rats results in intestinal bacterial proliferation, microbial penetration into lymph nodes, septicemia, and eventually death.[24–26,28,49–51] Bacterial penetration into normally sterile tissues during prolonged sleep deprivation implies the development of immune insufficiency and abnormal host defense, and suggests that long-term sleep loss increase susceptibility to infectious disease. Rats subjected to chronic sleep deprivation did not show changes in splenocyte responses to mitogens, although circulating lymphocyte numbers were reduced.[52] More extensive characterization revealed that as sleep deprivation progresses, rats develop neutrophilia and monocytosis, an evolving pro-inflammatory state, as reflected by serum cytokine levels, and increases in multiple serum immunoglobulin classes.[53] However, despite these indications of immune

activation, these animals do not clear bacteria and toxins,[53] suggesting the development of competing anti-inflammatory processes or interference with immune effector functions during sleep deprivation.

Other studies also suggest that sleep-deprived rodents undergoing antigenic challenge develop functionally significant immune perturbations. For example, secondary antibody responses to antigenic challenge are impaired in sleep-deprived mice and rats.[40,54] Sleep loss is also reported to retard both viral clearance and the development of a protective antibody response in influenza-infected mice,[54] but others have not confirmed this finding.[55,56] Loss of sleep may also modulate other physiologic responses related to immune or acute-phase responses. For example, sleep deprivation exacerbates fever in E. coli-inoculated rabbits,[57] non-pyrogenic doses of sheep red blood cells elicit fever when administered to sleep-deprived rats,[17] and intracerebroventricular administration of saline or immunoglobulins induces fever in sleep-deprived but not in rested rats.[58] Sleep deprivation is also reported to exacerbate anticoagulant-induced anemia[59] and to retard tumor growth in rats.[51] Sleep deprivation was recently reported to cause death in cyc^{01} mutant *Drosophila* in association with reduced expression of heat-shock genes after sleep loss.[60]

Taken together, the data that are accruing from both animal and human studies suggest that short-term sleep loss may be accompanied by enhanced non-specific host defense mechanisms, whereas chronic or prolonged sleep loss may result in immune impairment.[61,62] Similar arguments have been posed for the relationship between immune function and stress, particularly as reflected by elevations in circulating glucocorticoid levels.[63]

DOES INFECTIOUS DISEASE CHANGE SLEEP?

The quantitative and temporal changes that develop in sleep throughout the course of an infectious disease have been characterized in animals infected with various bacteria, viruses, and parasites. The precise characteristics of infection-related changes in sleep vary with the specific microorganism, the route of infection, the genetic background of the host, and differences in the disease process. For example, rabbits made septicemic by intravenous inoculation with *Pasteurella multocida* exhibit a different pattern of sleep responses than do rabbits that are infected intranasally, which causes pneumonia.[64] In general, rabbits with bacterial infections develop an initial increase and a subsequent decrease in the amount of time spent in SWS, whereas REMS is consistently reduced.[65] Infected rabbits also typically develop fevers. However, the fevers generally persist beyond the period of enhanced sleep. Thus, the temporal patterns of changes in sleep and temperature differ. The administration of killed bacteria and isolated bacterial components can elicit increased SWS, and treatment of animals with bacteriocidal antibiotics attenuates but does not eliminate the development of microbially induced changes in sleep.[19] Thus, viable bacteria and bacterial replication are not necessary to induce alterations in sleep.

The sleep patterns of rabbits infected with the fungal organism *C. albicans* are similar to those of rabbits with bacterial infections.[66] However, mice infected with *C. albicans* show qualitative and quantitative variation in both sleep and temperature, depending on the background strain of the infected mouse (Toth, LA, unpublished work). Mice also show strain variation in the sleep responses that develop during influenza infection.[67] The different sleep patterns that emerge during infection probably reflect activation of host defense systems.[15] Sleep–wake behavior may be more sensitive to the activation of host defense mechanisms than are the thermoregulatory or endocrine systems.[68]

The human condition known as fatal familial insomnia is associated with prion-related neuronal degeneration in the thalamus.[69] Animal studies also indicate that prions can influence sleep. Mice that genetically lack the prion protein gene demonstrate alterations in both sleep and circadian rhythms.[70,71] Rats inoculated with brain homogenate from scrapie-infected animals and cats inoculated with brain homogenate from a human with Creutzfeldt–Jakob disease gradually develop apparent drowsiness, increased SWS time, reduced wakefulness, and abnormal EEG and REMS patterns.[72–74]

Some studies have reported the effects of infection on sleep in humans. For example, volunteers who were inoculated with influenza virus or rhinovirus slept more during the symptomatic period, but their sleep quality was lower during the incubation period.[75] Children with HIV infection had significantly lower sleep efficiency than the control group.[76] Initial polysomnographic studies of asymptomatic adult men infected with HIV revealed a significant increase in the percentage of time spent in SWS during the second half of the night; frequent night-time awakenings and abnormal REMs architecture were also comon.[77–79] However, recent analyses suggest that pain and psychologic and psychosocial co-morbidity are major determinants of disturbed sleep in HIV infection.[80–82] Nonetheless, regardless of the proximal cause, sleep complaints are a common problem in HIV-infected populations.[83] Persons with trypanosomiasis ('sleeping sickness') develop fragmented nocturnal sleep and increased daytime sleep.[84] In rabbits, subcutaneous inoculation with *Trypanosoma brucei brucei* increases sleep after a latency of several days, coincident with the onset of fever and other clinical signs of illness.[27]

Somnolence continued to occur in association with the episodic recrudescence of parasitemia.[27] In addition to such episodes of hypersomnolence, loss of the normal circadian organization of sleep also develops during chronic trypanosomiasis in rabbits, rats, and humans.[27,84–86] The qualitative and temporal variation in sleep patterns after microbial infection may explain the apparently inconsistent changes in sleep reported in some studies of humans with spontaneous infections.[83–88] Administration of bacterial endotoxin affects sleep in both people and animals. In rats, endotoxin administration promotes non-REMS (NREMS) during the active (dark) phase and decreases REMS during both the rest and active (i.e., light and dark) phases of the diurnal cycle.[87–89] Endotoxin also suppresses REMS and prolongs REMS latency in humans,[90,91] but its effects on NREMS depend on the dose and time of administration.[91] Increases in the amount and intensity of nocturnal NREMS consistently develop only after the administration of subpyrogenic doses of endotoxin given shortly before the normal evening onset of sleep.[90,92] Administration of a mildly pyrogenic dose in the evening increases NREMS during the night;[93] however, administration of the same dose in the morning does not alter daytime NREMS.[90] Higher pyrogenic doses of endotoxin disrupt sleep and suppress NREMS.[91]

MEDIATORS OF SLEEP CHANGES IN RESPONSE TO IMMUNE CHALLENGE

As reviewed above, a substantial literature describes specific alterations in sleep amount and architecture during infections with a variety of pathogens. A compelling hypothesis is that the host response associated with microbial infections alters the expression of immune-modulatory substances that also regulate sleep. Various microbial components both trigger immune responses and elicit alterations in sleep during bacterial and viral infection (e.g., muramyl peptides and lipopolysaccharide in bacterial infections, and double-stranded (ds)RNA and envelope glycoproteins during viral infections). Research that began in the 1970s demonstrates that one class of immune effectors, cytokines, are powerful modulators of sleep–wake behavior. Observations that cytokine expression and protein levels change in response to microbial infection and that cytokines and their receptors are synthesized in the brain support a role for cytokines as mediators of infection-induced alterations in sleep. Most reports have focused on IL-1β and TNF-α.

Abundant evidence implicates IL-1 in the regulation of sleep. In general, substances or manipulations that induce IL-1 synthesis or release increase SWS, whereas substances that inhibit the synthesis or actions of IL-1 reduce SWS (reviewed in references 94 and 95). IL-1 receptors are widely distributed throughout the CNS, including important sleep-regulatory regions such as the hypothalamus.[96] IL-1 mRNA also occurs in many brain regions, and in rat brain varies diurnally, with its highest expression during the sleep phase of the diurnal cycle.[97] In humans, plasma IL-1 levels peak at sleep onset,[98] and measurable levels are detected more frequently in plasma samples collected during sleep rather than waking.[99] Prolonged wakefulness is associated with increased IL-1 mRNA,[100] and IL-1 protein is detected in plasma more frequently after sleep deprivation than during spontaneous sleep.[58] Anti-IL-1 treatments attenuate or prevent the rebound sleep that typically develops after sleep loss.[58,101,102] Collectively, these data provide strong evidence that IL-1 is involved in the regulation of sleep under normal conditions.

Evidence supporting a role for TNF in sleep regulation is similar to that for IL-1. TNF mRNA[103] and TNF protein concentrations[104] vary diurnally in rat brain, with peaks occurring during the sleep phase. In humans, peak plasma concentrations of TNF protein occur during sleep,[99] and plasma TNF-α concentrations correlate with EEG slow-wave activity.[105] Administration of TNF increases SWS time and EEG slow-wave amplitudes in a variety of species.[106–109] Direct disruption of the TNF system with antibodies, binding proteins, soluble receptors, or receptor fragments reduces normal spontaneous SWS,[110] the enhanced SWS that occurs after sleep loss,[111] and the sleep response to increased ambient temperature.[112] Mice that lack the 55 kDa TNF receptor sleep less than control mice.[106] Collectively, these data support a role for TNF in the regulation of sleep.

Accumulating evidence suggests that the cytokine IL-6 also modulates sleep, particularly during conditions of immune challenge. IL-6 is elevated in persons with conditions associated with excessive daytime sleepiness (e.g., narcolepsy and obstructive sleep apnea).[113] IL-6 concentrations vary in phase with sleep–wake behavior in humans[114,115] and in rats,[116] and prolonged wakefulness increased IL-6 concentrations in plasma of healthy humans[117,118] and in the brain and serum of rats.[116,119] In human volunteers, administration of IL-6 increased SWS during the latter half of the night.[120] Although initial studies of central or peripheral administration of human recombinant IL-6 in rabbits did not reveal changes in sleep,[121] a subsequent study in which rat IL-6 was administered centrally to rats revealed an initial increase and subsequent reduction in NREMS.[122] Central administration of anti-rat IL-6 did not alter sleep–wake behavior of normal rats.[122] However, IL-6 knockout mice respond to sleep loss with a delayed but quantitatively normal recovery of NREMS time[123] and show significantly less NREMS in response to lipopolysaccharide (LPS) administration than does the control strain.[124] Taken together, these data suggest that IL-6 may not be involved in the regulation of NREMS under normal conditions, but that elevated levels of IL-6 may alter sleep patterns during certain pathologic conditions or after immune challenge.

Type I (antiviral, or α/β) and type II (immunocyte, or γ) interferons (IFNs) are also sleep-modulatory cytokines. Type I IFNs have well-known antiviral properties and may be particularly important with respect to virally induced alterations in sleep. Almost all nucleated cells can produce type I IFNs in response to viral infection, and IFN-α receptors are present in the brain.[125] Viral components that induce IFN-α/β (e.g., dsRNA) also increase sleep.[126] IFN receptor I (IFN-RI) knockout mice spend less time in REMS than the control strain, with relatively minor changes in NREMS.[127] They also demonstrate a reduced sleep response to intratracheal challenge with a combination of synthetic dsRNA and IFN-γ.[128] Patients undergoing IFNα therapy report excessive sleepiness,[129,130] although their sleep may be disrupted rather than enhanced.[131] The administration of human recombinant IFN-α/β synchronizes the cortical EEG in

rats,[132] increases SWS in rabbits,[133,134] and reduces latency to REMS in monkeys.[135]

The degree to which sleep patterns change during viral infection may depend on the ability of the organism to mount a type I IFN response. In mice, IFN-α/β production is regulated in part by the *If1* gene. C57BL/6 mice produce relatively high levels of IFN-α/β in response to various challenges[136] and exhibit increased SWS in response to influenza infection.[137] In contrast, BALB/c mice produce lower levels in response to similar challenges[136] and do not show influenza-related sleep enhancement.[138] B6.C-*H28* mice, which have the BALB/c allele for low IFN-α/β production on the C57BL/6 genetic background, show C57BL/6-like sleep responses after challenge with influenza virus but BALB/c-like responses after challenge with Newcastle disease virus.[138] Thus, the critical factor mediating alterations in sleep can vary, depending on the challenge organism. However, because the *Ifl* allele also influences the expression of TNF-α and IL-6, as well as IFN-α/β,[139] the precise mediator of these effects on sleep remain uncertain.

PROPOSED MECHANISMS FOR TRANSMISSION OF PERIPHERAL IMMUNE SIGNALS TO THE BRAIN

The mechanisms by which proinflammatory cytokines produced by activated immune cells in the periphery signal the brain to elicit centrally mediated acute-phase responses is an important and unresolved question. Cytokines are large, hydrophilic proteins that would normally be unable to cross the blood–brain barrier. Several non-exclusive mechanisms have been proposed for cytokine-mediated immune-to-brain communication: 1. These are saturable transport systems;[140–142] 2. entry through sensory circumventricular organs that lack a functional blood–brain barrier;[143] 3. transduction by afferent sensory nerves, particularly the vagus;[144,145] and 4. transduction by perivascular cells and/or endothelial cells at the blood–brain interface.[146]

Studies evaluating immune–brain communication with respect to sleep have focused on transmission of cytokine signals via activation of the vagus nerve.[147–154] Several studies suggest that gastrointestinal peptides released after eating and cytokines released during an immune response may activate vagal afferents that then promote NREMS. Rats maintained on so-called 'cafeteria' diets develop increased NREMS[155] and increased IL-1β mRNA in liver and brain,[156] and subdiaphragmatic vagotomy prevents the change in NREMS.[148] that develops under this condition.[146] The increase in NREMS that occurs in rats after intraperitoneal administration of TNF-α[152] and LPS[151] is also attenuated by vagotomy. Similarly, vagotomy prevents the NREMS-promoting action of a low intraperitoneal dose of IL-1β, attenuates the effects of an intermediate dose, and does not alter the effects of a high dose.[149] Vagotomy also blocks the induction of IL-1β mRNA in the hippocampus and brainstem produced by IL-1 administration in rats and significantly attenuates the effect in the hypothalamus.[157] The presence of IL-1 receptor mRNA and IL-1-binding sites on glomus cells in the vagus nerve and increased afferent activity of the vagus after intraportal injection of IL-1 is consistent with a role for the vagus in generating the sleep changes that develop after peripheral administration of IL-1.[145,158,159] The finding that vagotomy attenuates but does not prevent the NREMS-promoting activity of IL-1 and TNF indicates that other mechanisms also relay peripheral cytokine signals to the brain.

SUMMARY AND CONCLUSIONS

The impact of peripheral immune signals on sleep undoubtedly depends on a wide variety of factors, including the route of administration of peripherally administered cytokines or infectious organisms, the anatomic location and nature of the immune response generated during various types of infectious disease, and host factors (e.g., stress, diet, and genetic background). Infectious disease and sleep appear to exert bidirectional influences on each other via effects on the immune system. Infection induces immune responses, which then impact sleep. Conversely, appropriate sleep promotes immune competence and perhaps promotes disease resistance. Sleep disorders that result in sleep loss and increased daytime sleepiness may be a risk factor for medical health problems.

ACKNOWLEDGMENTS

This work was supported in part by NIH Grants HL70522, NS40220, and RR16421, and by the Southern Illinois University School of Medicine.

REFERENCES

1. Barger LK, Cade BE, Ayas NT, et al. Extended work shifts and the risk of motor vehicle crashes among interns. N Engl J Med 2005; 352: 125–34.
2. Owens JA, Veasey SC, Rosen RC. Physician, heal thyself: sleep, fatigue, and medical education. Sleep 2001; 24: 493–5.
3. Tsai LL, Young HY, Hsieh S, Lee CS. Impairment of error monitoring following sleep deprivation. Sleep 2005; 28: 707–13.
4. Bursztyn M, Ginsberg G, Stessman J. The siesta and mortality in the elderly: effect of rest without sleep and daytime sleep duration. Sleep 2002; 25: 187–91.
5. Kripke DF, Garfinkel L, Wingard DL, Klauber MR, Marler MR. Mortality associated with sleep duration and insomnia. Arch Gen Psychiatry 2002; 59: 131–6.
6. Kripke DF, Simons RN, Garfinkel L, Hammond EC. Short and long sleep and sleeping pills. Is increased mortality associated? Arch Gen Psychiatry 1979; 36: 103–16.
7. Manabe K, Matsui T, Yamaya M, et al. Sleep patterns and mortality among elderly patients in a geriatric hospital. Gerontology 2000; 46: 318–22.
8. Nilsson PM, Nilsson J-A, Hedblad B, Berglund G. Sleep disturbance in association with elevated pulse rate for prediction of mortality – consequences of mental strain? J Intern Med 2001; 250: 521–9.
9. Pollak CP, Perlick D, Linsner JP, Wenston J, Hsieh F. Sleep problems in the community elderly as predictors

of death and nursing home placement. J Community Health 1990; 15: 123–35.

10. Wingard DL, Berkman LF. Mortality risk associated with sleeping patterns among adults. Sleep 1983; 6: 102–7.

11. Cirelli C, Bushey D, Hill S, et al. Reduced sleep in *Drosophila Shaker* mutants. Nature 2005; 434: 1087–92.

12. Amschler DH, McKenzie JF. Elementary students' sleep habits and teacher observations of sleep-related problems. J Sch Health 2005; 75: 50–6.

13. Savard J, Laroche L, Simard S, Ivers H, Morin CM. Chronic insomnia and immune functioning. Psychosom Med 2003; 65: 211–21.

14. Spiegel K, Sheridan JF, Van Cauter E. Effect of sleep deprivation on response to immunization. JAMA 2002; 288: 1471–2.

15. Benca RM, Quintans J. Sleep and host defense: a review. Sleep 1997; 20: 1027–37.

16. Dimitrov S, Lange T, Tieken S, Fehm HL, Born J. Sleep associated regulation of T helper 1/T helper 2 cytokine balance in humans. Brain Behav Immun 2004; 18: 341–8.

17. Brown R, Pang G, Husband AJ, King MG, Bull DF. Sleep deprivation and the immune response to pathogenic and non-pathogenic antigens. In: Husband AJ, ed. Behaviour and Immunity. Ann Arbor, MI CRC Press, 1992: 127–33.

18. Horne JA. A review of the biological effects of total sleep deprivation in man. Biol Psychol 1978; 7: 55–102.

19. Toth LA, Krueger JM. Alteration of sleep in rabbits by *Staphylococcus aureus* infection. Infect Immun 1988; 56: 1785–91.

20. Toth LA, Tolley EA, Krueger JM. Sleep as a prognostic indicator during infectious disease in rabbits. Proc Soc Exp Biol Med 1993; 203: 179–92.

21. Welsh DK, Richardson GS, Dement WC. Effect of age on the circadian pattern of sleep and wakefulness in the mouse. J Gerontol 1986; 41: 579–86.

22. Gourmelon P, Briet D, Court L, Tsiang H. Electro-physiological and sleep alterations in experimental mouse rabies. Brain Res 1986; 398: 128–40.

23. Gourmelon P, Briet D, Clarencon D, Court L, Tsiang H. Sleep alterations in experimental street rabies virus infection occur in the absence of major EEG abnormalities. Brain Res 1991; 554: 159–65.

24. Everson CA, Bergmann BM, Rechtschaffen A. Sleep deprivation in the rat: III. Total sleep deprivation. Sleep 1989; 12: 13–21.

25. Everson CA. Sustained sleep deprivation impairs host defense. Am J Physiol 1993; 265: R1148–54.

26. Rechtschaffen A, Gilliland MA, Bergmann BM, Winter JB. Physiological correlates of prolonged sleep deprivation in rats. Science 1983; 221: 182–4.

27. Toth LA, Tolley EA, Broady R, Blakely B, Krueger JM. Sleep during experimental trypanosomiasis in rabbits. Proc Soc Exp Biol Med 1994; 205: 174–81.

28. Everson CA. Clinical manifestations of sleep deprivation. In: Schwartz WJ, ed. Monographs in Clinical Neuroscience. Basel, Switzerland Larger, 1997: 34–59.

29. Suchecki D, Lobo LL, Hipólide DC, Tufik S. Increased ACTH and corticosteroid secretion induced by different methods of paradoxical sleep deprivation. J Sleep Res 1998; 7: 276–81.

30. Suchecki D. Paradoxical sleep deprivation and the hypothalamic–pituitary–adrenal axis. SRS Bull 2002; 8: 9–14.

31. Dinges DF, Douglas SD, Zaugg L, et al. Leukocytosis and natural killer cell function parallel neuro-behavioral fatigue induced by 64 hours of sleep deprivation. J Clin Invest 1994; 93: 1930–9.

32. Kollar EJ, Pasnau RO, Rubin RT, et al. Psychological, psychophysiological, and biochemical correlates of prolonged sleep deprivation. Am J Psychiatry 1969; 126: 488–97.

33. Moldofsky H, Lue FA, Davidson JR, Gorczynski R. Effects of sleep deprivation on human immune function. FASEB J 1989; 3: 1972–7.

34. Naitoh P, Kelly TL, Englund C. Health effects of sleep deprivation. Occup Med 1990; 5: 209–37.

35. Palmblad J, Cantell K, Strander H, et al. Stressor exposure and immunological response in man: interferon-producing capacity and phagocytosis. J Psychosom Res 1976; 20: 193–9.

36. Casey FB, Eisenberg J, Peterson D, Pieper D. Altered antigen uptake and distribution due to exposure to extreme environmental temperatures or sleep deprivation. J Reticuloendothel Soc 1974; 15: 87–95.

37. Kleitman N. Studies on the physiology of sleep. I. The effects of prolonged sleeplessness on man. Am J Physiol 1923; 66: 67–92.

38. Irwin M, Mascovich A, Willoughby R, Pike J. Partial sleep deprivation reduces natural killer cell activity in humans. Psychosom Med 1994; 56: 493–8.

39. Spiegel K, Sheridan JF, Van Cauter E. Effect of sleep deprivation on response to immunization. JAMA 2002; 288:1471–2.

40. Brown R, Price RJ, King MG, Husband AJ. Interleukin-1β and muramyl dipeptide can prevent decreased antibody response associated with sleep deprivation. Brain Behav Immun 1989; 3: 320–30.

41. Savard J, Laroche L, Simard S, Ivers H, Morin CM. Chronic insomnia and immune functioning. Psychosom Med 2003; 65: 211–21.

42. Uthgenannt D, Schoolmann D, Pietrowsky R, Fehm HL, Born J. Effects of sleep on the production of cytokines in humans. Psychosom Med 1995; 57: 97–104.

43. Boyum A, Wilk P, Gustavsson E, et al. The effect of strenuous exercise, calorie deficiency and sleep deprivation on white blood cells, plasma immunoglobulins and cytokines. Scand J Immunol 1996; 43: 228–35.

44. Hermann DM, Mullington J, Hinze-Selch D, et al. Endotoxin-induced changes in sleep and sleepiness during the day. Psychoneuroendocrinology 1998; 23: 427–37.

45. Kiecolt-Glaser JK, Glaser R, Gravenstein S, Malarkey WB, Sheridan JF. Chronic stress alters the immune response to influenza virus vaccine in older adults. Proc Nal Acad Sci USA 1996; 93: 3043–7.

46. Dunn CJ, Galinet LA, Gibbons AJ, Shields SK. Murine delayed-type hypersensitivity granuloma: an improved model for the identification and evaluation of different classes of anti-arthritic drugs. Int J Immunopharmac 1990; 12: 899–904.

47. Gabor JY, Cooper AB, Hanly PJ. Sleep disruption in the intensive care unit. Curr Opin Crit Care 2001; 7: 21–7.

48. Orr WC, Stahl ML. Sleep disturbances after open heart surgery. Am J Cardiol 1977; 39: 196–201.

49. Everson CA, Toth LA. Systemic bacterial invasion induced by sleep deprivation. Am J Physiol 2000; 278: R905–16.

50. Landis CA, Whitney JD. Effects of 72 hours sleep deprivation on wound healing in the rat. Res Nurs Health 1997; 20: 259–67.

51. Bergmann BM, Rechtschaffen A, Gilliland MA, Quintans J. Effect of extended sleep deprivation on tumor growth in rats. Am J Physiol 1996; 271: R1460–4.

52. Benca RM, Kushida CA, Everson CA, et al. Sleep deprivation in the rat: VII. Immune function. Sleep 1989; 12: 47–52.

53. Everson CA. Clinical assessment of blood leukocytes, serum cytokines, and serum immunoglobulins as responses to sleep deprivation in laboratory rats. Am J Physiol Regul Integr Comp Physiol 2005; 289: R1054–63.

54. Brown R, Pang G, Husband AJ, King MG. Suppression of immunity to influenza virus infection in the respiratory tract following sleep disturbance. Reg Immunol 1989; 2: 321–5.

55. Renegar KB, Floyd R, Krueger JM. Effects of short-term sleep deprivation on murine immunity to influenza virus in young adult and senescent mice. Sleep 1998; 21: 241–8.

56. Toth LA, Rehg JE. Effects of sleep deprivation and other stressors on the immune and inflammatory responses of influenza-infected mice. Life Sci 1998; 63: 701–9.

57. Toth LA, Opp MR, Mao L. Somnogenic effects of sleep deprivation and *Escherichia coli* inoculation in rabbits. J Sleep Res 1995; 4: 30–40.

58. Opp MR, Krueger JM. Interleukin-1 is involved in responses to sleep deprivation in the rabbit. Brain Res 1994; 639: 57–65.

59. Drucker-Colin RR, Jaques LB, Winocur G. Anemia in sleep-deprived rats receiving anticoagulants. Science 1971; 174: 505–7.

60. Shaw PJ, Tononi G, Greenspan RJ, Robinson DF. Stress response genes protect against lethal effects of sleep deprivation in *Drosophila*. Nature 2002; 417: 287–91.

61. Rogers NL, Sziba MP, Staab JP, Evans DL, Dinges DF. Neuroimmunologic aspects of sleep and sleep loss. Semin Clin Neuropsychiatry 2001; 6: 295–307.

62. Krueger JM, Fang J, Majde JA. Sleep in health and disease. In: Ader R, Felten DL, Cohen N, eds. Psychoneuroimmunology, 3rd edn. New York: Academic Press, 2001: 667–85.

63. Dhabhar FS, McEwen BS. Acute stress enhances while chronic stress suppresses cell-mediated immunity in vivo: a potential role for leukocyte trafficking. Brain Behav Immun 1997; 11: 286–306.

64. Toth LA, Krueger JM. Infectious disease, cytokines and sleep. In: Mancia M, Marini G, eds. The Diencephalon and Sleep. New York: Raven Press, 1990: 331–41.

65. Toth LA, Gardiner TW, Krueger JM. Modulation of sleep by cortisone in normal and bacterially infected rabbits. Am J Physiol 1992; 263: R1339–46.

66. Toth LA, Rehg JE, Webster RG. Strain differences in sleep and other pathophysiological sequelae of influenza virus infection in naive and immunized mice. J Neuroimmunol 1995; 58: 89–99.

67. Toth LA, Lyons S, Cox L. Sleep patterns during *Candida albicans*-induced renal disease in mice. Sleep 2003; 26: A365.

68. Bryant PA, Trinder J, Curtis N. Sick and tired: Does sleep have a vital role in the immune system? Nat Rev Immunol 2004; 4: 457–67.

69. Monari L, Chen SG, Brown P, et al. Fatal familial insomnia and familial Creutzfeld–Jakob disease: different prion proteins determined by DNA polymorphism. Proc Natl Acad Sci USA 1994; 91: 2839–42.

70. Tobler I, Gaus SE, Deboer T, et al. Altered circadian rhythms and sleep in mice devoid of prion protein. Nature 1996; 380: 639–42.

71. Tobler I, Deboer T, Fischer M. Sleep and sleep regulation in normal and prion protein-deficient mice. J Neurosci 1997; 17: 1869–79.

72. Bassant M-H, Cathala F, Court L, Gourmelon P, Hauw JJ. Experimental scrapie in rats: first electrophysiological observations. Electroenceph Clin Neurophysiol 1984; 57: 541–7.

73. Bassant M-H, Baron H, Gumpel M, Cathala F, Court L. Spread of scrapie to the central nervous system: study of a rat model. Brain Res 1986; 383: 397–401.

74. Gourmelon P, Amyx HL, Baron H, et al. Sleep abnormalities with REM disorder in experimental Creutzfeldt–Jakob disease in cats: a new pathological feature. Brain Res 1987; 411: 391–6.

75. Smith A. Sleep, colds, and performance. In: Broughton RJ, Ogilvie RD, eds. Sleep, Arousal and Performance. Boston, MA: Birkhauser, 1992: 233–42.

76. Franck LS, Johnson LM, Lee K, et al. Sleep disturbances in children with human immunodeficiency virus infection. Pediatrics 1999; 104: 1–5.

77. Darko DF, Mccutchan JA, Kripke DF, Gillin JC, Golshan S. Fatigue, sleep disturbance, disability, and indices of progression of HIV infection. AM J psychiat 1992; 149: 514–20.

78. Darko DF, Mitler MM, Henriksen SJ. Lentiviral infection, immune response peptides and sleep. Adv Neuroimmunol 1995; 5: 57–77.

79. Darko DF, Mitler MM, Miller JC. Growth hormone, fatigue, poor sleep, and disability in HIV infection. Neuroendocrinol. 1998; 67: 317–24.

80. Reid S, Dwyer J. Insomnia in HIV infection: a systematic review of prevalence, correlates, and management. Psychosom Med 2005; 67: 260–9.

81. Vance DE, Burrage JW, Jr. Sleep disturbances and psychomotor decline in HIV. Percept Mot Skills 2005; 100: 1004–10.

82. Vosvick M, Gore-Felton C, Ashton E, et al. Sleep disturbances among HIV-positive adults: the role of pain, stress, and social support. J Psychosom Res 2004; 57: 459–63.

83. Davis S. Clinical sequelae affecting quality of life in the HIV-infected patient. J Assoc Nurses AIDS care 2004; 15: 28S–33S.

84. Buguet A, Bert J, Tapie P, et al. Sleep–wake cycle in human African trypanosomiasis. J Clin Neurophysiol 1993; 10: 190–6.

85. Enanga B, Burchmore RJ, Stewart ML, Barrett MP. Sleeping sickness and the brain. Cell Mol Life Sci 2002; 59: 845–58.

86. Mhlanga JDM, Bentivoglio M, Kristensson K. Neurobiology of cerebral malaria and African sleeping sickness. Brain Res Bull 1997; 44: 579–89.

87. Lancel M, Cronlein J, Muller-Preuss P, Holsboer F. Lipopolysaccharide increases EEG delta activity within non-REM sleep and disrupts sleep continuity in rats. Am J Physiol 1995; 268: R1310–18.

88. Mathias S, Schiffelholz T, Linthorst AC, Pollmacher T, Lancel M. Diurnal variations in lipopolysaccharide-induced sleep, sickness behavior and changes in corticosterone levels in the rat. Neuroendocrinology 2000; 71: 375–85.

89. Schiffelholz T, Lancel M. Sleep changes induced by lipopolysaccharide in the rat are influenced by age. Am J Physiol Regul Integr Comp Physiol 2001; 280: R398–403.

90. Korth C, Mullington J, Schreiber W, Pollmacher T. Influence of endotoxin on daytime sleep in humans. Infect Immun 1996; 64: 1110–15.

91. Mullington J, Korth C, Hermann DM, et al. Dose-dependent effects of endotoxin on human sleep. Am J Physiol Regul Integr Comp Physiol 2000; 278: R947–55.

92. Pollmacher T, Schuld A, Kraus T, et al. Experimental immunomodulation, sleep, and sleepiness in humans. Ann NY Acad Sci 2000; 917: 488–99.

93. Pollmacher T, Schreiber W, Gudewill S, et al. Influence of endotoxin on nocturnal sleep in humans. Am J Physiol 1993; 264: R1077–83.

94. Opp MR, Kapás L, Toth LA. Cytokine involvement in the regulation of sleep. Proc Soc Exp Biol Med 1992; 201: 16–27.

95. Krueger JM, Toth LA. Cytokines as regulators of sleep. Ann NY Acad Sci 1994; 739: 299–310.

96. Cunningham ET, de Souza EB. Interleukin 1 receptors in the brain and endocrine tissues. Immunol Today 1993; 14: 171–6.

97. Taishi P, Bredow S, Guba-Thakurta N, Obal F, Krueger JM. Diurnal variations of interleukin-1β mRNA and β-actin mRNA in rat brain. J Neuroimmunol 1997; 75: 69–74.

98. Moldofsky H, Lue FA, Eisen J, Keystone E, Gorczynski R. The relationship of interleukin-1 and immune functions to sleep in humans. Psychosom Med 1986; 48: 309–18.

99. Gudewill S, Pollmächer T, Vedder H, et al. Nocturnal plasma levels of cytokines in healthy men. Eur Arch Psychiatr Clin Neurosci 1992; 242: 53–6.

100. Mackiewicz M, Sollars PJ, Ogilvie MD, Pack AI. Modulation of IL-1β gene expression in the rat CNS during sleep deprivation. NeuroReport 1996; 7: 529–33.

101. Opp MR, Krueger JM. Anti-interleukin-1β reduces sleep and sleep rebound after sleep deprivation in rats. Am J Physiol 1994; 266: R688–95.

102. Takahashi S, Fang J, Kapás L, Wang Y, Krueger J. Inhibition of brain interleukin-1 attenuated sleep rebound after sleep deprivation in rabbits. Am J Physiol 1997; 273: R677–82.

103. Bredow S, Guba-Thakurta N, Taishi P, Obal F, Krueger JM. Diurnal variations of tumor necrosis factor α mRNA and α-tubulin mRNA in rat brain. Neuroimmunomodulation 1997; 4: 84–90.

104. Floyd RA, Krueger JM. Diurnal variation of TNF α in the rat brain. NeuroReport 1997; 3: 915–18.

105. Darko DF, Miller JC, Gallen C, et al. Sleep electroencephalogram delta-frequency amplitude, night plasma levels of tumor necrosis factor α, and human immunodeficiency virus infection. Proc Natl Acad Sci USA 1995; 92: 12080–4.

106. Fang J, Wang Y, Krueger JM. Mice lacking the TNF 55 kDa receptor fail to sleep more after TNFα treatment. J Neurosci 1997; 17: 5949–55.

107. De Sarro G, Gareri P, Sinopoli A, David E, Rotiroti D. Comparative, behavioural and electrocortical effects of tumor necrosis factor-α and interleukin-1 microinjected into the locus coeruleus of rat. Life Sci 1997; 60: 555–64.

108. Kapás L, Krueger JM. Tumor necrosis factor-β induces sleep, fever, and anorexia. Am J Physiol 1992; 263: R703–7.

109. Shoham S, Davenne D, Cady AB, Dinarello CA, Krueger JM. Recombinant tumor necrosis factor and interleukin 1 enhance slow-wave sleep. Am J Physiol 1987; 253: R142–9.

110. Takahashi S, Kapas L, Fang J, Krueger JM. An anti-tumor necrosis factor antibody suppresses sleep in rats and rabbits. Brain Res 1995; 690: 241–4.

111. Takahashi M, Ogasawara K, Takeda K, et al. LPS induces NK1.1+ ab T cells with potent cytotoxicity in the liver of mice via production of IL-12 from Kupffer cells. J Immunol 1996; 156: 2436–42.

112. Takahashi S, Krueger JM. Inhibition of tumor necrosis factor prevents warming-induced sleep responses in rabbits. Am J Physiol 1997; 272: R1325–9.

113. Vgontzas AN, Papanicolaou DA, Bixler EO, et al. Elevation of plasma cytokines in disorders of excessive daytime sleepiness: role of sleep disturbance and obesity. J Clin Endocrinol Metab 1997; 82: 1313–16.

114. Bauer J, Hohagen F, Ebert T, et al. Interleukin-6 serum levels in healthy persons correspond to the sleep–wake cycle. Clin Investig 1994; 72: 315.

115. Vgontzas AN, Bixler EO, Lin HM, et al. IL-6 and its circadian secretion in humans. Neuroimmunomodulation 2005; 12: 131–40.

116. Guan Z, Vgontzas AN, Omori T, et al. Interleukin-6 levels fluctuate with the light–dark cycle in the brain and peripheral tissues in rats. Brain Behav Immun 2005; 19: 526–9.

117. Vgontzas AN, Papanicolaou DA, Bixler EO, et al. Circadian interleukin-6 secretion and quantity and depth of sleep. J Clin Endocrinol Metab 1999; 84: 2603–7.

118. Shearer WT, Reuben JM, Mullington JM, et al. Soluble TNF-α receptor 1 and IL-6 plasma levels in humans subjected to the sleep deprivation model of space flight. J Allergy Clin Immunol 2001; 107: 165–70.

119. Hu J, Chen Z, Gorczynski CP, et al. Sleep-deprived mice show altered cytokine production manifest by perturbations in serum IL-1ra, TNFα, and IL-6 levels. Brain Behav Immun 2003; 17: 498–504.

120. Spath-Schwalbe E, Hansen K, Schmidt F, et al. Acute effects of recombinant human interleukin-6 on endocrine and central nervous sleep functions in healthy men. J Clin Endocrinol Metab 1998; 83: 1573–9.

121. Opp M, Obál F, Cady AB, Johannsen L, Krueger JM. Interleukin-6 is pyrogenic but not somnogenic. Physiol Behav 1989; 45: 1069–72.

122. Hogan D, Morrow JD, Smith EM, Opp MR. Interleukin-6 alters sleep of rats. J Neuroimmunol 2003; 137: 59–66.

123. Morrow JD, Opp MR. Sleep–wake behavior and responses of interleukin-6-deficient mice to sleep deprivation. Brain Behav Immun 2005; 19: 28–39.

124. Morrow JD, Opp MR. Diurnal variation of lipopolysaccharide-induced alterations in sleep and body temperature of interleukin-6-deficient mice. Brain Behav Immun 2005; 19: 40–51.

125. Yamada T, Yamanaka I. Microglial localization of α-interferon receptor in human brain tissues. Neurosci Lett 1995; 189: 73–6.

126. Kimura-Takeuchi M, Majde JA, Toth LA, Krueger JM. The role of double-stranded RNA in induction of the acute-phase response in an abortive influenza virus infection model. J Infect Dis 1992; 166: 1266–75.

127. Bohnet SG, Traynor TR, Majde JA, Kacsoh B, Krueger JM. Mice deficient in the interferon type I receptor have reduced REM sleep and altered hypothalamic hypocretin, prolactin and 2′,5′-oligoadenylate synthetase expression. Brain Res 2004; 1027: 117–25.

128. Traynor TR, Majde JA, Bohnet SG, Krueger JM. Sleep and body temperature responses in an acute viral infection model are altered in interferon type I receptor-deficient mice. Brain Behav Immun 2005; 20: 290–9.

129. Smedley H, Katrak M, Sikora K, Wheeler T. Neurological effects of human recombinant interferon. BMJ 1983; 286: 262–5.

130. Mattson K, Niiranen A, Iivanainen M, et al. Neurotoxicity of interferon. Cancer Treat Rep 1983; 67: 958–61.

131. Spath-Schwalbe E, Lange T, Perras B, et al. Interferon-α acutely impairs sleep in healthy humans. Cytokine 2000; 12: 518–21.

132. Dafny N. Interferon modifies EEG and EEG-like activity recorded from sensory, motor, and limbic system structures in freely behaving rats. Neurotoxicology 1983; 4: 235–40.

133. Krueger JM, Dinarello CA, Shoham S, et al. Interferon α-2 enhances slow-wave sleep in rabbits. Int J Immunopharmacol 1987; 9: 23–30.

134. Kubota T, Fang J, Guan Z, Brown RA, Krueger JM. Vagotomy attenuates tumor necrosis factor-α-induced sleep and EEG δ-activity in rats. Am J Physiol Regul Integr Comp Physiol 2001; 280: R1213–20.

135. Reite M, Laudenslager M, Jones J, Crnic L, Kaemingk K. Interferon decreases REM latency. Biol Psychiatry 1987; 22: 104–7.

136. De Maeyer E, De Maeyer-Guignard J. A gene with quantitative effect on circulating interferon induction – further studies. Ann NY Acad Sci 1970; 173: 228–38.

137. Toth LA. Immune-modulatory drugs alter *Candida albicans*-induced sleep patterns in rabbits. Pharmacol Physiol Behav 1995; 51: 877–84.

138. Toth LA. Strain differences in the somnogenic effects of interferon inducers in mice. J Interferon Cytokine Res 1996; 16: 1065–72.

139. Raj NBK, Cheung SC, Rosztoczy I, Pitha PM. Mouse genotype affects inducible expression of cytokine genes. J Immunol 1992; 148: 1934–40.

140. Banks WA, Kastin AJ, Gutierrez EG. Penetration of interleukin-6 across the murine blood–brain barrier. Neurosci Lett 1994; 179: 53–6.

141. Banks WA, Tschop M, Robinson SM, Heiman ML. Extent and direction of ghrelin transport across the blood–brain barrier is determined by its unique primary structure. J Pharmacol Exp Ther 2002; 302: 822–7.

142. Banks WA, Farr SA, La Scola ME, Morley JE. Intravenous human interleukin-1α impairs memory processing in mice: dependence on blood–brain barrier transport into posterior division of the septum. J Pharmacol Exp Ther 2001; 299: 536–41.

143. Roth J, Harre EM, Rummel C, Gerstberger R, Hubschle T. Signaling the brain in systemic inflammation: role of sensory circumventricular organs. Front Biosci 2004; 9: 290–300.

144. Blatteis CM, Li S. Pyrogenic signaling via vagal afferents: What stimulates their receptors? Auton Neurosci 2000; 85: 66–71.

145. Goehler LE, Gaykema RPA, Hansen MK, et al. Vagal immune-to-brain communication: a visceral chemosensory pathway. Auton Neurosci Basic Clin 2000; 85: 49–59.

146. Schiltz JC, Sawchenko PE. Signaling the brain in systemic inflammation: the role of perivascular cells. Front Biosci 2003; 8: s1321–9.

147. Hansen MK, Krueger JM. Subdiaphragmatic vagotomy does not block sleep deprivation-induced sleep in rats. Physiol Behav 1998; 64: 361–5.

148. Hansen MK, Kapas L, Fang J, Krueger JM. Cafeteria diet-induced sleep is blocked by subdiaphragmatic vagotomy in rats. Am J Physiol 1998; 274: R168–74.

149. Hansen MK, Krueger JM. Subdiaphragmatic vagotomy blocks the sleep- and fever-promoting effects of interleukin-1β. Am J Physiol 1997; 273: R1246–53.

150. Hansen MK, Krueger JM. Gadolinium chloride pretreatment prevents cafeteria diet-induced sleep in rats. Sleep 1999; 22: 707–15.

151. Kapas L, Hansen MK, Chang HY, Krueger JM. Vagotomy attenuates but does not prevent the somnogenic and febrile effects of lipopolysaccharide in rats. Am J Physiol 1998; 274: R406–11.

152. Kubota T, Fang J, Guau Z, Brown RA, Krueger JM. Vagotomy attenuates tumor necrosis factor-alpha-induced sleep and EEG delta-activity in rats. AM J physiol Regul Integr Comp Physiol 2001; 280: R1213–20.

153. Malow BA, Edwards J, Marzec M, et al. Vagus nerve stimulation reduces daytime sleepiness in epilepsy patients. Neurology 2001; 57: 879–84.

154. Opp MR, Toth LA. Somnogenic and pyrogenic effects of interleukin-1β and lipopolysaccharide in intact and vagotomized rats. Life Sci 1998; 62: 923–36.

155. Danguir J. Cafeteria diet promotes sleep in rats. Appetite 1987; 8: 49–53.

156. Hansen MK, Taishi P, Chen Z, Krueger JM. Cafeteria feeding induces interleukin-1β mRNA expression in rat liver and brain. Am J Physiol 1998; 274: R1734–9.

157. Hansen MK, Taishi P, Chen Z, Krueger JM. Vagotomy blocks the induction of interleukin-1β (IL-1β) mRNA in the brain of rats in response to systemic IL-1β. J Neurosci 1998; 18: 2247–53.

158. Niijima A. The afferent discharges from sensors for interleukin 1 β in the hepatoportal system in the anesthetized rat. J Auton Nerv Syst 1996; 61: 287–91.

159. Goehler LE, Relton JK, Dripps D, et al. Vagal paraganglia bind biotinylated interleukin-1 receptor antagonist: a possible mechanisms for immune-to-brain communication. Brain Res Bull 1997; 45: 357–64.

14

Narcolepsy: Psychosocial, socioeconomic, and public health considerations

M Goswami, SR Pandi-Perumal

SYMPTOMS OF NARCOLEPSY

The earliest reported description of narcolepsy appears to be that recorded by Oliver in 1704.[1] Following reports of cases with symptoms of narcolepsy by Graves in 1851,[2] Caffé in 1862,[3] and Westphal in 1877,[4] it was Gelineau in 1880[5] who ascribed the term *narcolepsie* to describe a condition characterized by brief episodes of irresistible sleep and by falls (*astasias*) associated with emotional stimuli.

Narcolepsy is a chronic debilitating neurologic disorder, the hallmarks of which are hypersomnia and cataplexy (a sudden and transient decrement of muscle tone and loss of deep tendon reflexes, leading to muscle weakness, paralysis, or postural collapse, usually in response to an external stimulus).[6] Persons with narcolepsy often have intrusion of rapid eye movement (REM) sleep into wakefulness. Characteristically, patients report relief of discomfort from episodes of sleep attacks upon taking short naps. Cataplectic attacks, another form of REM intrusion, are usually evoked by a strong or deeply felt outburst of intense emotional expression such as laughter, joy, anger or fright, surprise, amusement, or excitement.[7,8] Yoss and Daly[9] described a classic tetrad of symptoms for the diagnosis of narcolepsy: excessive daytime somnolence (EDS – which is usually the first symptom), cataplexy (70–80%), hypnagogic or hypnopompic hallucinations (which can occur just prior to sleep onset or upon arousal (70%)), and sleep paralysis (loss of muscle tone at sleep onset or on awakening (60%)). However, each of these symptoms can appear at various stages of the disorder and in different combinations and degrees of severity.[8]

Cataplexy is characterized by a sudden bilateral loss of postural muscle tone – weakness with loss of deep tendon reflex often occurs in response to emotional triggers. During a cataplectic attack, a person loses muscular control but is aware of the environment. Hypnagogic hallucinations (vivid dream-like experiences), sleep paralysis, and automatic behaviors (the performance of routine tasks without awareness e.g., talking, driving, or writing) are auxiliary symptoms; fatigue, cognitive impairment, and disturbed nocturnal sleep are common complaints of narcolepsy patients.[10]

In most cases, sleepiness rather than cataplexy is the more perplexing and debilitating symptom; people with narcolepsy go through life feeling the way most of us would feel if we had been awake for 24 hours.[11] Nocturnal sleep is fragmented with reduction in slow-wave sleep (SWS); naps may offer some help, but sleepiness occurs following refreshing naps.[11] Thus, both nocturnal sleep and EDS pose a problem to these patients.[12,13]

DIAGNOSIS

If narcolepsy is suspected, polysomnography (PSG) and a Multiple Sleep Latency Test (MSLT) are often used to establish the diagnosis.[14] If sleep apnea and other excessive sleep problems can be ruled out, a daytime mean sleep onset latency (SOL) of less than 8 minutes (typically below 5 minutes) and the presence of rapid eye movement (REM) sleep in two or more of five daytime nap periods (MSLT) is abnormal and confirms the clinical laboratory diagnosis of narcolepsy. According to Stores,[8] a combination of EDS and definite cataplexy can be considered pathognomonic of narcolepsy.

PATHOPHYSIOLOGY

Narcolepsy is a neurologic condition, but its etiology and pathogenesis remain obscure,[15] although there have been recent advances in the understanding of the disease. A major milestone in narcolepsy research was the discovery of sleep-onset REM period (SOREM) sleep,[16] which led to a school of thought that cataplexy, hypnagogic hallucinations, and sleep paralysis might be due to alterations in REM sleep regulatory mechanisms.[17,18] In 1976, the dysfunction of REM sleep in narcolepsy was emphasized.[19] However, others supported the idea that narcolepsy is characterized by abnormalities of REM and non-REM (NREM) sleep activity.[20–22] The pathophysiology of narcolepsy appears to be related to abnormal expression and manifestations of REM sleep that intrude upon periods of wakefulness.[16,23–25]

Earlier studies of the genetics of narcolepsy showed that 98–100% of patients with narcolepsy are HLA-DR2-positive.[26–30] It is important to note that 20–25% of the normal Caucasian population may have this gene. In Israel, where only 11% of the control subjects in one study were DR2-positive, the prevalence rate of narcolepsy is about 1/100 of the rate of narcoleptics quoted in other studies.[31] Researchers in Japan demonstrated that HLA-DR2 and -DQWI were positive in most narcolepsy patients, and 30 patients were found to have the DRW15 subspecificity.[32] However, the incidence of HLA-DR15 varies among ethnic groups and is lower in the African–American population. Later, it was discovered that HLA-DQ6 occur more frequently in persons with narcolepsy with cataplexy than in those without cataplexy, and subjects were also found to be DQA1*0102-positive. Also, there is a positive correlation between DQB1*0602 positivity and the severity of cataplexy.[33,34] This gene appears to confer susceptibility to narcolepsy; however, several DQB1*0602-negative families have narcolepsy with cataplexy.[35] A multifactorial model, in which exogenous factors may precipitate symptoms in predisposed individuals, may be helpful in explaining the development of the symptoms. Experiments carried out on monozygotic twins point to environmental factors.[35] However, the appearance of symptoms at puberty may indicate a hormonal effect. Some authors have proposed an autoimmune mechanism behind narcolepsy.[36–38] The role of the neuropeptide hypocretin/orexin in the pathophysiology is a recent discovery. This neuropeptide was deficient in some cases of narcolepsy,[39] and the brains of persons with narcolepsy have shown an absence of hypocretin neurons in the hypothalamus.[40,41] Hypocretin neurons project to the locus coeruleus and are excitatory. They also project to regions of the brain that are important in producing and maintaining arousal. Changes in neurotransmission in these areas due to a defect in the hypocretin system may explain the EDS of persons with narcolepsy.[42]

PREVALENCE

The prevalence of narcolepsy is estimated at 0.05% and 0.067% in the San Francisco Bay area and Los Angeles County, respectively, and about 250 000 people are estimated to have narcolepsy in the USA.[43,44] Epidemiologic studies suggest that narcolepsy occurs in approximately 1 in 2000 individuals.[8,45,46] It is not as rare as was noted in the earlier literature, and may in fact affect as many people in the USA as multiple sclerosis.[47] Similar prevalence rates have been observed in Europe.[48]

Sex does not appear to be a discriminating variable. A higher rate for men noted by some researchers may reflect a different pattern of utilization of services or the inclusion of cases of sleep apnea, which is reported to be more prevalent among men than women. Socioeconomic status and race have not been reported as differentiating variables in the USA. However, a low prevalence rate (0.0002%) has been observed in Israel, probably because of a concurrent low rate of the HLA-DR2 gene in the population.[31]

DISEASE ONSET

While frequently undiagnosed or misdiagnosed, the peak age of onset of narcolepsy is in adolescence and young adulthood, and is generally between 15 and 30 years.[49,50] However, it can occur at any age, including early childhood or late adulthood. For example, some authors have reported the onset of narcolepsy before the age of 11 years.[51–53]

TREATMENT: NON-PHARMACOLOGIC AND PHARMACOLOGIC

Presently, there is no cure for this condition; however, the symptoms of EDS and cataplexy can be ameliorated with medications. A comprehensive treatment plan must be adopted, to help allay the clinical symptoms as well as improve health-related quality of life (HRQOL) of affected individuals. Individual needs of patients and their reactions to medications play an important role in the treatment strategy. Non-medical management includes modifying sleep–wake schedules, napping at strategic times of the day, balancing nutritional intake, and exercising to reduce excessive weight and to increase subjective feelings of alertness. Support and counseling may be needed, as will be seen in the ensuing discussion, to cope with the effects of narcolepsy on the lives of patients.

The pharmacologic management of narcolepsy entails the use of stimulants for EDS, tricyclic antidepressants for the secondary symptoms, and benzodiazapines to consolidate disturbed nocturnal sleep.[54,55] Other sleep disorders, if present, must also be treated. Stimulants such as amfetamines, methylphenidate, mazindol, and wakefulness-promoting medications such as modafinil are prescribed for EDS. Commonly reported side-effects of these medications include tremors, irritability, sweating, gastrointestinal symptoms, headache, nausea, and, in rare cases, dyskinesia, hypertension, tachycardia, and psychosis. Tricyclic antidepressants such as imipramine, clomipramine, and protriptyline are prescribed for cataplexy. Side-effects include anticholinergic effects, weight gain, sexual dysfunction, orthostatic hypotension, and antihistaminic symptoms. Selective serotonin reuptake inhibitors (SSRIs) such as fluoxetine and venlafaxine are effective in reducing cataplexy and have fewer side-effects than tricyclics.[42]

It has been shown that γ-hydroxybutyrate (GHB), an endogenous hypnotic chemical, consolidates night-time sleep and improves sleep disruption, cataplexy, daytime sleepiness, and other secondary symptoms of narcolepsy. It is reported to promote both REM sleep and slow-wave sleep.[56] A multicenter study was conducted on 136 narcolepsy patients who experienced 3–249 (median 21) cataplexy attacks weekly. Three doses of GHB (as sodium oxybate 3, 6, or 9 g) or placebo were taken by the subjects in equally divided doses at bedtime. Compared with placebo, a dose-related response was observed in the occurrence of cataplexy, sleep attacks, and naps. Weekly cataplexy attacks were reduced at the 6 g dose and significantly at the 9 g dose ($p = 0.0008$). The results of the Epworth Sleepiness Scale (ESS) showed a reduction at all doses, which was significant at the 9 g dose ($p = 0.0001$). The Clinical Global Impression of Change (CGI-c) was significant at the 9 g dose ($p = 0.0002$). Naps and sleep attacks were also significantly reduced at the 9 g dose ($p = 0.0035$). Sodium oxybate was well tolerated at all three doses. Commonly reported side-effects were nausea, headache, dizziness, and enuresis.[57] Another study on 25 patients with narcolepsy–cataplexy demonstrated dose-related decrease in nocturnal awakenings and increase in daytime SOL. There was an increase in slow-wave sleep (SWS) and delta power, and a reduction in REM sleep. Significant improvements in sleep architecture coincided with significant improvements in daytime functioning.[58]

An unsettling observation made by several investigators is that, in many cases, even with medications, the symptoms of EDS cannot be controlled. Consequently, patients must learn to live with it and its profound effects on their lives.[54,59,60]

IMPACT OF NARCOLEPSY ON HEALTH AND WELFARE: QUALITY OF LIFE ISSUES

It is significant that, whereas strides have been made in the study of the biomedical aspects of narcolepsy, it is only recently that scientific consideration has been given to the social and psychologic aspects of narcolepsy. There is a lack of knowledge about narcolepsy among professionals and lay people. Narcolepsy may be misdiagnosed as depression or hypothyroidism; the symptoms of hypnagogic hallucinations may be mistaken for schizophrenia. In many cases, narcolepsy may remain undiagnosed for several years, and schoolteachers or parents may mistake the symptoms of EDS for laziness, lack of interest, or drug addiction. Thus, contact with an appropriate professional may be delayed by as long as 10 years from the time of inception of symptoms. During this time, the affected individual may drop out of school or become unemployed because of the inability to keep awake.

A strong denial mechanism is often operative, in which case the affected individual may delay an initial contact with a professional for diagnosis and treatment. Denial also poses difficulty in making role transition from well to impaired state, thereby precipitating personal and interaction problems for the individual with family and friends.

The socioeconomic effect impinging on the lives of patients has been reported.[61] International studies, which included Canada, Japan, and Czechoslovakia, have shown that work (performance, income, and job loss), education, driving (accidents or loss of license), interpersonal relationships, social life, and personality were adversely affected.[62] Patients attributed most of these effects to EDS, although some were due to the adverse reaction of medications (e.g., loss of libido and impotence). Based on the clinical presentation and the natural history of narcolepsy, it is suggested that the effects were not influenced by ethnic, cultural, or genetic factors, but were disease-attributed. EDS is characterized in most patients by its unrelenting chronicity, marked intensity, and poor response to treatment.[63] Even in treated patients, their functional status is poor compared with continuous positive airway pressure (CPAP)-treated and untreated obstructive sleep apnea/hypopnea syndrome (OSAHS) patients.[60] The compound effects of narcolepsy were noted in one study in New York City. Unemployment and divorce rates were high in narcolepsy in comparison with the US national rates.[64]

A study in Germany[65] has documented the economic burden of narcolepsy on 75 patients diagnosed with narcolepsy. Information on the symptoms of narcolepsy and their economic impact was obtained through a standardized telephone interview. A mailed questionnaire was utilized to assess HRQOL (SF-36 and EQ-5D). The study measured direct and indirect costs in 2002 Euros. All values were converted from Euros to 2002 US dollars (1 US$ = 0.96 Euros) and are presented in US dollars. Direct medical costs covered medications, inpatient care (hospital), outpatient care (doctor visits), and diagnostic testing. Direct non-medical costs included treatment such as physiotherapy and home equipment. Nursing and sickness benefits were included in this category. In Germany, employees receive sickness benefits if they are out of work for more than 30 days. None of the patients needed nursing care and none was out of work for more than 30 days. Indirect costs included days off from work due to narcolepsy and early retirement.

Direct costs amounted to $3310. Drug costs were $1060, more than 50% of which were attributed to new wake-promoting medications. Annual indirect costs amounted to $11 860 per patient due to early retirement because of narcolepsy. Out of 75 patients, 32 reported narcolepsy as the cause of unemployment. The high economic burden of narcolepsy is comparable to that of diseases such as Parkinson's disease, Alzheimer's disease, epilepsy, and stroke.[65] (Annual direct costs ($3310) plus indirect costs ($11 860) equals $15 170.)

If we examine this issue of impact from a public health perspective, it is pertinent to note that, according to public health reports, automobile accidents are the third leading cause of death and injury in the USA.[66] It has been reported that sleepiness is a risk factor for automobile accidents.[67–71] A study of the hazards of sleep-related motor vehicle accidents showed that the proportion of individuals with sleep-related accidents was 1.5–4 times greater in the hypersomnolent patient group than in the control group. Patients with sleep apnea and narcolepsy accounted for 71% of all sleep-related accidents. The proportion of patents with sleep-related accidents was highest in the narcolepsy group.[72] Motor vehicle crash drivers show significantly more driver sleepiness, slower reaction times, and a trend for greater objective sleepiness compared with matched controls.[73] A recent analysis of responses from 10 870 drivers showed that 23% of all respondents experienced one or more accident. Among respondents who reported four or more accidents, a strong association existed for the most recent accident to include injury ($p < 0.0001$). Sleep disorders were reported by 22.5% of all respondents, with a significantly higher prevalence (35%; $p = 0.002$) for drivers who had been involved in three or more accidents. Thus, sleepiness was strongly associated with a greater risk of automobile accidents.[74] Early diagnosis and education about the impact of sleepiness could reduce automobile accidents; however, most physicians receive little education in the diagnosis and management of sleep disorders.[75]

Other psychosocial areas of investigation are described in a comparison study with epilepsy.

It showed that narcolepsy patients were more affected at work, had poorer driving records, higher accident rates from smoking, and greater problems in planning recreation. Epilepsy patients showed greater problems in educational achievement and maintaining a driver's license.[76] The negative impact of narcolepsy due to EDS and impaired alertness was reaffirmed in 1990.[77] In 1982, McMahon et al.[78] used the Human Service Scale to study need satisfaction in 114 persons with narcolepsy compared with 2406 disabled individuals in order to gain information for rehabilitation planning. This scale is designed to measure physiologic (health), emotional, family, social needs, economic security, economic self-esteem, and vocational self-actualization. A high proportion of those who had narcolepsy scored below the average of the disabled group in needs satisfaction: social needs (35%), physiologic needs (25%), emotional needs (23%), and family needs (21%). On the other hand, persons with narcolepsy had higher scores than the disabled group in vocational self-actualization, economic security, and economic self-esteem. The authors concluded that the feasibility of employment of persons with narcolepsy is high; however, the psychologic aspects of narcolepsy require treatment. Thus, the wide ramifications of having narcolepsy are evident and devastating.

In addition to the social or community-level influence of narcolepsy on health, many studies have examined the role of narcolepsy on psychologic and mental health. Difficulty with concentration, memory, and depression; high anxiety levels; and apathetic demeanor are described by several investigators.[62,64,79,80] Sours[49] described problems of adjustment in overall functioning in narcolepsy. Krishnan et al[81] reviewed the charts of 24 ambulatory male veterans with narcolepsy and found that these patients showed poor adjustment to illness, high unemployment rates, and disturbed family relationships. Sixteen of the patients had adjustment disorder, depression, alcohol dependence, or personality disorder. There were no psychotic diagnoses in the group. Although the sample is highly selected, the devastating impact of narcolepsy is obvious.

In 1982, Kales et al[82] found obsessive–compulsiveness, depression and anxiety, a tendency to internalize and control feelings, feelings of frustration in emotional fulfillment, and impaired interpersonal relationships among 50 patients with narcolepsy.

In 1986, Baker et al[83] reported high scores of hypochondriasis, depression, and hypomania. It was suggested by the authors that these high scores were probably due to difficulties in coping with the symptoms of hypersomnolence. High scores on schizophrenia may have been related to symptoms of hypnagogic hallucinations and other auxiliary symptoms of narcolepsy.[84]

Another devastating effect of narcolepsy is the complaint of decreased libido or impotence or both among male patients with narcolepsy.[62,81,85] It has been reported that impotence is a well-documented side reaction of the tricyclic antidepressants that are prescribed for cataplexy.[85] Depression in narcolepsy may be another factor accounting for sexual dysfunction. Cataplexy or sleep attacks during sex are likely to impair the sexual relationship of partners.

The problem of untoward side-effects of medications poses a dilemma for many patients. Adverse drug reactions of stimulant medications may occur, especially if prescribed in high doses for prolonged periods of time for severe cases of narcolepsy. Amfetamines may cause irritability, mood changes, headaches, palpitations, sweating, and tremors,[86] paranoia, or psychosis with visual hallucinations and paranoid delusions.[87–90] Dyskinesias may also result from prolonged use of amfetamines.[91] Thus, patients may cease treatment because of the negative effects of medications on the quality of their personal and social lives.[92] Cessation of treatment may in turn render the person totally incapacitated, and unable to work or to participate in meaningful social activities.

The frequency of alcohol abuse or dependence was reported in 1989.[93] Patients with disorders of excessive somnolence (DOES) abused alcohol more frequently than did patients with other sleep disorders or controls. A Self-Administered Alcohol Screening Test (SAAST) showed that 26.8% in the narcolepsy group scored greater than 7%, which indicates possible or probable alcoholism, compared with 13.2% of the entire DOES group or 5.4% of the controls. The cause of this dependence on alcohol is not known, and may be correlated with personality type or frustrations in coping with the negative life effects of narcolepsy. Management must include careful screening, treatment, and support by appropriate professionals.

Despite the well-known and long-recognized impact of narcolepsy on psychosocial functioning and health in general,[94,95] only a limited number of studies have addressed the HRQOL issues.[96] The first clinical trial in narcolepsy to include HRQOL was conducted to study the effects of modafinil (Provigil).[97] Data were collected in two similar 9-week double-blind studies. A total of 558 subjects from 38 centers were randomized into one of three groups: placebo, 200 mg modafinil, or 400 mg modafinil. Several validated instruments were used to measure the extent of sleepiness and alertness. A questionnaire comprising the 36-item Short Form Survey (SF-36) and supplemental narcolepsy-specific scales was administered to assess quality-of-life changes with treatment. These instruments were pretested on narcolepsy patients in two sleep centers.[98]

Compared with the general population, subjects with narcolepsy were more affected in vitality, social functioning, and ability to perform usual activities due to physical and emotional problems. People with narcolepsy experienced HRQOL effects as bad as or worse than those with Parkinson's disease and epilepsy in several HRQOL areas. HRQOL effects were worse among people with narcolepsy than among those with migraine headaches, with one exception: bodily pain.

The 400 mg modafinil group showed improvement over placebo in 10 of the 17 HRQOL scales. When compared with the placebo group, the 400 mg modafinil group had fewer limitations in everyday activities due to physical or emotional problems, more energy, and less interference with normal social activities due to health. In addition, the 400 mg modafinil group had fewer narcolepsy symptoms and higher attention/concentration, productivity, self-esteem, and overall health perceptions compared with placebo. The 200 mg modafinil group showed better results than placebo in the following 9 of the 17 HRQOL scales: physical functioning, role limitations due to physical problems, vitality, mental health summary scale, narcolepsy symptoms, attention/concentration, productivity, self-esteem, and driving limitations.

The profound effect of narcolepsy on children warrants special attention. Alertness levels and performance in young people are significantly compromised when sleepiness results in sleep attacks during task performance. Attention, memory, motor, and cognitive skills are affected by sleepiness.[99,100] Due to the inability to wake up early, school-aged youth often miss the morning hours at school or their school performance may be inconsistent. Quite often, narcolepsy or other sleep disorders are not considered, and the child is viewed by teachers and school administrators as lazy or having a behavioral problem. Many children suffering from symptoms of excessive daytime sleepiness get placed in special education classes, are seen as hyperactive, and have conflicts with teachers. Socially, these youngsters suffer because they want to hide their illness from peers and teachers. The falls that can occur in cataplexy are especially embarrassing. These children benefit by meeting others with the same sleep disorder. Family members often do not understand the condition or its symptoms, and this results in interpersonal problems with the child. Prompt diagnosis and management will reduce the frustrations, self-doubt, and lack of self-confidence often experienced by those who are afflicted with this impairment.

NEEDS OF PERSONS WITH NARCOLEPSY

Although an estimated 250 000 people in the USA have narcolepsy, no study has attempted to assess their total health service needs and access to relevant services. Traditionally, the needs of patients are determined by medical professionals who focus on the physical aspects of a disorder and its medical management. This highly commendable service by physicians in the face of rising pressures by patients and third-party payment systems must be supported and respected. Today, however, complex arrays of factors operate that make it necessary to reexamine the traditional methods of patient care and their beneficial effects on the patient. It must be noted that, with increasing prevalence of chronic illness and an aging population, coupled with uncertain and unanticipated consequences of long-term use of medications, alternative modes of management have gained increasing significance. The proliferation of self-help groups and support groups across the country in the management of various diseases is testimony that, in addition to the medical management of disease, the non-medical aspects of care are a needed component of treatment. The beneficial effects of social support in stressful life events have been examined by several authors;[101–103] its buffering effect has been demonstrated in pregnancy,[104] mental health,[105,106] and unemployment.[107,108]

In view of this demand by patients for supplemental/alternative care in addition to the medications prescribed by physicians, it was felt that a survey to assess the perceived needs of narcolepsy patients would yield useful information for program development and patient management. The Narcolepsy Project conducted such a survey in 1986 to assess the employment status and psychosocial support needs of persons with narcolepsy in New York State who had registered with the Project.[64] Of the 120 patients who received the questionnaire (80 were returned because of change of address), 68 completed responses were received, eliciting a response rate of 57%. When respondents and non-respondents were compared, no statistically significant differences were observed in age, sex, or marital status ($p < 0.05$). Therefore, age, sex, and marital status do not appear to bias the results.[10] The following perceived needs were reported in descending order: information and referral center for narcolepsy (84%); group counseling (65%); assistance in making career transitions (50%); transportation (34%); homemaker services (25%); and homecare services (18%).

With regard to employment status, 16% were unemployed and seeking work – a rate higher than the US average of 7.5%.[109]

In personal interviews, respondents expressed fear of traveling alone or in the dark, embarrassment about symptoms of daytime sleepiness and automatic behavior, and fear of being mistaken for drug addicts, or being labeled as 'lazy'. Untreated patients manifested a low level of motivation and an apathetic demeanor. Problems with memory, a low level of energy, and pervasive feelings of tiredness or weakness were common complaints.[10]

Thus, the major perceived needs of persons with narcolepsy were psychosocial support services, assistance in making career transitions, and transportation services, indicating the need to develop programs tailored to these patients' expressed needs.

IS NARCOLEPSY A DISABILITY OR A DEVELOPMENTAL DISABILITY?

Let us now consider the definition of narcolepsy in terms of its functional status. What is the difference between a disability and impairment? According to the American Medical Association (AMA) Guide to the Evaluation of Permanent Impairment, (page x of Foreword)[110] permanent medical impairment is related to the health status of the individual, whereas disability may be determined within the context of the personal, social, or occupational demands or the statutory or regulatory requirements that the individual is unable to meet as a result of the impairment. Again (p 215),[110] 'Impairment is a medical determination. It involves any anatomical or functional abnormality or any clinically significant behavior changes', whereas 'disability' refers to 'the functional, social, or vocational level of an individual that has been altered by an impairment'.

Because narcolepsy does not cause physical disfigurement or a discernable handicap, many professionals, as well as patients, do not realize that the federal and state governments classify narcolepsy legally as a 'disability'.

The laws and regulations that protect people with disabilities and specifically narcolepsy are described in detail by Sundram and Johnson.[111] Here, we briefly present these laws. The Rehabilitation Act of 1973 prohibits discrimination on the basis of disability under any program or activity receiving federal financial assistance[112] and defines an 'individual with handicaps' as a person who has:[113]

(a)   a physical or mental impairment that substantially limits one or more of the major life activities of such individuals

(b)   a record of such impairments, or

(c)   has been regarded as having such an impairment

Narcolepsy, being a neurologic disorder, falls within this definition. The Americans with Disabilities Act of 1990 (ADA) uses the same definition of disability as individuals with handicaps under the Rehabilitation Act, which includes narcolepsy.[111] The ADA protects individuals with disabilities and provides equal opportunities in employment, public accommodations, transportation, state and local government services, and telecommunication.[111] Narcolepsy is also considered a disability under the New York State Human Rights Law, which bars discrimination against the handicapped. Thus, individuals with narcolepsy are eligible for services through the state developmental disabilities programs. Most providers of care as well as consumers are unaware of the rights of individuals with a disability such as narcolepsy.

What is a developmental disability? An advisory from the New York State Office of Mental Retardation and Developmental Disabilities states that under Section 1.03(22) of the New York State Mental Hygiene Law, which is the legal base for eligibility determination, a developmental disability is defined as a disability of a person that:

(a)   (1)   is attributable to mental retardation, cerebral palsy, epilepsy, neurological impairment, or autism

        (2)   is attributable to any other condition of a person found to be closely related to

mental retardation because such condition results in similar impairment of general intellectual functioning or adaptive behavior to that of mentally retarded persons or requires treatment and services similar to those required for such persons; or

(3)   is attributable to dyslexia resulting from a disability described in (1) or (2)

(b)   originates before such person attains age 22 year

(c)   has continued or can be expected to continue indefinitely, and

(d)   constitutes a substantial handicap to such a person's ability to function normally in society

Functional limitations constituting a substantial handicap are defined in this document as significant limitations in adaptive functioning that are determined from the findings of assessment by using a nationally normed and validated, comprehensive, and individual measure of adaptive behavior administered by a qualified practitioner. Some patients with narcolepsy qualify for services and benefits following this definition of a developmental disability.

IMPLICATIONS FOR PATIENTS, FAMILY, AND COMMUNITY

The consequences of narcolepsy on the life of the patient are several and often pervasive. Because people with narcolepsy look normal, their tendency to fall asleep in socially unacceptable situations is perceived by others as lack of drive or interest. This causes relationship problems with family members, teachers, and employers. The individual, often unaware of the problem, strives unusually hard to meet the expectations of a highly success-oriented society. Unable to fulfill these expectations, the person experiences a considerable amount of role strain and role conflict. Most of the person's time and energy are expended in resolving these conflicts, with little time for rewarding social activities.

Repeated failures in fulfilling role obligations lead to disrupted relationships, poor self-esteem, lack of confidence, and a sense of vulnerability to all kinds of stressful situations. Alienation (a sense of isolation) is often observed in personal interviews with patients.

Individuals with narcolepsy, it was noted earlier, also tend to manifest symptoms of depression and anxiety. Cataplectic attacks are avoided by keeping away from situations that precipitate such attacks, thus depriving the individual of many enriching activities. Anticipation of such attacks is likely to lead to high levels of anxiety. Depression may result from dysfunctional relationships and frustrations in achieving life's goals.

In personal interviews, patients with narcolepsy report fear of being mistaken for drug addicts by others; therefore, they are afraid of revealing the nature of their illness to anyone, especially in the work environment. In severe and prolonged uncontrolled cases these patients may find themselves without a family or a job, quite destitute, and lonely.

At a global level, an undiagnosed case of narcolepsy is a loss to the community, since most individuals with narcolepsy, when proper treatment is instituted, can function normally within the framework of the family and the work environment. Lack of awareness of the impact and management of narcolepsy can result in ineffective utilization of human resources with a subsequent drain on the national economy.

RECOMMENDATIONS

Management of narcolepsy

Once a diagnosis has been established, efforts should be directed toward secondary preventive measures. This would entail medical and non-medical strategies for slowing the disease process and reducing its negative impact. It is clear that, along with the medications prescribed by physicians, the psychosocial management of the impact of the clinical symptoms, diagnosis, and treatment needs to be provided by special counselors. For example, the psychologic effects, problems in interpersonal relations, education, and employment need the skills of a professional who has a background in the social sciences. Moreover, medical professionals must consider very seriously the problem of iatrogenesis. Ideal management of the patient should integrate the medical and non-medical aspects of care to treat the whole person and not just the disease. This comprehensive approach to patient care would improve the quality of health services, increase patient and provider satisfaction, and improve health outcomes.

Counseling and support services provided by professionals must encompass emotional and social support to enhance coping skills of affected individuals as well as advocacy to get timely referrals, diagnosis, treatment, and, when applicable, disability benefits. Additionally, support that is more instrumental in nature (financial benefits for disability status, homecare services, homemaker services, and transportation) is an expressed need of narcolepsy patients.

A sociomedical model of healthcare delivery that would integrate the medical and psychosocial basis of care is recommended. In this model, the medical and social science professionals are envisioned as working in a synergistic relationship toward the twin goals of ameliorating the impact of a disability and increasing patient satisfaction – an important component of quality of healthcare services.

The importance of self-help groups led by patients must not be underestimated. These groups, however, must include diagnosed cases of narcolepsy and not suspected or questionable cases. Self-help groups, as well as support groups led by professionals, must be incorporated into the existing healthcare delivery system to provide feedback from patients and to avoid fragmentation of services – another crucial component of quality of healthcare services.

Public health measures

Narcolepsy is a lifelong illness that calls for comprehensive yet sustained care. In light of our observation that there are delays in seeking professional help for sleepiness, problems of misdiagnosis, and

lack of awareness about the psychosocial ramifications of having narcolepsy, we infer that diffusion of knowledge about narcolepsy has not occurred at the community level. It is therefore recommended that public health measures for prevention be adopted. Information about sleep, alertness, and narcolepsy must be disseminated to employers, parent groups, schools, and healthcare professionals. Screening devices that are simple and inexpensive need to be developed for use in schools and colleges. Appropriate diagnosis and treatment instituted early in the life cycle of the condition can save the youngster and the family much frustration. Physicians have an important role in educating their patients about the risks of accidents due to EDS. They must have the tools for diagnosis and management of sleep disorders and be familiar with the laws and regulations governing driving conditions. Educational programs for the public, physicians, and drivers are needed. The AMA has recommended continued research on devices and technologies to detect EDS and prevent the deterioration of driver alertness and performance.[114]

Education of professionals

Information about sleep, alertness, and narcolepsy must be provided in medical schools, as well as to primary care physicians, so that accurate diagnosis and referral to sleep disorder specialists can be made. Medical board examinations could include questions on sleep. This recommendation is based on the observation that many cases are undiagnosed or misdiagnosed by primary care physicians. Difficulties in getting medications from pharmacists, expressed by many patients, may be alleviated by directing an educational campaign toward pharmacists and involving them in symposia and conferences on sleep.

A sociomedical model of healthcare delivery would call for the training of a professional with a background in public health medicine, genetics, and the social sciences. This professional must also have excellent communication skills and coordinate patient management strategies with medical professionals involved in the treatment process.

Furthermore, awareness of the laws and regulations governing the rights of patients with narcolepsy will enable professionals to make appropriate referrals and become effective advocates.

Finally, professionals must be cognizant of the menacing effects of such seemingly benign symptoms as hypnagogic hallucinations, sleep paralysis, and automatic behaviors. These symptoms may cause severe psychologic distress and interpersonal difficulties. Accidents may result due to automatic behavior. With awareness of these factors, appropriate therapy can be instituted to improve the quality of life of narcolepsy patients.

Employment

Work lends structure, discipline, personal satisfaction, and dignity to life. It is also more cost-effective to support the disabled to engage in work or to volunteer their talents rather than live solely on disability benefits. The course of action to be taken will depend on the level of severity of the disability. In view of the American values of independence and self-help, health policy must recommend the promotion of functioning in society rather than merely treating a disorder. Individuals may be transitioned from a disability status into a functional status by the support of healthcare workers. Incentives may be offered to the disabled, such as a training program or an adjusted job with pay, so that financial rewards are available during the training period or a part-time job experience while still on disability benefits.

Advocacy in the work environment is needed so that structural changes may be instituted in the form of flexible work hours, work sharing, part-time jobs, napping periods at work, and the opportunity to have a home-based office.

Research priorities

Our review of existing literature reveals several drawbacks in research. Investigations are based on selected diagnosed cases of narcolepsy, often without comparison groups. A major selection bias is introduced, since only the insured or those who can afford the high costs of diagnosis are included in studies. The lower socioeconomic groups, the unemployed, and minority groups may be underrepresented in estimates of prevalence rates and unmet needs. The small numbers available for research tend to reduce the statistical power of the study. Often the diagnostic categories are not clearly defined; for instance, cases without a PSG and MSLT evaluation may be included in the study. Heterogeneity within diagnostic categories (e.g., sleep apnea cases) is likely to suppress the relationship between variables. Moreover, the symptom categories of narcolepsy are often not clearly defined. Lastly, the confounding effects of medications on memory, depression, and hypnagogic hallucinations need consideration.

An enactment of a national plan to pool resources for research in a manner that is integrative and beneficial to all participants is needed. More studies with comparison groups and clearly defined diagnostic categories must be encouraged. Operational definitions of symptoms of narcolepsy must be developed to standardize measures and make meaningful comparisons between studies. Population surveys using statistical sampling techniques would yield more accurate prevalence and incidence rates. Operational definitions of disability status and levels of severity specific for narcolepsy would provide fair and objective methods of determining disability benefits and eligibility for work incentives. An international study of correlations between diet, climate, napping habits, coping mechanisms, and narcolepsy may reveal useful data in understanding the precipitating factors and cultural differences in coping techniques in narcolepsy. Finally, the following research questions need to be addressed:

- What are the predictors of narcolepsy?

- What role would one ascribe to the environment in the pathophysiology of narcolepsy?

- What are the predictors of the levels of severity in narcolepsy?

- What is the impact of support in narcolepsy?

- By what mechanism do support groups provide benefits to patients?

- What kind of work environment and occupations are ideal for those who have disorders of EDS or narcolepsy?

Until researchers can discover the cause and cure for narcolepsy, optimum management strategy should focus on the integration of the biologic, psychologic, social, and spiritual dimensions of health. This laudable task can only be accomplished by medical and social science professionals working in a symbiotic relationship in the delivery of healthcare and public health research.

More reliable state and national policy initiatives need to be developed, and they in turn must focus on the strategies for financing and structuring the delivery of evidence-based services to the patient population.

REFERENCES

1. Oliver WA. Relation of an extraordinary sleepy person, at Tinsbury, near Bath. Philosophical Transactions of the Royal Society. London, 1704; 24: 2177–82.
2. Graves RJ. Observations on the nature and treatment of various diseases. Dublin Q J Med 1851; 11: 1–20.
3. Caffé M. Maladie du sommeil. J Connais Med Pharmaceut 1862; 29: 323.
4. Westphal C. Eigenthumliche mit Einschafen verbundene Anfalle. Arch Psychiat Nervenkr 1877; 7: 631–5.
5. Gelineau J. De La Narcolepsie. Gazette de l' Hopital (Paris) 1880; 53: 626–8; 635–7.
6. Bassetti C. Narcolepsy. Curr Treat Options Neurol 1999; 1: 291–8.
7. Bassetti C, Aldrich MS. Narcolepsy. Neurol Clin 1996; 14: 545–71.
8. Stores G. The protean manifestations of childhood narcolepsy and their misinterpretation. Dev Med Child Neurol 2006; 48: 307–10.
9. Yoss RE, Daly D. Criteria for the diagnosis of the narcoleptic syndrome. Mayo Clin Proc 1957; 3: 320–8.
10. Goswami M. The influence of clinical symptoms on quality of life in patients with narcolepsy. Neurology 1998; 50(2 Suppl 1): S31–6.
11. Siegel JM. Narcolepsy: a key role for hypocretins (orexins). Cell 1999; 98: 409–12.
12. Guilleminault C, Brooks SN. Excessive daytime sleepiness: a challenge for the practicing neurologist. Brain 2001; 124: 1482–91.
13. van den Pol AN. Narcolepsy: a neurodegenerative disease of the hypocretin system? Neuron 2000; 27: 415–18.
14. Roth T, Roehrs TA. Etiologies and sequelae of excessive daytime sleepiness. Clin Therapeutics 1996; 18: 562–76.
15. Dauvilliers Y, Billiard M, Montplaisir J. Clinical aspects and pathophysiology of narcolepsy. Clin Neurophysiol 2003; 114: 2000–17.
16. Vogel G. Studies in psychophysiology of dreams III. The dream of narcolepsy. Arch Gen Psychiatry 1960; 3: 421–8.
17. Rechtschaffen A, Wolpert EA, Dement WC, Mitchell SA, Fischer C. Nocturnal sleep in narcoleptics. Electroenceph Clin Neurophysiol 1963; 15: 599–609.
18. Takahashi H, Jimbo M. Polygraphic study of narcoleptic syndrome with special reference to hypnogogic hallucinations and cataplexy. Folia Psychiatrica et Neurologica Japonica 1963; 7: 343–7.
19. In: Guilleminault C, Passouant P, Dement WC, eds. Narcolepsy, Vol 1. New York: Spectrum, 1976: 4.
20. Dement WC, Rechtschaffen A. Narcolepsy: polygraphic aspects, experimental and theoretical considerations. In: Gastaut H, Lugaresi E, Berti-Ceroni G, Coccagna G, eds. The Abnormalities of Sleep in Man. Bologna, Italy: Aulo Gaggi, 1968: 147–64.
21. Broughton RJ. Narcolepsy. CMAJ 1974; 110: 7.
22. Montplaisir J, DeChamplain J, Young S, Missala K, Sourkes T. Narcolepsy and idiopathic hypersomnia: biogenic amines and related compounds in CSF. Neurology 1982; 32: 1299–302.
23. Aldrich MS. The neurobiology of narcolepsy–cataplexy syndrome. Int J Neurol 1991/92; 25/26: 29–40.
24. Krahn LE, Black JL, Silber MH. Narcolepsy: new understanding of irresistible sleep. Mayo Clin Proc 2001; 76: 185–94.
25. Scammell TE. The neurobiology, diagnosis, and treatment of narcolepsy. Ann Neurol 2003; 53: 154–66.

26. Honda Y, Juji T, Matsuki K, et al. HLA-DR2 and DW2 in narcolepsy and in other disorders of excessive somnolence without cataplexy. Sleep 1986; 9: 133–42.

27. Langdon N, Welsh KI, Dam WV, Vaughan RW, Parkes JD. Genetic markers in narcolepsy. Lancet 1984; ii: 1178–80.

28. Billiard M, Seignalet J, Besset A, Cadilhac J. HLA-DR2 and narcolepsy. Sleep 1986; 9: 149–52.

29. Pollack S, Peled R, Gideoni O, Lavie P. HLA-DR2 in Israeli Jews with narcolepsy–cataplexy. Isr J Med Sci 1988; 24: 123–5.

30. Lock CB, So AK, Welsh KI, Parkes JD, Trowsdale J. MHC class II sequences of an HLA-DR2 narcoleptic. Immunogenetics 1988; 27: 449–55.

31. Peled R, Lavie P. Narcolepsy–cataplexy: an extremely rare disorder in Israel. Sleep Res 1987; 16: 404–6.

32. Honda Y, Matsuki K. Genetic aspects of narcolepsy. In: Thorpy MJ, ed. Handbook of Sleep Disorders. New York: Marcel Dekker, 1990: 217–34.

33. Mignot E, Hayduk R, Black J, et al. HLA DQB1*0602 is associated with cataplexy in 509 narcoleptic patients. Sleep 1997; 20: 1012–20.

34. Mignot E, Ling L, Rogers R, et al. Complex HLA-DR and -DQ interactions confer risk of narcolepsy–cataplexy in three ethnic groups. Am J Hum Genet 2001; 68: 686–99.

35. Mignot E. Genetic and familial aspects of narcolepsy. Neurology 1998; 50(2 Suppl 1): S16–22.

36. Lin L, Hungs M, Mignot E. Narcolepsy and the HLA region. J Neuroimmunol 2001; 117: 9–20.

37. Black JL 3rd. Narcolepsy: a review of evidence for autoimmune diathesis. Int Rev Psychiatry 2005; 17: 461–9.

38. Overeem S, Verschuuren JJ, Fronczek R, et al. Immunohistochemical screening for autoantibodies against lateral hypothalamic neurons in human narcolepsy. J Neuroimmunol 2006; 6: 6.

39. Nishino S, Ripley B, Overeem S, Lammers GJ, Mignot E. Hypocretin (orexin) deficiency in human narcolepsy. Lancet 2000; 355: 39–40.

40. Peyron C, Faraco J, Rogers W, et al. A mutation in a case of early onset narcolepsy and a generalized absence of hypocretin peptides in human narcoleptic brains. Nat Med 2000; 6: 991–7.

41. Thannical TC, Moore RY, Nienhuis R, et al. Reduced number of hypocretin neurons in human narcolepsy. Neuron 2000; 27: 469–74.

42. Brooks SN, Mignot E. Narcolepsy and idiopathic hypersomnolence In: Lee-Chiong TL Jr, Sateia MJ, Carskadon MA, eds. Sleep Medicine. Philadelphia, PA: Hanley and Belfus, 2002: 193–202.

43. Dement WC, Zarcone V, Varner V, et al. The prevalence of narcolepsy. Sleep Res 1972; 1: 148.

44. Dement WC, Carskadon M, Ley R. The prevalence of narcolepsy II. Sleep Res 1973; 2: 147.

45. Hublin C, Kapiro J, Partinen M, et al. The prevalence of narcolepsy: an epidemiological study of the Finnish twin cohort. Ann Neurol 1994; 35: 709–16.

46. Silber MH, Krahn LE, Olson EJ, et al. The epidemiology of narcolepsy in Olmsted County, Minnesota: a population based study. Sleep 2002; 25: 197–202.

47. Uryu N, Maeda M, Nagata Y, et al. No difference in the nucleotide sequence of the DQB B1 domain between narcoleptic and healthy individuals with DR2 DW2. Hum Immunol 1989; 24: 175–81.

48. Ohayon MM, Priest RG, Zulley J, Smirne S, Paiva T. Prevalence of narcolepsy symptomatology and diagnosis in the European general population. Neurology 2002; 58: 1826–33.

49. Sours JA. Narcolepsy and other disturbances in the sleep–waking rhythms. A study of 115 cases with review of the literature. J Nerv Ment Dis 1963; 137: 523–42.

50. Passouant P, Billiard M. The evolution of narcolepsy with age. In: Guilliminault C, Dement WC, Passouant P, eds. Narcolepsy. New York: Spectrum, 1976: 179–97.

51. Roth B. Narcolepsy and Hypersomnia. Basel: S Karger, 1980.

52. Guilleminault C, Anders TF. Sleep disorders in children. Adv Pediatr 1976; 22: 155–74.

53. Guilleminault C. Narcolepsy syndrome. In: Kryger MH, Roth TA, Dement WC, eds. Principles and Practice of Sleep Medicine. Philadelphia, PA: WB Saunders, 1989: 338.

54. Thorpy MJ, Goswami M. Treatment of narcolepsy. In: Thorpy MJ, ed. A Handbook of Sleep Disorders. New York: Marcel Dekker, 1990: 235–58.

55. Houghton WC, Scammell TE, Thorpy M, Houghton WC. Pharmacotherapy for cataplexy. Sleep Med Rev 2004; 8: 355–66.

56. Lammers GJ, Arends J, Declerk AC, et al. Gamma-hydroxybutyrate and narcolepsy: A double-blind placebo-controlled study. Sleep 1993; 16: 216–20.

57. U.S. Xyrem Multicenter Study Group. A randomized, double blind, placebo-controlled multicenter trial comparing the effects of three doses of orally administered sodium oxybate with placebo for the treatment of narcolepsy. Sleep 2002; 25: 42–9.

58. Mamelak M, Black J, Montplaisir J, Ristanovich R. A pilot study on the effects of sodium oxybate on sleep architecture and daytime alertness in narcolepsy. Sleep 2004; 27: 1327–34.

59. Mitler MM, Hajdukovic R, Erman M, Koziol JA. Narcolepsy. J Clin Neurophysiol 1990; 7: 93–118.

60. Teixeira VG, Faccenda JF, Douglas NJ. Functional status in patients with narcolepsy. Sleep Med 2004; 5: 477–83.

61. Broughton WA, Broughton RJ. Psychosocial impact of narcolepsy. Sleep 1994; 17: 545–9.

62. Broughton R, Ghanem Q, Hishikawa Y, et al. Life effects of narcolepsy in 180 patients from North America, Asia and Europe compared to matched controls. Can J Neurol Sci 1981; 8: 299–304.

63. Broughton R, Ghanem Q, Hishikawa Y, Sugita Y, Nevismalova S, Roth B. Life effects of narcolepsy: relationships to geographic origin (North American, Asia or European) and to other patient and treatment variables. Can J Neuro Sci 1983; 10: 100–4.

64. Broughton R, Ghanem Q. The impact of compound narcolepsy on the life of the patient. In: Guilleminault C, Dement WC, Passouant P, eds. Narcolepsy. New York: Spectrum, 1976: 201–19.

65. Dodel R, Peter H, Walbert T, et al. The socioeconomic impact of narcolepsy. Sleep 2004; 27: 1123–8.

66. US Bureau of the Census. Statistical Abstract of the United States: 1990. Washington, DC: US Department of Commerce, 1990: 606.

67. Findley LJ, Fabrizio M, Thommi G, Surratt PM. Severity of sleep apnea and automobile crashes. N Engl J Med 1989; 320: 868–9.

68. Mitler M, Carskadon M, Czeisler C, et al. Catastrophies, sleep and public policy: consensus report. Sleep 1988; 11: 100–9.

69. National Commission on Sleep Disorders Research Report. Vol 1. Executive Summary and Executive Report. Bethosda, MD: National Institutes of Health, 1993.

70. Horne J, Reyner L. Vehicle accidents related to sleep: a review. Occup Environ Med 1999; 56: 289–94.

71. Maclean AW, Davies DR, Thiele K. The hazards and prevention of driving while sleepy. Sleep Med Rev 2003; 7: 507–21.

72. Aldrich MS. Automobile accidents in patients with sleep disorders. Sleep 1989; 12: 487–94.

73. Kingshott RN, Jones DR, Smith AD, Taylor DR. The role of sleep-disordered breathing, daytime sleepiness, and impaired performance in motor vehicle crashes – a case control study. Sleep Breath 2004; 8: 61–72.

74. Powell NB, Schechtman KB, Riley TW, Li K, Guilleminault C. Sleepy driving: accidents and injury. Otolaryngol Head Neck Surg 2002; 126: 217–27.

75. Rosen RC, Rosekind M, Rosevear C, Cole WE, Dement WC. Physician education in sleep and sleep disorders. Sleep 1993; 16: 249–54.

76. Broughton R, Guberman A, Roberts J. Comparison of the psychosocial effects of epilepsy and of narcolepsy/cataplexy: a controlled study. Epilepsia 1984; 25: 423–33.

77. Rosenthal L, Merlotti L, Young DK, et al. Subjective and polysomnographic characteristics of patients diagnosed with narcolepsy. Gen Hosp Psychiatry 1990; 12: 191–7.

78. McMahon ST, Walsh JK, Sexton K, Smitson SA. Need satisfaction in narcolepsy. Rehab Liter 1982; 43: 82–5.

79. Ganado W. The narcolepsy syndrome. Neurology 1958; 8: 487–96.

80. Roth TA, Merlotti L. Advances in the diagnosis of narcolepsy. Presented at 3rd International Symposium on Narcolepsy, San Diego, CA, June 1988.

81. Krishnan RR, Volow MR, Miller PP, Carwile ST. Narcolepsy: preliminary retrospective study of psychiatric and psychosocial aspects. Am J Psychiatry 1984; 141: 428–31.

82. Kales A, Soldatos CR, Bixler EO, et al. Narcolepsy–cataplexy II. Psychosocial consequences and associated psychopathology. Arch Neurol 1982; 139: 169–71.

83. Baker TL, Guilleminault C, Nino-Murcia G, Dement WC. Comparative polysomnographic study of narcolepsy and idiopathic central nervous system hypersomnia. Sleep 1986; 9: 232–42.

84. Kishi Y, Konishi S, Koizumi S, et al. Schizophrenia and narcolepsy: a review with a case report. Psychiatry Clin Neurosci 2004; 58: 117–24.

85. Karacan I. Erectile dysfunction in narcoleptic patients. Sleep 1986; 9: 227–31.

86. Parkes JD. Amphetamines and other drugs in the treatment of daytime drowsiness and cataplexy. In: Parkes JD, ed. Sleep and its Disorders. London: WB Saunders, 1985: 459–82.

87. Zarcone V. Narcolepsy. N Engl J Med 1973; 288: 1156–66.

88. Pfefferbaum A, Berger P. Narcolepsy, paranoid psychosis, and tardive dyskinesia: a pharmacological dilemma. J Nerv Ment Dis 1977; 164: 293–7.

89. Schrader G, Hicks EP. Narcolepsy, paranoid psychosis, major depression, and tardive dyskinesia. J Nerv Ment Dis 1984; 172: 439–41.

90. Young D, Scoville WB. Paranoid psychosis in narcolepsy and possible danger of benzedrine treatment. Med Clin North Am 1938; 22: 637–46.

91. Mattson RH, Calverley JR. Dextroamphetamine-sulfate-induced dyskinesias. JAMA 1968; 204: 400–2.

92. Gillin JC, Horowitz D, Wyatt RJ. Pharmacologic studies of narcolepsy involving serotonin, acetylcholine and monoamine oxidase. In: Guilleminault C, Dement WC, Passouant P, eds. Narcolepsy. New York: Spectrum, 1976: 585–604.

93. Fredrickson PA, Kaplan J, Richardson J, Esther M. Prevalence of alcohol abuse in narcolepsy and other disorders of excessive somnolence. Arch Found Thanatol 1989; 16: No.12.

94. Broughton WA, Broughton RJ. Psychosocial impact of narcolepsy. Sleep 1994; 17: S45–9.

95. Bruck D. The impact of narcolepsy on psychosocial health and role behaviours: negative effects and comparisons with other illness groups. Sleep Med 2001; 2: 437–46.

96. Reimer MA, Flemons WW. Quality of life in sleep disorders. Sleep Med Rev 2003; 7: 335–49.

97. Beusterien KM, Rogers AE, Walsleben JA, et al. Health-related quality of life effects of modafinil for treatment of narcolepsy. Sleep 1999; 22: 757–65.

98. Stoddard RB, Goswami M, Ingalls KK. The development and validation of an instrument to evaluate quality of life in narcolepsy patients. Drug Information Journal 1996. Amber, PA: Drug Information Association, 1996: 850.

99. Kashden J, Wise M, Avarado I, et al. Neurocognitive functioning in children with narcolepsy. Sleep Res 1996; 25: 262.

100. Nevšímalová Sona. Narcolepsy in children. Sleep Res 1999; (2 Suppl 1): 410.

101. Cohen S, Wills TA. Stress, social support and the buffering hypothesis. Psychol Bull 1985; 98: 310–57.

102. Leavy RL. Social support and psychological disorder: a review. J Community Psychol 1983; 11: 3–21.

103. Gottlieb BH. Social Networks and Social Support. Beverly Hills, CA: Sage, 1981.

104. Nuckolls KG, Gassell J, Kaplan BH. Psychosocial assets, life crises and the prognosis of pregnancy. Am J Epidemiol 1972; 95: 431–41.

105. Wilcox BL. Social support, life stress and psychological adjustment: a testing of the buffering hypothesis. Am J Community Psychol 1981; 9: 371–87.

106. Lin N, Woefel MW, Light SC. The buffering effect of social support subsequent to an important life event. J Health Soc Behav 1985; 26: 247–63.

107. Gore SL. The effects of social support in moderating the health consequences of unemployment. J Health Soc Behav 1978; 19: 157–65.

108. Pearlin LI, Lieberman M, Menaghan E, Mullen J. The stress process. J Health Soc Behav 1981; 22: 337–57.

109. US Bureau of the Census. Characteristics of the Civilian Labor Force, by State: 1984. In: Statistical Abstract of the United States. Washington, DC: US Department of Commerce, 1986: 393.

110. American Medical Association. Guide to the Evaluation of Permanent Impairment, 2nd edn. Chicago, IL: American Medical Association, 1984.

111. Sundram CJ, Johnson PW. The legal aspects of narcolepsy. In: Goswami M, Pollak PC, Cohen FL, et al, eds. Psychosocial Aspects of Narcolepsy. New York: Haworth Press, 1992: 175–92.

112. The Rehabilitation Act of 1973, 29, U.S.C. S 701 et seq.

113. The Rehabilitation Act of 1973, 29, U.S.C. S 706 (7) (b).

114. Lyznicki JM, Doege TC, Davis RM, Williams MA, for the Council of Scientific Affairs AMA. Sleepiness, driving, and motor vehicle crashes. JAMA 1998; 279: 1908–13.

15

Stress and sleep

Vadim Rotenberg

The restricted space available here does not allow coverage of all of the important aspects of such a broad and polydimensional topic as the relationship between stress and sleep (animal models of stress outcome on sleep are discussed in Chapter 17). Thus, the present chapter deals only with data collected in humans, and will concentrate on contradictions among the data, proposing an integral theoretical approach to the problem.

SLEEP: A VICTIM OF STRESS OR COPING MODERATOR?

Alteration of sleep structure under stressful conditions may reflect a number of different and even opposite processes. On the one hand, brain mechanisms of sleep, like any other physiologic system, may be damaged by stress. In such cases, sleep disturbances not only represent a negative outcome of stress, they also contribute to this outcome. On the other hand, alterations of sleep may represent an attempt to compensate for the negative outcome of stress on the psychophysiologic state of the subject, contributing to the coping mechanisms that protect health. In both cases, sleep structure became different from that typical of the normal healthy subject under non-stressful conditions, and it may be difficult for researchers to discriminate these two types of sleep alteration despite their opposing tendencies. At the same time, if different subjects in the same otherwise similar group display these

opposite reactions during an investigation, this can mask differences in the sleep outcome of stress and make the average sleep structure undistinguishable from normal sleep structure. This may be why some investigators have failed to show any substantial changes in sleep structure, particularly in rapid eye movement (REM) sleep variables after definitely stressful events such as examinations[1] and skydiving.[2]

Individual differences in stress reactions that neutralize and mask the specific features of sleep alteration were elucidated in an investigation of healthy young students on a post-examination night compared with a post-holiday night in a restful condition without stress.[3] In order to check whether the examination was really stressful for students and how stable was their physiologic reaction, heart rate, arterial blood pressure, and bioelectrical activity (electromyogram, EMG) of mimic muscles were registered 30 minutes before and 30 minutes after the examination. Control data on the same indices were collected under restful conditions after holiday at the same time of day. Before sleep and after awakening on the post-examination and control nights students were asked to solve some logical tasks (in a modification of the Raven test). The time spent on the solution of these tasks as well as the number of mistakes were evaluated. In addition, a Cattell test was carried out before the sleep investigation in the restful (control) condition.

When the averaged data on sleep structure were compared under experimental and control conditions

Table 15.1 Dynamics of autonomic variables and electromyography (EMG) of mimic muscles and sleep variables before and after examination and in a control state in students of groups I and II

Heart rate, EMG and sleep stages	Group I			Group II		
	Control	Examination		Control	Examination	
		Before	After		Before	After
Heart rate (beats/min)	73	82	70	75	85	89
EMG amplitude (μV)	9.5	20.9	12.8	10.3	28.0	36.0
SWS (%)	27.3 ± 1.6	—	30.9 ± 2.6	22.2 ± 1.8	—	21.7 ± 3.2
REM (%)	20.8 ± 2.1	—	19.8 ± 1.6	19.5 ± 1.6	—	25.2 ± 1.8

SWS, slow-wave sleep; REM, rapid eye movement sleep

for both groups of students, no significant differences between the two conditions were found, seemingly confirming the above-mentioned investigations.[1] However, the sleep structure after stress, in contrast to that after holidays, demonstrated a high variability: students exhibited different alterations in sleep structure that neutralized each other. At the same time, they displayed two opposite patterns in the dynamic of EMG and autonomic variables from pre- to post-examination state (Table 15.1). In some students (group 1), heart rate, blood pressure, and muscle tone significantly decreased just after the examination, while in others (group 2), the level of these variables had no tendency to decrease and even demonstrated a small tendency to increase after the examination, when the stressful situation had already passed. Interestingly, the two groups showed no differences in either the objective marks of the examination or the subjective evaluation of these results. These two groups also displayed a different style in the solution of logical tasks (however, only before the night sleep after the examination). Group II, which contained students with persistent emotional tension, were faster and less accurate in solving the tasks in comparison with group I and in comparison with their own results after morning awakening as well as in comparison with the control investigations after the restful period. It appears that the solution of the tasks by the group II

students in the evening after examination was determined by the state of irritation, and this state diminished after sleep.

The night sleep just after the examination was different in these two groups. While the sleep of the group I students was similar after examination and after rest (there was only a non-significant tendency for slow-wave sleep (SWS) to increase after examination), the students of group II displayed an increase in REM sleep percentage after examination (from 19.5% on the control night to 25.2%; $p < 0.01$). In group II, the REM sleep percentage after examination was also higher than the REM sleep percentage of both nights in group I, while in the control investigation, the REM sleep percentage was similar to that in group I. In group II, the SWS percentage in both nights was lower than in group I, and for the night after examination, this difference was significant (21.7% vs 30.9%; $p < 0.05$). Only the subjects of group II displayed on the post-examination night a high (0.74) positive correlation between the total duration of sleep and the REM sleep percentage and a negative correlation (-0.6) between SWS and REM sleep duration. The heart rate on the post-examination night was higher in REM sleep in subjects of group II in comparison with subjects of group I, whereas the control night investigation revealed no differences between the two groups. The activation shifts that followed spontaneous body movements were more prominent in the subjects of group II at all stages of sleep on the post-examination night.

The main differences between the two groups were concentrated in the first two sleep cycles after the examination. In the first cycle, subjects of group I displayed a significantly higher amount of SWS in comparison with subjects of group II, while subjects of group II displayed a higher amount of REM sleep. In the subsequent sleep cycles, the difference between the groups diminished, although subjects of group I, in contrast to those of group II, displayed a tendency for SWS to appear in the last cycles.

What is the implication of the difference between the groups in their reaction to stress? We have suggested that emotional tension before the examination, although represented by similar alterations in EMG and autonomic variables, is qualitatively different in these groups:[4]

(1) Subjects of group I exhibited a normal, adaptive emotional tension that ensured physiologic and psychologic mobilization for coping and active overcoming of the stressful situation. This emotional tension is task-oriented and for this reason diminishes after the achievement of the goal when the examination has been passed. This emotional tension is functional and has no roots in the subjects' previous psychological problems, and for this reason does not need any special additional mechanisms for its reduction.

(2) The emotional tension of the subjects of group II is different in nature. It is a neurotic-like anxiety that does not mobilize, and even

suppresses personal resources and constructive efforts. It is very possible that this emotional tension before examination reflects the subjects' fearful imaginations of failure during examination and its negative consequences, and presumably is based on the restoration in memory, on a conscious or unconscious level, of some previous traumatic failures. This causes frustration and predisposes the subject to a 'giving-up' reaction. The self-esteem of the subject is reduced, resulting in the inner conflict and a disordered self-image. In this condition, the solution of a real task (such as passing an examination) does not help to reduce the emotional tension produced by the psychodynamic problem. This problem requires the activation of defense mechanisms, and REM sleep is an important component of these mechanisms. Investigations by Cartwright and co-workers[5,6] and Greenberg's Boston group[7–10] have shown that REM sleep and dreams are involved in defense mechanisms, and the effect of REM deprivation is very much related to the removal of these mechanisms.

Another investigation was performed in sportsmen in a game situation (Table 15.2). Polysomnography was registered in a group of sportsmen a few days before the collective game and after the end of the game. Column (A) represents the average data of REM sleep before the game; (B) represents REM sleep percentage after a loss in those sportsmen who have been troubled with the loss; (C) represents REM sleep percentage in sportsmen who did not take the loss close to heart; and

Table 15.2 REM sleep percentage in sportsmen in a game situation

(A) Before game	(B) After a loss with frustration	(C) After a loss with disinterest	(D) After a win
19.3	37.2	20.3	19.4

(D) represents REM sleep in a group who won. The difference between groups is in the same direction as that between students: REM sleep percentage increased after the traumatic loss.

Although maladaptive emotional tension requires sleep, and particularly REM sleep, for its compensation (and in healthy subjects such as group II students, REM sleep increases in stressful conditions), if this emotional tension exceeds normal limits and the functional efficiency of REM sleep is not high enough, this tension disturbs sleep, including REM sleep, thus producing a vicious circle.[11] However, usually in such cases, SWS is even more suppressed than REM sleep. Therefore, we have suggested a special indicator in sleep for characterizing the quality of stress-related presleep emotional tension, namely the ratio of the duration of REM sleep to that of delta sleep in the first two cycles, where in healthy subjects under normal conditions, delta sleep is usually most prominent and REM sleep is relatively low in comparison with subsequent cycles (REM/SWS).[4] This method has the advantage of minimizing the significance of the absolute duration of the delta sleep (SWS) and REM sleep: even if maladaptive anxiety reduces REM sleep (due to frequent awakenings and disorganization of night sleep), it usually reduces SWS still further, and the resulting REM/SWS ratio increases anyway. In patients with neurotic (maladaptive) anxiety, the REM/SWS ratio was 0.8; in depressed patients, it was 1.9; in healthy subjects, it was 0.54; and in group I students after examination, it was 0.41, while in group II students, it was 0.72.

It can be suggested that the maladaptive emotional tension that characterizes group II corresponds to emotion-focused coping.[12,13] Sadeh et al[14] have shown that in young undergraduate students in the high-stress period of their life (in comparison with low-stress periods), high emotion-focused coping scores were associated with reduced sleep time, while high problem-focused coping scores (the most adaptive way of coping) were associated with longer sleep periods. Participants with low emotion-focused coping scores increased their true

sleep time on average by more than half an hour on moving from a low- to a high-stress period, whereas the true sleep time of participants with high emotion-focused coping scores decreased by 23 minutes. Individuals with high emotion-focused coping reported decreased perceived sleep quality during the high-stress period in comparison with the low-stress period, whereas the opposite was true with low emotion-focused coping.

This confirms data on shortened sleep and insomnia in subjects with high emotion-focused coping.[15,16] It may be a sign of disturbed adaptation under a high emotional load due to ineffective coping. This conclusion corresponds with data suggesting that emotion-focused coping is ineffective in stressful situations.[17] It is worth emphasizing that insomnia accompanied by many complaints during wakefulness (regarding sleepiness, emotional tension, decreased attention, etc.) has nothing in common with normal short sleeping that is not accompanied with any subjective complaints and usually characterizes well-defended subjects with high behavioral activity.[18]

High emotion-focused coping predicted increased anxiety during examination, associated with a poor adaptation to stress.[19] Morin et al[16] also confirmed that increased reported anxiety and arousal level are linked to emotion-focused coping and insomnia.

'General anxiety' (factor F1 of the Cattell test) is a stable characteristic of personality, and, according to our investigation, it is not similar to maladaptive anxiety. One-third of students in the above-mentioned investigation[3] displayed a low or moderate level of factor F1 (group A), while other students displayed a high level of this factor (group B). In terms of group membership, groups A and B did not correspond to groups I and II. The sleep variables of groups A and B are presented in Table 15.3. In subjects with prominent general anxiety, REM sleep percentage without stress was significantly lower than in subjects with a moderate level of this variable, while after the examination the former subjects displayed an increase in REM sleep percentage in comparison

Table 15.3 Sleep stages in students with a low level of general anxiety (A) and in students with a high level of anxiety (B) in a quiet state and after examination

Sleep stages%	Group A		Group B	
	Control	Examination	Control	Examination
SWS	27.4 ± 1.4	20.5 ± 3.3	22.7 ± 2.6	29.6 ± 3.0
REM	23.6 ± 1.7	22.6 ± 1.6	16.6 ± 1.7	21.5 ± 2.4

SWS, slow-wave sleep; REM, rapid eye movement sleep

to the restful period. However, in group B, the REM sleep percentage after examination did not exceed the level of group A after examination and did not achieve the level in group II with stable emotional tension after examination. According to these data, it is possible to assume that Cattell factor F1 reflects high sensitivity and that in persons with increased sensitivity, the functional REM sleep system is flexible and can produce an increase or decrease in REM sleep, depending on the reaction to stressful conditions. In particular, subjects with high sensitivity may display a prominent first-night effect (FNE) which is exactly what happened in group B in restful conditions after holiday. The FNE is a normal reaction of the healthy subject in the unfamiliar sleep environment of the sleep laboratory, which produces stress. Compared with subsequent nights, sleep on the first night is characterized by decreased sleep efficiency, increased sleep onset latency (SOL) and REM sleep latency, decreased REM sleep percentage or at least a moderate REM sleep reduction in the first part of the night,[20] SWS reduction (not universal), and an increased number of sleep-stage shifts and awakenings.[21] FNE presumably reflects the natural increase in the subject's state of vigilance in an unfamiliar sleeping environment as part of the adaptive orientation in the new (stressful) situation. Healthy subjects sleeping at home, in a familiar environment, showed no FNE and no habituation of sleep structure from the first to subsequent nights of sleep investigation. FNE is a normal reaction of healthy subjects, while depressed patients

often do not show evidence of FNE.[22,23] This absence of FNE is presumably related to the decreased adaptability of depressed patients, and reflects the lack of an orienting reaction in the new environment. According to our data,[24,25] depressed patients who do not display FNE (according to REM sleep variables) present more mood-congruent psychotic features in their clinical picture, are resistant to antidepressive medication, and require electroconvulsive therapy (ECT) for a positive treatment outcome. Thus, according to REM sleep alterations, FNE represents a reaction to stress quite opposite to that of group II students after examination, especially taking into consideration that the night after examination was the first night in the sleep laboratory. It is worth emphasizing that the stress of the first night, as well as the reaction to the stress of examination, is characterized by an increased alertness that displays itself in an increased number of sleep-stage shifts and awakenings, and sometimes in SWS reduction. This means that the adaptive emotional tension not only does not require activation of the REM sleep system (group I students), but even causes a decrease in REM sleep requirement if this emotional tension arises during sleep investigation. We suggest that this can explain the data[26] on the influence of acute social stress on sleep structure. The experimental group in this investigation was instructed to give public speeches in the morning, with the evaluation of the subjects' performance. Stress rating and mean arterial blood pressure were higher in this group after task notification compared with baseline, and REM count in the sleep before the speeches displayed a tendency to be lower from cycle to cycle in comparison with the control group. This difference became significant in the last REM sleep period.

All of the above-mentioned data are related to sleep alteration under acute stress. Data on alterations of sleep under chronic stress represented by post-traumatic stress disorders (PTSDs) are also very ambiguous and contradictory. Sleep architecture in PTSD patients in their chronic state is characterized on average by a subtle increase in alertness, and differs only mildly from normal (sleep latency is longer, sleep efficiency is lower, and awake time is longer[27]). SWS varied from extremely decreased to extremely increased, with the latter being in contradiction with the symptoms of depression and anxiety typical of these patients. However, this corresponds to the sleepwalking and night terrors that usually accompany SWS, as well as to an elevated awakening threshold.[27–30]

In comparison with healthy control subjects, REM latency in PTSD patients has been reported to be either shortened or lengthened,[27,31–34] and REM sleep is either increased[35] or decreased.[32] Kaminer and Lavie[36] have shown that less-adjusted Holocaust survivors with PTSD had more anxiety dreams than well-adjusted survivors or normal controls. At the same time, artificial awakenings from REM sleep resulted in a lower dream recall than in controls. This confirms data of Kramer et al[37] that PTSD patients who complain of bad dreams recall only about half as many dreams after REM awakenings as control subjects do, although REM sleep in PTSD is characterized by an increased number of REMs. According to REM sleep variables (especially REM latency), PTSD inpatients are bidirectionally sensitive to the degree of familiarity they associate with the sleep laboratory conditions. In comparison with healthy controls, inpatients familiar with the laboratory environment demonstrate a reduced FNE while patients unfamiliar with this environment demonstrate enhanced FNE.[38]

The difference in sleep structure in PTSD is presumably related to the different clinical features

of this disease, in a way similar to acute stress. The clinical picture of PTSD includes, on the one hand, a persistent reexperiencing of past traumatic events (images, thoughts, perceptions, nightmares, illusions, and hallucinations), accompanied by increased physiologic reactivity on exposure to internal and external cues that symbolize or resemble the traumatic event as well as persistent symptoms of increased arousal (irritability, hypervigilance, exaggerated startle reaction, prominent orienting reaction, FNE, and difficulty falling and staying asleep). On the other hand, these patients display persistent avoidance of stimuli associated with the trauma (avoidance and repression of thoughts, feelings, and memories associated with the trauma; apathy and diminished activity; and hopelessness).

Recently, we have attempted to integrate these different symptoms into a holistic framework.[39] The central point of the clinical picture is the feeling of helplessness caused by traumatic events. It is possible to consider a persistent reexperiencing of traumatic events and increased arousal as an unsuccessful attempt to cope with this helplessness by trying to win back this traumatic event. Because the event has already passed, this goal cannot be achieved, no matter how active is the subject, and as a result symptoms of avoidance and helplessness return. The continuous oscillations between unsuccessful attempts to cope and giving up can explain the complicated picture of sleep in PTSD.

SHIFTWORK STRESS AND SLEEP

The biologic clock of our body is adapted to the circadian rhythm related to the regular 24-hour shifts of the light and dark periods. Autonomic and endocrine functions correspond to this rhythm, and when a person changes the schedule of their activity by working during the night and resting during the day, the routine biologic rhythms do not usually follow the new schedule. As a result, the person makes efforts to be active in periods that are naturally predisposed for sleep and rest and to rest in periods predisposed for the most productive activity. This dissociation causes stress. For the biologic clock, it is especially difficult to adapt to the regularly rotating unstable shifts. Even after several years on such a job, the temporal profile of cortisol shows only partial adaptation to the work schedule.[40] Work during the 'wrong' phase of the circadian rhythm increases the risk of stress-related psychosomatic diseases: ischemic heart disease, gastrointestinal disorders, and reduced immune function.[41–43]

In this chapter, the discussion of this topic will be restricted to the possibility of estimating the level of adaptation to the stress of shiftwork on the basis of sleep structure.

In our investigation,[44,45] polysomnography was performed in 30 train dispatchers during daytime sleep after nightwork (8 PM–8 AM), the subsequent night sleep, the night sleep after the day of rest, and the night sleep after the day shift. The level of

subjective adaptation to shiftwork was estimated based on general satisfaction with job and sleep, the presence/absence of neurotic and somatic complaints, the average level of mood, and the level of social activity during rest. A special questionnaire estimated the quality of wakefulness that preceded sleep (the degree of fatigue and sleepiness, the number of naps, and the level of emotional tension during the shift), and another questionnaire was presented just after the polysomnography in order to estimate the quality of sleep. See Table 15.4.

A positive rank correlation was found between the subjective estimation of sleep quality and SWS duration in night sleep. The correlation increased when fatigue and sleepiness in the previous wakefulness was high. Subjects estimated their sleep as excellent (point 5) only when SWS exceeded 70 minutes and stage 4 exceeded 40 minutes per night. All subjects who exhibited more than

Table 15.4 Sleep structure in dispatchers with different adaptations to shiftwork stress: 1, sleep during the day after the nightshift; 2, sleep on the first night after the nightshift; 3, sleep on the second night after the nightshift; 4, sleep after the dayshift

Sleep variables	Adapted subjects				Maladapted subjects				Intermediate group			
	1	2	3	4	1	2	3	4	1	2	3	4
Sleep duration (min)	162	410	379	401	97	391	358	396	93	366	380	386
Sleep latency (min)	10	4	4	4	4	6	11	8	15	5	16	12
Latency to stage 2	5	4	7	5	8	6	8	5	4	7	6	5
REM latency (min)	66	64	66	66	59	72	61	53	67	72	77	72
Number of REM sleep episodes	2	5	4	5	2	4	4	5	1	3	4	7
REM sleep (min)	20	83	89	91	16	90	76	90	10	82	80	95
Stage 1 (min)	14	23	28	30	11	30	80	24	16	26	45	40
Stage 2 (min)	63	199	173	182	45	240	223	233	37	206	193	188
Stage 3 (min)	13	32	24	31	10	20	20	24	8	30	21	20
Stage 4 (min)	52	73	65	68	15	11	9	16	21	22	40	43
No. of awakenings	1	1	1	0.5	1	1	1	1	0.5	0.2	1	1
Wakefulness (min)	56	8	1	6	7	10	7	10	10	1	11	18

REM, rapid eye movement

70 minutes of SWS every night (group 1) were adapted to shiftwork according to the above-mentioned markers, while most subjects who exhibited an SWS deficit every night (group 2) were maladapted to shiftwork. In group 1, SWS reached its maximum (105 minutes) in the first night after the nightshift, and was reduced to a minimum (85 minutes) in the night after the day of rest. In group 2, SWS reached its peak (37 minutes) after the dayshift. In most of the group 1 subjects, REM sleep reached its peak on the second night after the nightshift, and when it reached its peak on the first night in parallel, SWS increased prominently. Conversely, in more than half of the subjects in group 2, REM sleep was more prominent on the first night after the nightshift, when the SWS amount was low. In group 2, the sum of REM sleep amount during day sleep and in the first night after the nightshift in some subjects was twice the amount of REM sleep after the day of rest.

In group 2, there was a negative correlation between SWS and REM sleep in the first night and a positive correlation between REM sleep and total sleep duration in the night after the dayshift. SWS increased and REM sleep reduced in day sleep in group 1 in comparison with group 2. Subjects in group 2 more often perceived their emotional tension as being high.

Thus, in group 1 subjects who adapted to the shiftwork without signs of distress, the change in sleep structure from night to night is similar to the rebound effect after single sleep deprivation in healthy subjects with a normal rest–work schedule: namely an initial rebound of SWS and a secondary rebound of REM sleep. In maladapted subjects, REM sleep exceeded SWS in day sleep as well as in the first recovery night sleep after the nightshift, and was most prominent on the first recovery night. This means that maladapted subjects after the nightshift display competition between the increased SWS requirement (which is common for all subjects irrespective of their adaptation to shift-work) and an increased REM sleep requirement that presumably characterized only these subjects. This competition is resolved in favor of REM sleep.

In healthy well-adapted and non-sensitive subjects, the competition between the relatively moderate REM sleep requirement and the high SWS requirement that are normal after sleep deprivation is easily resolved in favor of SWS,[46] and the REM sleep requirement is satisfied with a delay in the subsequent night sleep. Short sleepers are characterized by a low REM sleep requirement,[18] and they were found to be the most adapted to shift-work stress.[47] On the contrary, persons with low ego strength who need REM sleep for its restoration are especially sensitive to sleep deprivation.[48] We are coming to the conclusion that the main cause of the maladaptation to the stress of shiftwork is a strong psychologically determined requirement for REM sleep, and this requirement is regularly frustrated by shiftwork. This is the same requirement that characterized those students who demonstrated a stable maladaptive emotional tension under examination stress or sportsmen who failed and were frustrated by failing, and PTSD patients who display giving up.

THEORETICAL INTEGRATION OF DATA

We believe that the search activity (SA) concept[49–51] provides an explanation of all these data. SA is activity that is oriented to changing a situation (or at least a subject's attitude to it) in the absence of a precise prediction of the outcome of such activity but taking into consideration the results at each stage of the activity. SA is a component of many different forms of behavior: self-stimulation in animals and creative behavior in humans, as well as exploratory and active defense (fight/flight) behavior in all species. The opposite of search activity is renunciation of search, which encompasses depression and neurotic anxiety in humans, freezing in animals, and learned helplessness in both species. Panic and stereotyped activity are also different from SA: a subject in a state of panic does not consider the real outcome of activity, and stereotyped behavior is based on precise prediction of the outcome. The difference between adaptive emotional tension, which mobilizes all psychologic and physiologic resources in the face of stress, and maladaptive, unproductive emotional tension, which hampers successful and relevant activity, is determined by the presence or absence of SA.[52]

All forms of behavior that include SA increase body resistance, while the absence of search decreases body resistance and predisposes a person to mental and psychosomatic disorders.[53–55] It is a process of SA in itself, independent of the pragmatic results of such activity, that prevents somatic disorders. SA is an important mechanism of development and evolution, stimulating subjects and populations in the search for novel approaches and at the same time restoring physiologic resources for this risky and potentially exhausting behavior.

If search activity is so important for survival and development, and renunciation of search is so destructive and dangerous for health, it would be reasonable to assume a natural and fundamental biologic mechanism that can restore search activity after temporary renunciation of search. There is much evidence that dreams in REM sleep compensate for the renunciation of search in previous wakefulness and restore SA in subsequent wakefulness. Dreams provide a good opportunity for SA after giving up. The subject is separated from reality while sleeping, including those stressful circumstances that caused renunciation of search, and is free to start searching from the beginning. In addition, within his or her dream, the dreamer can make attempts to solve the current or any other problem by means of very flexible imagary, since the final aim of the dreamwork is only restoration of the SA process. However, it is necessary to take into consideration that REM sleep may be efficient or inefficient with respect to this function, and the difference between these two states can determine whether sleep will be a stress moderator or a victim of stress.

If the functional load on the REM sleep system exceeds its resources, the emotional tension, accompanied by increased alertness, disturbs the whole sleep structure, including REM sleep.

We have investigated sleep structure in parallel with psychologic examination (MMPI) in 132 healthy subjects and patients with neurotic anxiety and anxious depression.[56] Neurotic MMPI scales – hypochondria (Hs), anxiety/depression (D), and hysteria (Hy) – were divided into the following groups according to their level: (1) <65 T-points (low); (2) 65–74 T-points (moderate); (3) >74 T-points (high). The lowest REM sleep percentage (<15%) occurred least often in subjects with the leading D-score in group 3. The highest REM sleep percentage (>25%) was found in all subjects with the leading D-score in group 2 (65–74 T-points). However, when the absolute value of the leading D-score exceeded 75 T-points, the highest REM sleep percentage occurred relatively seldom (in 17% of such cases). This is a direct sign of the nonlinear relation between the level of the pathologic emotional tension and REM sleep percentage.

If the function of REM sleep is to compensate (reduce) maladaptive emotional tension, then the increase in REM sleep in subjects with a moderate level of anxiety/depression is not only an effect of this state, but also a cause of the prevention of its further increase – until REM sleep function is sufficient. Incidentally, 65–74 T-points on scale D reflects increased sensitivity, which is inherent in individuals known as healthy long sleepers, and they are characterized by a high REM sleep percentage.[18] Like our group II students, they regularly go to sleep in a state of emotional tension, and sleep with a high proportion of REM sleep helps them to release this tension. However, it follows from this that the excessive increase in emotional disturbances under longlasting stressful conditions is a consequence of a functional insufficiency of REM sleep.

This functional insufficiency displays itself initially by an alteration of its qualitative characteristics and only secondarily by its reduction. Moreover, in some cases, REM sleep percentage may even be increased; however, this does not help to compensate for the maladaptive emotional tension if the REM sleep quality is deficient. The latter manifests itself first of all as a reduction in dream recall after awakening in REM sleep. For instance, in insomnia (which is a very common outcome of emotional stress[57]), dream recall occurred in less than 60% of all awakenings from REM stage,[58] while in healthy highly sensitive subjects, dream recalls occurred even more often than in healthy non-sensitive subjects – in more than 85% of all awakenings. Both according to the author's observation and according to data in the literature, in healthy subjects, mental activity in dreams grows simultaneously with increasing sensitivity to life events estimated as stressful. Dreams of highly sensitive persons contain more images and are more vivid in comparison with those of less sensitive persons, dream recalls are longer, and dreams show a greater number of active actions. Thus, in healthy subjects, the increase in emotional sensitivity up to a certain limit is accompanied by an intensification of dream activity that prevents further increase and stabilization of the maladaptive emotional tension (distress). Patients with emotional disturbances are usually more sensitive than even the most sensitive healthy test subjects; however, they display a drop of mental activity in dreams that we are considering as a sign of functional inefficiency of REM sleep.[11,59] Only in healthy subjects does the intensity of the REMs in REM sleep correlate with the degree of the subject's active participation in dream actions – while in patients, it correlates with negative emotionality.[59]

According to some investigations of sleep alteration under stressful events,[60] the dynamic is as follows: the first step is an intensification of REM sleep mental activity, sometimes in parallel with an increase of REM duration; in the second step, the intensification of dream activity achieves its maximum and REM sleep duration grows further; in the third step, the first signs of disturbed compensation appear, with the dream content becoming impoverished while the REM sleep percentage is still high; finally, emotional tension, not being compensated, disturbs all sleep and causes a reduction in REM sleep. This is a state of insomnia that is such a typical outcome of stress. According to Drake et al,[61] individuals with higher scores on the Ford Insomnia Response-to-Stress Test (which measures stress-related vulnerability to sleep disturbances) had lower sleep efficiency, increased latency to stage 1 sleep, and increased arousal on the Multiple Sleep Latency Test (MSLT). Neuroticism and internalization of stressful events may predispose to insomnia. Fuller et al[62] have shown that high-anxiety subjects of different natures (PTSD, panic disorders, and general anxiety disorders) display decreased sleep efficiency and disrupted sleep continuity, they take longer to fall asleep, they have lower SWS percentages and greater stage 1 percentages, and they show more arousals during the first half of the sleep period. The relationship of insomnia to stressful events was established by Healey et al.[57] In this investigation, it was shown that although usually sleep problems developed slowly, 74% of poor sleepers reported that a major life event was related to the onset of their sleep problem. The difference between poor and good sleepers in Life Change Unit Scores was significant only for the year of onset of insomnia. This investigation also showed that there are some predispositions to such a maladaptive reaction to stress. Poor sleepers recalled more frequent nightmares and problems with sleep in childhood, and they were more emotionally upset and had less contact with their parents. In adulthood before insomnia, they had a feeling of inferiority, low affiliation. They considered themselves to be more passive and had more health complaints than good sleepers. The authors suggested that poor sleepers internalize their reaction to stressful life events rather than externalizing their response through overt behavior. In our terms, this means that they do not display search activity under stressful conditions, and this may relate to the lack of emotional support in childhood. A long-lasting load on REM sleep defense mechanisms from childhood makes these subjects vulnerable to the development of maladaptive emotional tension.

REFERENCES

1. Holdstock TL, Verschoor GJ. Student sleep patterns before, during and after an examination period. South African J Psychol 1974; 4: 16–24.

2. Knowless J, Beaumaster E, MacLean A. The sleep of skydivers: a study of stress. In: Proceedings of Second International Sleep Research Congress, Edinburgh 1975: 119.

3. Goncharenko AM, Schakhnarovich VM, Rotenberg VS. Changes of sleep in various types of reactions to an emotional stress. Zhurnal Visshey Nervnoy Deyatelnosti 1977; 27: 837. [in Russian]

4. Rotenberg VS, Arshavsky VV. REM sleep, stress and search activity. Waking Sleeping 1979; 3: 235–44.

5. Cartwright RD, Monroe LJ, Palmer C. Individual differences in response to REM deprivation. Arch Gen Psychiatry 1967; 16: 297–302.

6. Cartwright RD. Night Life. Englewood Cliffs, NJ: Prentice-Hall.

7. Greenberg R, Fingar R, Kantrowitz J, Kawliche S. The effects of REM deprivation: implications for a theory of the psychological function of dreaming. Br J Med Psychol 1970; 43: 1–11.

8. Greenberg R, Pillard R, Pearlman C. The effect of dream (stage REM) deprivation on adaptation to stress. Psychosom Med 1972; 34: 257–62.

9. Greenberg R, Pearlman C. Cutting the REM nerve: an approach to the adaptive role of REM sleep. Perspect Biol Med 1974; 17: 513–21.

10. Grieser C, Greenberg R, Harrison R. The adaptive function of sleep: the differential effects of sleep and dreaming on recall. J Abnormal Psychol 1972; 80: 280–6.

11. Rotenberg VS. The Adaptive Function of Sleep: Reasons for and Signs of its Dysfunction. Moscow: Nauka, 1982. [In Russian]

12. Lazarus RS, Folkman S. Stress, Appraisal and Coping. New York: Springer-Verlag, 1984.

13. Lazarus R. Emotion and Adaptation. New York: Oxford University Press, 1991.

14. Sadeh A, Keinan G, Daon K. Effects of stress on sleep: the moderating role of coping style. Health Psychol 2004; 23: 542–5.

15. Hicks RA, Marical CM, Conti PA. Coping with a major stressor: differences between habitual short and long sleepers. Percept Motor Skills 1991; 72: 631–6.

16. Morin CM, Rodrigue S, Ivers H. Role of stress, arousal and coping skills in primary insomnia. Psychosom Med 2003; 65: 259–67.

17. Martelli MF, Auerbach SM, Alexander J, Mercuri LG. Stress management in the health care setting: matching interventions with patient coping styles. J Consult Clin Psychol 1987; 55: 201–7.

18. Hartmann E. The Functions of Sleep. New Haven, CT: Yale University Press, 1973.

19. Zeidner M. Personal and contextual determinants of coping and anxiety in an evaluative situation: a prospective study. Person Individ Differ 1994; 16: 899–918.

20. Agnew H, Webb W, Williams R. The first night effect: an EEG study of sleep. Psychophysiology 1996; 2: 263–6.

21. Browman C, Cartwright R. The first night effect on sleep and dreams. Biol Psychiatry 1980; 15: 809–12.

22. Akiskal HS, Lemmi H, Yerevanian B, King D, Belluomoni J. The utility of the REM latency test in psychiatric diagnosis: a study of 81 depressed out-patients. Psychiatry Res 1982; 7: 101–10.

23. Ansseau M, Kupfer DJ, Reynolds CF III. Internight variability of REM latency in major depression: implications for the use of REM latency as a biological correlate. Biol Psychiatry 1985; 20: 489–505.

24. Rotenberg VS, Hadjez J, Kimhi R, et al. First night effect in depression: new data and a new approach. Biol Psychiatry 1997; 42: 267–74.

25. Rotenberg VS, Kayumov L, Indursky P, et al. REM sleep in depressed patients: different attempts to achieve adaptation. J Psychosom Res 1997; 42: 565–75.

26. Germain A, Buysse DJ, Ombao H, Kupfer DJ, Hall M. Psychophysiological reactivity and coping styles influence the effects of acute stress exposure on rapid eye movement sleep. Psychosom Med 2003; 65: 857–64.

27. Pillar G, Malhotra A, Lavie P. Post-traumatic stress disorder and sleep – what a nightmare! Sleep Med Rev 2000; 4: 183–200.

28. Dagan Y, Lavie P, Bleich A. Elevated awakening thresholds in sleep stage 3–4 in war-related post-traumatic stress disorder. Biol Psychiatry 1991; 30: 618–22.

29. Lavie P, Katz N, Pillar G, Zinger Y. Elevated awakening thresholds during sleep: characteristics of chronic war-related posttraumatic stress disorder patients. Biol Psychiatry 1998; 44: 1060–5.

30. Schoen LKM, Kinney L. Auditory thresholds in the dream disturbed. Sleep Res 1984; 13: 102.

31. Greenberg R, Pearlman C, Campel D. War neuroses and the adaptive function of REM sleep. Br J Med Psychol 1972; 45: 27–33.

32. Schlosberg A, Benjamin M. Sleep patterns in three acute combat fatigue cases. J Clin Psychiatry 1978; 9: 546–9.

33. Hefez A, Metz L, Lavie P. Long-term effects of extreme situational stress on sleep and dreaming. Am J Psychiatry 1987; 144: 344–7.

34. Glaubman H, Mikulincer M, Porat A, Wsserman O, Birger M. Sleep of chronic post-traumatic patients. J Traumatic Stress 1990; 3: 255–63.

35. Van Kammen WB, Christiansen C, van Kammen DP, Reynolds CF. Sleep and the prisoner-of-war experience – 40 years later. In: Giller IR, ed. Biological Assessment and Treatment of Posttraumatic Stress Disorder. Washington, DC: American Psychiatric Association Press, 1990: 159–72.

36. Kaminer H, Lavie P. Sleep and dreams in well adjusted and less adjusted Holocaust survivors. In: Stroebe MS, Stroebe W, Hansson RO, eds. Handbook of Bereavement. New York: Cambridge University Press, 1993: 331–4.

37. Kramer M, Schoen LS, Kinney L. Psychological and behavioral features of disturbed dreamers. Psychiatry J Univ Ottawa 1983; 9: 102–6.

38. Woodward SH, Bliwise DL, Friedman MJ, Gusman FD. First night effects in post-traumatic stress disorder inpatients. Sleep 1996; 19: 312–17.

39. Rotenberg VS. The psychophysiology of REM sleep in relation to mechanisms of psychiatric disorders. In: Golbin AZ, Kravitz HM, Keith LG, eds. Sleep Psychiatry. London: Taylor & Francis, 2004: 35–64.

40. Weibel L, Spiegel K, Follenius M, Ehrhart J, Brandenberger G. Internal dissociation of the circadian markers of the cortisol rhythm in night workers. Am J Physiol 1996; 270: E608–13.

41. Van Reeth O, Weibel L, Spiegel K, et al. Interactions between stress and sleep: from basic research to clinical situations. Sleep Med Rev 2000; 4: 201–19.

42. Koller M. Health risk related to shift work. Int Arch Occup Environ Health 1983; 53: 59–75.

43. Knutsson A, Akerstedt T, Jonson BG, Orth-Gomer K. Increased risk of ischaemic heart disease in shift workers. Lancet 1986; ii: 89–92.

44. Rotenberg VS, Schachnarovich VM, Kandror IS, et al. The structure of night and day sleep in shift workers according to the problem of adaptation to shift work. Fiziologia Cheloveka 1975; 1: 756–62. [in Russian]

45. Rotenberg VS. The competition between SWS and REM sleep as index of maladaptation to shift work. Homeostasis 1991; 33: 235–8.

46. Brunner DP, Dijk D-J, Tobler L, Borbely AA. Effect of partial sleep deprivation on sleep stages and EEG power spectra: evidence for non-REM and REM sleep homeostasis. Electroenceph Clin Neurophysiol 1990; 74: 492–9.

47. Cherepanova VA, Putilov AA. Sleep–wake pattern type and objective physiological characteristics during day and night wakefulness. Abstract presented at 20th International Conference on Chronobiology, Tel-Aviv, 1991: 71.

48. Lester J, Knapp T, Roessler R. Sleep deprivation, personality and performance on a complex vigilance task. Waking Sleeping 1976; 3: 238–48.

49. Rotenberg VS. Search activity in the context of psychosomatic disturbances, of brain monoamines and REM sleep function. Pavlovian J Biol Sci 1984; 10: 1–15.

50. Rotenberg VS. Sleep after immobilization stress and sleep deprivation: common features and theoretical integration. Crit Rev Neurobiol 2000; 14: 225–31.

51. Rotenberg VS. Sleep deprivation in depression: an integrative approach. Int J Psychiatry Clin Pract 2003; 7: 9–16.

52. Rotenberg VS, Boucsein W. Adaptive vs. maladaptive emotional tension. Genet Soc Gen Psychol Monogr 1993; 119: 207–32.

53. Rotenberg VS, Arshavsky VV. Search activity and its impact on experimental and clinical pathology. Activitas Nervosa Superior (Praha) 1979; 21: 105–15.

54. Rotenberg VS, Shattenstein AA. Neurotic and psychosomatic disorders: psychophysiological approach based on search activity concept. Homeostasis 1994; 35: 265–8.

55. Rotenberg VS, Sirota P, Elizur A. Psychoneuroimmunology: searching for the main deteriorating psychobehavioral factor. Genet Soc Gen Psychol Monogr 1996; 122: 329–46.

56. Rotenberg VS. The nature of non-linear relationship between the individual's present psychic state and his sleep structure. Dyn Psychiatry 1986; 101: 516–24.

57. Healey ES, Kales A, Monroe LJ, et al. Onset of insomnia: role of life-stress events. Psychosom Med 1981; 43: 439–51.

58. Rotenberg VS. The estimation of sleep quality in different stages and cycles of sleep. J Sleep Res 1993; 2: 17–20.

59. Rotenberg VS. Functional deficiency of REM sleep and its role in the pathogenesis of neurotic and psychosomatic disturbances. Pavlovian J Biol Sci 1988; 23: 1–3.

60. Cartwright RD, Lloyd SR. Early REM sleep: a compensatory change in depression? Psychiatry Res 1994; 51: 245–52.

61. Drake C, Richardson G, Roehrs T, Scofield H, Roth T. Vulnerability to stress-related sleep disturbance and hyperarousal. Sleep 2004; 27: 285–91.

62. Fuller KH, Waters WH, Binks PG, Anderson T. Generalized anxiety and sleep architecture: a polysomnographic investigation. Sleep 1997; 20: 370–6.

16

Sleep and attachment disorders in children

Karl Heinz Brisch

INTRODUCTION

An infant's quiet night of sleep is a source of happiness and empowerment for parents. In prenatal classes, many parents worry that their baby might develop a sleep disorder and that night-time could become an intense scene of crying and responses. Indeed, quite a percentage of infants and children develop sleep disorders, and nocturnal wakings and bed sharing are quite common during early childhood. During infancy, the frequency of night-wakings increases with maturation of locomotion.[1] Nocturnal awakings have been reported in 20–30% of 1- to 3-year-olds.[2,3] These findings appear despite the fact that methodologic problems exist in assessing sleep problems in infants, and it is well documented that maternal reports do not objectively reflect the sleep pattern of their infants.[4] Although a sleep disorder does not necessarily lead to an attachment disorder, an infant's crying through the night can be the start of a disturbed parent–infant relationship that may conclude with this result. Conversely, attachment disorders in children are also associated with a range of psychosomatic problems, one of which is sleep problems. If a sleep disorder and an attachment disorder are a baby's predominant symptoms, then the parent–infant and, later, parent–child relationship will be stressful and in the worst case can progress to a vicious circle of crying and physical abuse. Therefore, it is necessary to understand more about the association of sleep and attachment and their disorders in children, and to strategize prevention measures that can help parents and infants establish sleep patterns and regulate sleep rhythms from the beginning.[5–12]

ATTACHMENT THEORY AND DISORDERS

Attachment is a fundamental human motivation that helps the infant to survive. During the first year, an infant develops a specific, exclusive attachment relationship to an attachment figure that serves as a secure base for the infant and provides protection. Once the baby's attachment system starts to develop, which can be observed from 12 weeks onward, the infant reacts on separation with attachment behavior, such as crying to protest against separation from the attachment figure followed by seeking physical contact and reunion.[13] We can distinguish three different patterns of attachment quality. A securely attached infant will protest after separation from his or her attachment figure and will calm down quickly after reunion. An insecurely avoidant attached infant will appear not to be stressed by separation and will not actively seek physical contact with the attachment figure after reunion, whereas an insecurely anxious–ambivalent attached infant will react with extreme arousal and will take a long time to settle down after his or her attachment figure has returned. It is typical that the attachment system of the infant, once activated, can be preferentially calmed by physical contact with the attachment figure. Only if the primary attachment figure, for example the mother, is not present, does the infant allow a secondary attachment figure, such as the father, to soothe him or her.[14–18]

Attachment disorders are caused by an infant's early experiences of repeated separation and multiple traumas. Such disorders commonly evolve from traumatic events such as physical, sexual, or emotional violence and severe deprivation, often perpetrated by attachment figures. In addition, if an attachment figure is sometimes a source of emotional availability and protection for the child and at other times a source of violence and anxiety, it will be difficult for the child to organize these disparate experiences into a coherent internal working model of attachment.[18,19]

On a behavioral level, attachment disorders may emerge as strange patterns. Two forms of attachment disorders are included in the International Classification of Diseases (ICD-10)[20] and the Diagnostic and Statistical Manual of Mental Disorders, 4th edition (DSM-IV).[21] One pattern involves non-selective, undifferentiated attachment behavior. Children possessing this pattern exhibit promiscuous attachments, rapidly and seemingly randomly seeking physical contact with strangers. They are indiscriminately friendly toward strangers, who by definition can never be real attachment figures. Other children display a type of disorder characterized by inhibited attachment behavior: these children, although anxious, do not show their attachment behavior, instead suppressing their attachment activities, which results in a continuous state of high arousal. Additional types of attachment disorders have been classified, including attachment disorders with psychosomatic symptoms (e.g., sleep problems).[18] Further types of attachment disorders (such as non-attachment behavior in an attachment-relevant situation, aggressive behavior, role reversal, and a hyperactivation of attachment behavior) also show pathologic behavior patterns in attachment-relevant situations.[22]

Separation at night for sleep is one of the attachment-related situations leading to activation of the attachment system. Children with different types of attachment disorders may have disturbed sleep patterns or even sleep disorders. For example, some attachment-disordered children cannot calm down easily at night or wake up often and suffer from nightmares and night walking. These disorders may manifest through hyperactivity of their attachment system, or the children may have difficulty separating before sleep. Other children may suffer from an inhibited attachment disorder and will anxiously lie in bed, and not cry at night to seek the attachment figure. Caregivers of these latter children may thus think the infants are easily cared for, whereas the babies are instead lying in bed in a state of hyperarousal. Their hyperarousal and inhibition of showing attachment may cause them to complain of stomach aches or headaches, vomit, or develop an elevated temperature. If attachment figures do not understand these signals and prefer children who do not cry at night, children may develop chronic psychosomatic symptoms. Still other children may suffer from undifferentiated attachment disorders (as most foster infants do) and will be happy when anyone picks them up from bed. They might calm down for a short while, but will again cry until another person comes along. No secure attachment representation results from this undifferentiated attachment behavior, so that while the children may receive physical contact from various people, there is no decrease in the level of arousal.

Infants or children with hyperactivation of their attachment system normally cannot separate until they fall asleep in close physical contact with their parents in the children's or the parents' bed. It is important to note that many parents also have attachment problems and have difficulty separating, and sometimes it is not clear who is clinging to whom. Some parents, especially those with prior trauma experiences, also have their own sleep problems. Attachment anxiety has been associated with self-reported sleep difficulties in men and women; even with depressed affect being included as a control variable, the effect of attachment anxiety remained significant.[23] If a mother has an attachment disorder with role reversal, she may carry her infant into her bed and take the infant as a secure base to help herself fall asleep. Mothers with panic disorders, when describing parenting behaviors concerning infant sleep, reported less sensitivity toward their infants, who showed more ambivalent/resistant attachment, higher salivary cortisol levels, and more sleep problems.[24] Mothers with high symptoms of depression and anxiety more likely had ambivalent attached infants and used high levels of active physical comforting, and their infants developed high initial levels of sleep problems that continued in infant sleep disturbances over time.[25] Benoit et al[26] have shown that a mother's own insecure status of attachment is strongly correlated with attachment and sleep disturbances in her infant: every insecurely attached mother in their study had a child or children with sleep disturbances. Therefore, at the start of treatment, it is vital that the therapist learns something about the parents' own histories of attachment and their experiences of unresolved loss and separation, so that treatment can also address their needs – or the therapy of the sleep-disordered child will not be successful. The importance of focusing on parents' status of attachment when treating their infant's sleep problem cannot be overstated.

Finally, sleep disturbances and sleep disorders of infants caused by traumatizing experiences with insensitive care by attachment figures can lead to attachment disorders, but if a child is securely attached during the day, then inconsistent caregiving or unresponsiveness to attachment signals at night will not necessarily lead to a complete attachment disorder but perhaps only to subtle irritations in the attachment system. It may be that infants with insensitive night-time care become more clingy or ambivalent in their daytime attachments, which makes separation for sleep more difficult and may result in long-lasting behavioral problems.[27,28]

The presence of parents when an infant separates for sleep and sleeps during the night may support him or her in developing a secure attachment representation. Children from kibbutzim who were home sleepers with their parents developed a secure attachment relationship with their parents, while infants who slept in the group setting without their parents available at night developed attachment relationships with their metapelet (caregiver in the kibbutzim).[29–32]

ATTACHMENT, SEPARATION, AND SLEEP

Looking at attachment behavior from an evolutionary point of view, most infants around the world have slept and continue to sleep in close physical contact with their parents for the first year of life and possibly longer, so these infants do not experience separation at sleeping hours.[33] Thus, a crying baby at night is not a question in most countries. Only in Western countries and especially in Europe and North America do parents expect an infant to separate at night and sleep in his or her own bed or own room. This form of separation between infants and attachment figures during the night is not consistent with evolutionary development. In former times, when human beings were nomads, survival required that an infant remained in close physical contact with the attachment figure, usually the biologic mother, during the daytime and even more so during nighttime. Since an infant is dependent on the attachment figure for all of his or her physical, social, and emotional needs, close physical contact was a great advantage for survival. It is likely that the attachment system in humans developed within the context of evolution, as those infants who showed attachment behavior when separated from the attachment figure and when experiencing anxiety had a higher survival rate than those who did not. This might explain why many children in Western countries do not stay in their beds at night, especially when they experience anxiety and initiate co-sleeping in the parents' bedroom once they can walk.[3] Through the lens of attachment, it is not surprising that once arrived and snuggling up to their parents, the children can fall asleep within seconds.

Considered in the context of evolution, then, it is quite natural that an infant reacts to nightly separation from his or her attachment figure with alarm, crying, and signaling a desire to be picked up. If the attachment figure does not arrive to soothe the infant, the attachment arousal can escalate to hyperarousal in the autonomous nervous system, leading to an increase in bowel movements, as with colicky infants, or to vomiting when the gastrointestinal tract reacts. Therefore, night-time crying, seeking physical contact with the attachment figure, and protesting against separation from the attachment figure are correct evolutionarily based behavior.[34–36]

Nonetheless, an infant can learn to sleep through the night without his or her attachment figure. If Western cultural standards indicate that it is proper for parents and children to sleep apart, parents must train children to tolerate this type of separation, even though it is contrary to evolution. Parents must listen for sounds from the baby after separating and leaving the room and be ready to provide the child with a positive, attachment-oriented experience. Whenever the infant starts crying energetically and increasingly loudly, the parent should return to the room and try to console the infant. The child will sometimes need physical contact to calm down, especially if he or she has become hyperaroused. Returning rapidly to the room when the child starts to cry intensely is key to not having the child's arousal escalate to hyperarousal. Parents may have to enter the room repeatedly during the first nights, but this frequency will decrease. If parents respond promptly to an infant's crying at night, the baby will cry less during the next few weeks. In contrast, if parents delay in answering the cry signal and consoling the child by physical contact – perhaps because of their philosophy not to spoil the baby – the child will cry for longer periods in the future.[36] It has been found that each time the parents come in and respond, the infant learns that he or she is not lost, separate, and alone, but that the attachment figure is available and sensitive to his or her signaling. When parents consistently and reliably respond in this way, an infant will make an important discovery: even while separated at night when it is dark and anxiety can become intense, attachment figures are present and emotionally and physically available. This comes to signify an important attachment representation within the context of sleep and night-time separation, implying security and safety despite separation from the parents.[37]

THERAPY OF ATTACHMENT-RELATED SLEEP DISORDERS

Sleep problems in babies can be subtle indicators of difficulties in parent–infant relationships. If a baby cries for several hours day after day, it is important to seek help with a specially trained psychotherapist, who can quickly treat the dyad with an eye toward assessing the attachment and trauma experiences of the mother and father in addition to the interactional irritability of the infant.[18,38,39] The aim of attachment-related therapy for sleep disorders in infants is to enable these children to separate from the attachment figures in the evening, fall asleep, and remain in their own bed overnight without nightmares, anxiety, or panic attacks.

As mentioned earlier, attachment and separation concerns are present for parents as well as infants and children, and thus treatment must involve both parties. As in any attachment-related therapy, the therapist must become a therapeutic bonding figure; i.e., he or she must become a safe place for the parents as well as for the infant or child. In the same way that parents' 'sensitive behavior' is required for the positive development of a baby's secure attachment,[40] a therapist must become a secure base for parents – a framework for trust and a springboard for change.[14,18] Highly interactive therapeutic sensitivity – in which the therapist comes to recognize family signals (especially the parents'), interprets these signals correctly, and reacts conscientiously and promptly – will lead to the development of such a therapeutic bond, which will become a model for the parent–child relationship. The therapist fosters the development of a secure therapeutic bonding with the parents, and, as a result, parents can become a safe haven for their infants.[41]

The therapist can then help the parents to understand the night-time needs of their infants, be sensitive about a child's anxiety, and react appropriately by going into the infant's bedroom and trying to soothe him or her. If the baby is in an elevated state of arousal, the parents should take the child out of bed and provide physical contact. Most hyperaroused children will quickly relax with physical contact. Securely attached infants will need more and longer periods of physical contact to calm down than insecurely avoidant attached infants, but securely attached infants will have longer sleep durations than avoidant attached infants.[34] Some parents may allow a child to sleep briefly with them to calm down, after which the child can be placed back in his or her bed.

CASE STUDY

A mother, T., was referred by her pediatrician and telephoned that she urgently needed help to deal with the night-time needs of her 6-week-old infant. Every night, Baby S. had awakened for a feeding session. After being fed and put back to bed, the infant started to whine and cry, whereupon the mother would go into S.'s bedroom, lift her out of bed, cuddle and soothe her, rock her, and lay her back down in bed. Despite these ministrations, the baby continued to cry. This interaction went on several times each night, with the mother walking around and rocking S. for hours until the two fell asleep on the sofa during the morning hours. The whole family, especially the mother, was exhausted and did not know 'how to survive'. The partnership was in danger, as the husband threatened to leave the family. The couple's first child, now 6 years old, had also cried at night for 2 years, but the parents had decided to have another child despite their first 'catastrophic' experience. For these parents, the first years of having a child were equated with regular nightmares and

sleepless nights. As a result, the whole family was in an acute alarm state, and the children were at risk of harm from their parents. This is the moment when parents might start shaking babies. Things were worst at night, but similar difficult sleeping interactions took place during Baby S.'s morning and afternoon sleep. Several pediatric examinations had established a normal developmental pattern for her, with no indications of somatic disease to explain the symptom of sleep disturbance. Therefore, the sleep problem seemed to be a psychosomatic sleep disturbance.

A video diagnostic session of the mother changing diapers and playing with the infant as she would have done at home revealed an interesting interactional pattern. At first, the mother interacted sensitively, with eye contact, fine vocal attunement, and touch, responding to cues from the infant and engaging in a very nice dialogue of rhythmic interaction. But in between were switches in behavior and affect attunement: suddenly the mother would stop, avert her gaze, and anxiously and sadly examine the child's feet. Her affect became simultaneously shut down, depressed, and highly aroused. This lasted about 20 seconds, after which she again attended to the infant, interacting vocally and visually, then switching back and examining the child's feet, saying that the feet were too cold. In 2 minutes of videotaping, there were several switches back and forth between mother and child. When the mother shut down eye contact with S. and became preoccupied with the infant's feet, the child's gaze also shifted.

When we watched the video recording with the mother and tried to understand what we saw and how to interpret this, she told us she was not aware of these switches but remarked that she was checking the child's feet for signs of disability. T. related that, because of her age, she had undergone amniocentesis to check for possible fetal abnormalities. The first result of amniocentesis indicated an abnormal set of chromosomes and a handicapped child. T. and her husband were deeply shocked, and the gynecologist took another blood sample from the umbilical cord that revealed a normal set of chromosomes and a normal child. Of course, this double diagnosis of contrary results led to extreme arousal and stress for the parents. The mother was highly ambivalent about attaching prenatally to the child or holding back in case the baby was born disabled. After birth, externally and physically, baby S. appeared normal, so the mother declined a third, postnatal, chromosome test. Nevertheless, she began constantly to check the child for signs of abnormality, such as the special foot or hand folds found in children with Down syndrome, which she had learned about on the Internet and in books about disabled children. Although she did not find any such signs, the absence of abnormalities did not calm her, and she compulsively checked her child over and over. She had also read that disabled children sometimes exhibit a particular type of crying and wondered whether S.'s crying at night was the special kind of whimpering and crying called the cri-du-chat syndrome. On top of the erroneous prenatal diagnosis, S.'s crying was a trigger for anxiety and bonding ambivalence on the part of the mother, alarming her and leading her to worry that the symptom was part of a disability as yet undiagnosed.

During the process of diagnostics, we routinely perform an Adult Attachment Interview (AAI)[42] or an Adult Attachment Projective test (AAP),[43] as well as a Caregiving Interview (CGI)[44] for any mother presenting an infant with early interactional problems. These three interviews give us a lot of information about parents' own attachment representations and perhaps unresolved trauma experiences. During the AAI, the mother was asked when she was first separated from her own parents. She remembered quite vividly that at the age of 3 year, she was admitted to a hospital for a tonsillectomy. Her mother sent both baby S.'s mother and her 8-year-old brother for tonsillectomies, with the idea that the brother might calm her down when feelings of being lost and separated at night-time would come up. Baby S.'s mother felt very lonely at night in her unfamiliar bed in the hospital, and experienced a tremendous, sick feeling in her stomach, which she did not interpret as anxiety and arousal. At this point in the AAI, I realized

that the mother had previously told me that she felt sick to her stomach when little S. cried at night, and she took the baby out of her bed and started walking about the apartment. The mother of baby S. had also experienced a second separation shortly after her discharge from the hospital, when her mother gave birth to another child and all the children left home to stay with a grandmother. Again, she felt lonely and separated from her mother and had the same gastrointestinal symptoms. From that point onward, she could never tolerate separation and stay elsewhere overnight. Any attempt at an overnight separation such as in kindergarten or during school excursions failed because she became sick and her parents had to pick her up during the night.

Attachment dynamics of the sleeping disorder

Within the context of attachment-oriented psychodynamic theory, the mother's history and Baby S.'s sleep problem become more understandable. When the mother and her husband were confronted with the possibility of expecting a disabled child, triggers of anxiety and preoccupation emerged. The mother was highly ambivalent about bonding with her infant, and became preoccupied with searching for signs of disability after birth. Thus, the mother was in a permanent status of arousal, which did not help to bring the child into a relaxed state and help her fall asleep. Baby S. might have sensed the mother's ambivalence – clinging to her infant on the one hand and being preoccupied and emotionally distant on the other – which might have led S. to cry louder and search for physical contact with the mother, as the child experienced emotional separation and detachment from her mother. Furthermore, the AAI revealed that the mother retained her own separation problems from childhood and had a high psychosomatic arousal and trigger when she had to separate from her infant: The 3-year-old within the mother's own representational world needed an attachment figure. Because of her own experiences, the mother could not be a secure attachment base for her own infant. S.'s crying at night had triggered the mother's own separation experience from the past and brought the mother into a helpless state. Parents who become triggered by their infant's night-time crying and whose own traumatic experiences are reactivated have a high probability of acting out at night or becoming hyperaroused and needing their own attachment figure, thus not being emotionally available to their infants.

Treatment

Using an attachment-oriented approach, the following treatment procedure was arranged. During the daytime just before putting little S. to sleep, the mother telephoned me, and we talked about her feelings of anxiety and feeling lost. This therapeutic phone contact helped her to feel reassured and secure and to separate more easily from the child. During the night-time, there was still a great sleep disturbance, so we explained the attachment problem to the husband and asked him to get up at night with his wife. This led to the following situation. When the mother had nursed the infant at night and put her to bed, the infant was still awake, whining a bit but not crying. The husband took the mother's hand and helped her separate from the infant, providing a secure base and becoming an attachment figure for her. While the mother became calmer, little S. was already sound asleep.

Baby S.'s sleep problem disappeared rapidly, and it became quite clear that the infant's sleep problem was an entangled reenactment of acute insecurity because of the prenatal diagnosis and the early unresolved trauma of the mother. After the acute situation with Baby S. eased, the mother came for further therapeutic sessions to work on her unresolved trauma. The result was quite remarkable, and the mother made an astonishing recovery. For

the first time in her life, she could drive away for holidays and sleep in an unfamiliar bed. Furthermore, she was able, without hyperarousal and anxiety, to cross bridges and drive through tunnels, locations previously to be avoided. After termination of the treatment, she phoned me only once, after her son's first day of school. The morning after the first day, her son told her he wanted to go to school with his friends and without her, and he separated quite easily with a quick goodbye. Standing at the window and watching him walk along the road, she experienced the same sick feeling and remembered that it was related to her experience of early separation. At that moment, she decided to phone me, and we talked about how the situation came about and how it was triggered. She was aware of it, and did not need to reenact that situation by holding back or accompanying her son, hindering his autonomy and individuation.

DISCUSSION

Sleep problems of infants and even older children can be highly related to attachment problems. Children and adults with attachment disorders may have problems at night falling asleep, staying in their bed in darkness, or going back to sleep after waking from anxiety or nightmares. Depending on the attachment disorder, they long for physical contact, or, in contrast, may not want physical contact and instead stay in bed in a hyperaroused state, suppressing their attachment needs and developing psychosomatic symptoms.*

Children who have experienced early trauma such as deprivation or violence are likely to develop attachment disorders. Typically, those children do not have an inner representation of security, and if they have to separate and sleep in the dark apart from any person, anxiety arises and activates the attachment system. Depending on the

---

*In addition to gastrointestinal symptoms, respiratory symptoms (e.g., asthmatic symptoms with coughing and wheezing) are quite common and should be considered outside diagnoses of allergies. A convincing study has shown how asthma attacks and separation problems are associated.[45]

type of attachment disorder, they will start crying, shouting, fighting, or entering dissociative states and not showing signs of attachment behavior.

Since a baby cannot crawl or walk to search for the attachment figure, the only way to signal an attachment need is to cry through the night. If an infant is to form a secure attachment during the night, the parents must help the child to calm down by walking into the room and soothing the child, going away to help him or her to tolerate a short period of separation, and returning if the child is aroused again. This helps the baby to learn a form of separation training in which the attachment figure is available and will consistently arrive to soothe him or her when anxiety becomes intolerable and the crying escalates to a panic state. This training requires more time, emotional and physical availability, and sensitivity in a consistent and reliable way than leaving the child to cry through the night and get used to sleeping on his or her own.

Ultimately, if the child cannot calm down, a temporary period of having the child sleep with the parents may be wise, provided that there is no contraindication for co-sleeping such as drug addiction, alcoholism, smoking, elevated temperature in the parents' room, or a very soft mattress. Most children who bed in between the mother and father fall asleep fairly soon at night or after waking from nightmares, as the space between their attachment figures seems to provide the most security and reassurance.

PREVENTION

Many parents in Western countries themselves did not have the stressful experience of initially sleeping apart from their own parents, and so started co-sleeping with their infants, as most parents and children throughout the world still do.[46] Insufficient research is currently available that examines how parental status of attachment, correlated with co-sleeping and bedding-in, influences the emotional development of infants. Studies on sleep patterns in earlier days, which did not include attachment concerns in the research, showed that co-sleeping mothers and infants had the same sleep pattern in terms of depth and alertness. When the child became uneasy and irritable, the mother awoke and fed it, and both fell asleep again. Co-sleeping mothers were in tune with their babies and did not feel irritated during the night. In contrast, if the infant slept in a bed next to the mother's, their sleep rhythms were not as well tuned together, and if the child slept in a different room, the sleep rhythms of mother and infant were completely uncoordinated. Those mothers were the most exhausted in the morning.[*,46–48]

Children who can reestablish close physical contact with their parents at bedtime or even sleep together in the same room may form more secure relationships than those who are separated from their parents at night (parenthetically, this is one reason why admittance of parents with their infants in children's hospitals should be the norm). If parents do not want to co-sleep or room-in with their infant, they must consider attachment theory and attachment needs and realize that they are subjecting the child to a behavior that is contrary to evolution. If parents want children to sleep on their own, then the separation in the evening hours and calming down at night have to be done delicately and with the awareness that the evening and night separations are the most sensitive phases for attachment needs. Parents have to reassure children again and again that they are physically and

---

*Coincidentally, bedding-in during the weeks after delivery seems to protect against postpartum depression, as the incidence of postpartum depression is much lower in Asian countries, where bedding-in is the traditional form of caring. Some researchers recommend that bedding-in after delivery should be practiced everywhere as a preventive method against maternal postpartum depression.[49,50] In addition, we hypothesize that if mothers and children do not co-sleep or bed-in, then perhaps mothers become depressed because they cannot see their infants and worry about whether the children are still breathing and alive. Co-sleeping promotes breastfeeding, and might (consciously or unconsciously) reassure a mother during the night that her baby is breathing, side by side with her in physical contact, and so she might relax and sleep more quietly. In addition, the child would feel secure about the mother's closeness.[51,52]

emotionally available and help make the separation tolerable. Here, significant teaching and training are necessary for parents. In our parent groups, one of the biggest fears is that if the child is brought to the parents' bed as a co-sleeper, he or she might 'stay for 25 years'. Of course, this will not happen, and most parents find places and times for sexual activity outside of the parental bed at night, so that, among other things, co-sleeping need not be an obstruction to parental sexuality.

All these subjects are part of our new prevention program SAFE® (Secure Attachment Formation for Educators). Parents participate in this preventive program of four prenatal and six postnatal full-day workshops from the 20th week of gestation until the end of the child's first year. In addition to receiving many instructions and having personal experiences, all parents are given the AAI. Parents with unresolved traumas receive supportive psychotherapy before birth and trauma-centered therapy after birth. The goals of this prevention program are to uncover parental unresolved traumas that could be risk factors leading to a reenactment with the infant and to treat these problems before and after birth so that harm to the infant is prevented.

CONCLUSIONS

Sleep problems in infants and children can be difficult psychologic problems that always need early attention and treatment. Diagnosis should focus on the whole family – i.e., psychosocial and partnership problems, individual attachment problems and traumatic experiences of the mother and father, and the infant's own experiences of attachment or trauma. Children with attachment disorders are high-risk candidates for sleep problems, because separation and sleeping at night are important markers of the attachment relationship with the attachment figure. On the other hand, sleeping through the night does not mean that no attachment problems exist. The infant may have learned that no-one is available at night, no matter how loud he or she might cry.

In addition to markedly helping individual families, education about attachment theory, attachment figures, and attachment relationships holds the potential to effect dramatic social change. Such information can be obviously and directly useful to parents of infants with sleep disorders, as we have seen in this chapter. Moreover, many powerful societal benefits could also accrue if knowledge about the concrete ramifications of attachment theory were disseminated more widely, to adult clients, clinics, schools, and society at large.

ACKNOWLEDGMENTS

I am most grateful to the parents who allowed me to learn about their attachment problems and to increasingly understand the psychodynamics within families with infants who cry at night. Through these case histories and treatment experiences, I learned about the attachment-related problems of sleep disturbances in children with normal family backgrounds and those with attachment disorders and trauma-related experiences. Without these experiences, this chapter would not have been possible.

REFERENCES

1. Scher A, Cohen D. Locomotion and night waking. Child Care Health Dev 2005; 31: 685–91.
2. Jenni OG, Zinggeler Fuhrer H, Iglowstein I, Molinari L, Largo R. A longitudinal study of bed sharing and sleep problems among Swiss children in the first ten years of life. Pediatrics 2005; 115: 223–40.
3. Thunström M. Severe sleep problems among infants in a normal population in Sweden: prevalence, severity, and correlates. Acta Paediatr 1999; 88: 1356–63.
4. Sazonov E, Sazonova N, Schuckers S, Neuman M, CHIME Study Group. Activity-based sleep–wake identification in infants. Physiol Meas 2004; 25: 1291–304.

5. Moore SM. Disturbed attachment in children: A factor in sleep disturbance, altered dream production, and immune dysfunction. J Child Psychother 1989; 15: 99–111.

6. Anders TF. Infant sleep, nighttime relationships, and attachment. Psychiatry 1993; 57: 11–20.

7. Anders TF, Keener M, Bowe TR, Shoaff BA. A longitudinal study of nighttime sleep-wake patterns in infants from birth to one year. In: Call JD, Galenson E, Tyson PI, eds. Frontiers of Infant Psychiatry. New York: Basic Books, 1983: 150–70.

8. Sadeh A, Anders TF. Infant sleep problems: origins, assessment, interventions. Infant Mental Health J 1993; 14: 17–34.

9. Minde K. Sleep problems in toddlers: effects of treatment on their daytime behavior. J Am Acad Child Adolesc Psychiatry 1994; 33: 1114–21.

10. Wolke D, Meyer R, Ohrt B, Riegel K. Co-morbidity of crying and feeding problems with sleep problems in infancy: concurrent and predictive associations. Early Dev Parenting 1995; 4: 191–207.

11. Zucherman B, Stevenson J, Bailey V. Sleep problems in early childhood: continuities, predictive factors, and behavioral correlates. Pediatrics 1987; 80: 664–71.

12. Von Hofacker N, Papouseck M. Disorders of excessive crying, feeding, and sleeping: The Munich Interdisciplinary Research and Intervention Program. Infant Mental Health J 1998; 19: 180–201.

13. Ainsworth MDS, Blehar M, Waters E, Wall S. Patterns of Attachment: A Psychological Study of the Strange Situation. Hillsdale, NJ: Lawrence Erlbaum, 1978.

14. Bowlby J. A Secure Base: Clinical Implications of Attachment Theory. London: Routledge, 1988.

15. Bowlby J. Attachment and Loss. Vol 1: Attachment. New York: Basic Books, 1969.

16. Bowlby J. Attachment and Loss. Vol 2: Separation, Anxiety and Anger. New York: Basic Books, 1973.

17. Bowlby J. Attachment and Loss. Vol 3: Loss: Sadness and Depression. New York: Basic Books, 1980.

18. Brisch KH. Treating Attachment Disorders: From Theory to Therapy. New York: Guilford, 2002.

19. Bretherton I. In pursuit of the internal working model construct and its relevance to attachment relationships. In: Grossmann KE, Grossmann K, Waters E, eds. Attachment from Infancy to Adulthood: The Major Longitudinal Studies. New York: Guilford, 2005: 13–47.

20. World Health Organization ICD-10 Classification of Mental and Behavioural Disorders: Diagnostic Criteria for Research. Geneva: 1992.

21. Diagnostic and Statistical Manual of Mental Disorders – Text Revision, 4th edn. Washington, DC: American Psychiatric Association, 2000.

22. Zeanah CH, Boris NW. Disturbances and disorders of attachment in early childhood. In: Zeanah CH, ed. Handbook of Infant Mental Health, 2nd edn. New York: Guilford, 2000: 353–68.

23. Carmichael CL, Reis HT. Attachment, sleep quality, and depressed affect. Health Psychol 2006; 24: 526–31.

24. Warren SL, Gunnar MR, Kagan J, et al. Maternal panic disorders: infant temperament, neurophysiology, and parenting behavior. J Am Acad Child Adolesc Psychiatry 2003; 42: 814–25.

25. Morrel J, Steel H. The role of attachment security, temperament, maternal perception, and caregiving behavior in persistent infant sleeping problems. Infant Mental Health J 2003; 24: 447–68.

26. Benoit D, Zeanah CH, Boucher C, Minde K. Sleep disorders in early childhood: Association with insecure maternal attachment. J Am Acad Child Adolesc Psychiatry 1992; 31: 86–93.

27. Scher A, Zuckerman S, Epstein R. Persistent night waking and settling difficulties across the first year: early precursors of later behavioural problems? J Reprod Infant Psychol 2005; 23: 77–88.

28. Thunström M. Severe sleep problems in infancy associated with subsequent development of attention-deficit/hyperactivity disorder at 5.5 years of age. Acta Paediatrica 2002; 91: 584–92.

29. Sagi A, Lamb ME, Lewkowicz KS, et al. Security of infant–mother, –father, and –metapelet attachments among kibbutz-reared Israeli children. In: Bretherton I, Waters E, eds. Growing Points of Attachment Theory and Research. Chicago, IL: University of Chicago Press, 1985: 357–75.

30. Sagi A, van Ijzendoorn MH. Multiple caregiving environments: the kibbutz experience. In: Harel S, Shonkoff JP, eds. Early Childhood Intervention and Family Support Programs: Accomplishments and Challenges. Jerusalem: JDC–Brookdale Institute, 1996: 143–62.

31. Sagi A, van Ijzendoorn MH, Aviezer O, Donnell F, Mayseless O. Sleeping out of home in a kibbutz communal arrangement: it makes a difference for

infant– mother attachment. Child Dev 1994; 65: 992–1004.

32. Sagi-Schwartz A, Aviezer O. Correlates of attachment to multiple caregivers in kibbutz children from birth to emerging adulthood: the Haifa Longitudinal Study. In: Grossmann KE, Grossmann K, Waters E, eds. Attachment from Infancy to Adulthood: The Major Longitudinal Studies. New York: Guilford, 2005: 165–97.

33. Latz S, Wolf AW, Lozoff B. Cosleeping in context: sleep practices and problems in young children in Japan and the United States. Arch Pediatr Adolesc Med 1999; 153: 339–46.

34. Scher A. Attachment and sleep: a study of night waking in twelve-month-old infants. Dev Psychobiol 2001; 38: 274–85.

35. Scher A. Mother–child interaction and sleep regulation in one-year-olds. Infant Mental Health J 2001; 22: 515–28.

36. St James-Roberts I, Alvarez M, Csipke E, et al. Infant crying and sleeping in London, Copenhagen, and when parents adopt a 'proximal' form of care. Pediatrics 2006; 117: 1146–55.

37. Hayes MJ, Roberts SM, Stowe R. Early childhood co-sleeping: parent–child and parent-infant nighttime interactions. Infant Mental Health J 1998; 17: 348–57.

38. Daws D. Through the Night: Helping Parents and Sleepless Infants. London: Free Association Books, 1993.

39. Daws D. Family relationships and infant feeding problems. Health Visitor 1994; 67: 162–4.

40. Grossmann K, Grossmann KE, Spangler G, Suess G, Unzner L. Maternal sensitivity and newborns' orientation responses as related to quality of attachment in northern Germany. In: Bretherton I, Waters E, eds. Growing Points of Attachment Theory and Research. Chicago: University of Chicago Press, 1985: 231–56.

41. Orlinsky DE, Grawe K, Parks BK. Process, and outcome in psychotherapy – noch einmal. In: Bergin AE, Garfield SL, eds. Handbook of Psychotherapy and Behavior Change, 4th edn. New York: Wiley, 1994: 270–376.

42. George C, Kaplan N, Main M. The Attachment Interview for Adults. Berkeley, CA: University of California unpublished manuscript, 1985.

43. George C, West M, Pettem O. The Adult Attachment Projective: disorganization of adult attachment at the level of representation. In: Solomon J, George C, eds. Attachment Disorganization. New York: Guilford, 1999: 318–46.

44. George C, Solomon J. Representational models of relationships: links between caregiving and representation. Infant Mental Health J 1996; 17: 198–216.

45. Sandberg S, Paton JY, Ahola S, et al. The role of acute and chronic stress in asthma attacks in children. Lancet 2000; 356: 982–7.

46. Jenni OG, O'Connor BB. Children's sleep: an interplay between culture and biology. Pediatrics 2005; 115: 204–16.

47. Louis J, Cannard C, Bastuji H, Challamel MJ. Sleep ontogenesis revisited: a longitudinal 24-hour home polygraphic study on fifteen normal infants during the first two years of life. Sleep 1997; 20: 323–33.

48. Minard KL, Freudigman K, Thoman EB. Sleep rhythmicity in infants: index of stress or maturation. Behav Processes 1999; 47: 189–203.

49. Nelson EAS, Schiefenhoevel W, Haimerl F. Child care practices in nonindustrialized societies. Pediatrics 2000; 105: e75.

50. Strobl CW. Postpartale Dysphorie (Baby-Blues) und Wochenbettdepression. Eine katamnestische Untersuchung an 585 Müttern aus Kliniken in München und Starnberg. [Postpartum dysphoria (baby-blues) and postpartum depression. A follow-up study on 585 mothers from clinics in Munich and Starnberg.] Munich: Ludwig-Maximilians-Universität, 2002.

51. McKenna J, Mosko S, Richard C, et al. Experimental studies of infant–parent co-sleeping: mutual physiological and behavioral influences and their relevance to SIDS (sudden infant death syndrome). Early Hum Dev 1994; 38: 187–201.

52. Gay CL, Lee KA, Lee SY. Sleep patterns and fatigue in new mothers and fathers. Biol Res Nurs 2004; 5: 311–18.

17

Animal models of insomnia

Paula A Tiba, Sergio Tufik, Deborah Suchecki

INTRODUCTION

The influence of stress on sleep has been recognized for millennia. Hippocrates stated that sleeplessness is a sign of pain and suffering that may lead to mental illness, whereas excessive daytime sleepiness is an indication of illness. The philosopher also emphasized the importance of sleep as a remedy for psychologic and physical stress.[1]

The most referred to stress-related sleep disorder is insomnia. Several epidemiologic studies have pointed to stress as a triggering factor in the development of insomnia, although individual vulnerability has a major influence. Numerous reports indicate that stress profoundly influences sleep. Although it is common listening to people complaining of a bad night of sleep under stressful situations, insomnia results from the individual vulnerability to these events. Cartwright and Wood[2] showed that subjects undergoing the process of divorce exhibit less time in delta sleep. After completion of the divorce process, sleep is normalized; however, those individuals for whom the process was prolonged showed a depression-type sleep pattern, including augmented percentage of rapid eye movement (REM) sleep.

Insomniacs frequently exhibit symptoms of anxiety, which are exacerbated at bedtime. In addition, these patients also present dysregulation of the hypothalamic–pituitary–adrenocortical (HPA) axis – so much so, that adrenocorticotropic hormone (ACTH) and cortisol levels are higher than those of healthy volunteers during the cortisol-quiescent period.[3] However, it has not yet been established whether the hyperactivity of the HPA axis is a preexistent condition or a consequence of the poor sleep quality. So far, the latter may be a stronger possibility, since numerous studies in both animals and humans have shown that sleep deprivation or sleep restriction result in changes of HPA-axis activity, resulting in increased secretion of ACTH and corticosterone (or cortisol in humans) after prolonged paradoxical sleep deprivation.[4,5] Sleep restriction in rats induces a daily elevation of ACTH and corticosterone, but at the end of 8 days of sleep restriction, restrained stress-induced ACTH secretion is attenuated, suggesting either a reduced hypothalamic stimulation of and/or an increased negative feedback at the pituitary level.[6] In humans, 24-hour sleep deprivation leads to increased cortisol levels on the evening following the manipulation,[7] and prolonged sleep restriction results in augmented cortisol levels and sympathetic activity.[8]

EFFECTS OF STRESS HORMONES ON SLEEP

Stress as much as sleep is a phenomenon that involves the whole central nervous system (CNS). Many neurotransmitters participate in the regulation of both sleep and stress response. For instance, norepinephrine (noradrenaline), serotonin, and acetylcholine stimulate the paraventricular nucleus of the hypothalamus, the site of corticotropin-releasing factor (CRF) synthesis, whereas γ-aminobutyric acid (GABA) inhibits it.[9] These neurotransmitters work in concert to regulate sleep such that norepinephrine is involved in waking and GABA induces sleep; acetylcholine in specific areas of the CNS stimulates REM sleep, and serotonin is involved with the generation of slow-wave sleep (SWS).[10] Therefore, the interaction between sleep and stress is a complex one and cannot be considered a direct or straightforward relationship.

Since it is a global phenomenon, it is only natural to believe that stress alters numerous neurotransmitter and hormonal systems in and out of the CNS. The major hormones that participate in the stress response are those of the HPA axis, the locus ceruleus (LC)–adrenal medulla system, and other hypophysiary hormones such as prolactin (PRL). A close relationship between these hormones and sleep has been determined, especially in humans, who exhibit a monophasic pattern of sleep. Major pulses of growth hormone secretion occur during delta sleep, when the lowest levels of HPA and epinephrine (adrenaline) activity are observed. Therefore, a negative relationship between cortisol, epinephrine, and delta sleep has been established.[11] Of particular interest is stress-induced PRL secretion and its relationship with REM sleep. It has been well established in human beings that a rise in PRL levels is observed after sleep onset and that maximal values occur in the early morning hours.[12] The REM sleep-promoting effects of PRL have been demonstrated in cats, rats, and rabbits, although they seem to be period-dependent, in as much as REM sleep is induced only when PRL is administered in the light period (the resting period for these species), whereas injection during the dark period inhibits REM sleep.[13] More recently, intracerebroventricular (i.c.v.) administration of low doses of PRL-releasing peptide was shown to increase PRL levels and to induce REM sleep.[14] Moreover, intact rats exposed to ether stress exhibit increased levels of PRL and of REM sleep, but animals previously hypophysectomized do not, suggesting that PRL may be involved in the augmented REM.[15]

The hormones of the HPA axis are involved with waking. This is not difficult to understand – because who could feel asleep in face of a stressful stimulus? Release of CRF, ACTH, glucocorticoids and norepinephrine increases stimulus-driven attention, cognition and the metabolic machinery necessary for the fight-or-flight response (Figure 17.1).[16] Accumulating evidence has shown that CRF is one of the mediators of wakefulness. The i.c.v. administration of CRF in rats decreases slow-wave sleep (SWS) and results in a waking-like electroencephalograph (EEG) pattern.[17] Moreover, blockade of CRF receptors also reduces waking and increases SWS. These effects seem to be mediated, at least in

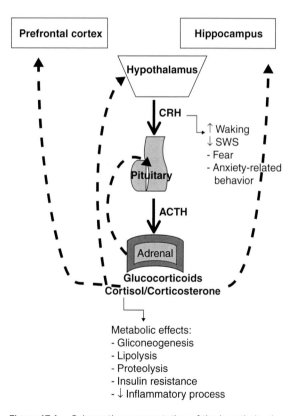

Figure 17.1 Schematic representation of the hypothalamic–pituitary–adrenocortical (HPA) axis and the main effects of corticotropin-releasing factor (CRF) and glucocorticoids. Filled arrows represent stimulation and dashed arrows represent inhibition. The main sites of glucocorticoid negative feedback are the prefrontal cortex, hippocampus, hypothalamus, and pituitary (adapted from Arborelius L et al. J Endocrinol 1999; 160: 1–12[16])

part, by interleukin-1 (IL-1), since administration of a CRF antagonist inhibits corticosterone secretion and increases mRNA for IL-1α and IL-1β.[18] Exogenous administration of IL-1 during the animal's active phase results in increased time in SWS and reduced waking time.[19] In humans, administration of metyrapone results in a significant reduction of the time spent in delta sleep.[20] This effect can be explained by the fact that as a cortisol synthesis inhibitor, metyrapone suppresses the negative-feedback system, leading to increased ACTH plasma levels, which reflects an increase in CRF secretion.

Administration of corticosterone to rats increases the time of waking and reduces the time of deep SWS.[21] However, it is worth mentioning that the doses used in this study result in plasma levels far higher than physiologic stress levels. Adrenalectomized rats exhibit shorter sleep episodes, with less SWS and longer waking periods during the light phase, whereas the opposite is observed during the dark phase. When corticosterone replacement results in basal plasma levels (5 μg/dl), normal sleep pattern is restored, but when replacement results in higher than basal levels (approximately 10 μg/dl), SWS is inhibited.[22]

These finely tuned glucocorticoid effects on sleep are likely mediated by the balance between the two well-known glucocorticoid receptors: mineralocorticoid and glucocorticoid (MRs and GRs, respectively). MRs exhibit high affinity for the natural ligands (corticosterone/cortisol and aldosterone) and are located predominantly on the limbic system. From 80% to 90% of MRs are occupied throughout the day, including the nadir of the circadian rhythm. GRs, in contrast, show a much lower affinity for the natural ligand (one-tenth of the MR affinity), but a high affinity for synthetic corticosteroids. They are widely distributed in the brain and periphery, and are only occupied during the bursts of corticoid secretion, i.e., during the peak of circadian rhythm and stress response. Therefore, MRs are involved with the control of circadian activities of the glucocorticoids, and GRs restore the disruption of homeostasis resulting

from exposure to stressful situations, although both receptors work in a concerted manner to maintain appropriate balance of body functions.[23]

ANIMAL MODELS FOR THE STUDY OF STRESS-INDUCED SLEEP CHANGES

The use of experimental models of human diseases is advantageous insofar as many of the mechanisms involved in the installation of the disease can be disclosed, not to mention potential therapeutic agents and preventive actions. Nonetheless, there is special difficulty in modeling human psychopathologies, because these involve higher cognitive functions that cannot yet be tested in animals. Still, these models are extremely useful to unveil the neurobiology and, in some cases, even conditions that may trigger or prevent the development of such pathologies.

Insomnia results from the interaction between environmental conditions (stressful situations) and individual vulnerability.[3,24] Therefore, it is not only the stimulus but also how it is processed by the subject that determines how much and for how long neurotransmitters and hormones will be released in response to the challenge. In addition, as has been already mentioned, it is not possible, as yet, to determine whether increased ACTH and cortisol levels observed in patients are a cause or consequence of insomnia. The use of animal models is a suitable strategy to try to answer these questions.

Changes in sleep pattern induced by stressful events result from an integration of genetic, neuroendocrine, and neurophysiologic mechanisms. Therefore, the initial behavioral responses that animals exhibit when confronted with stressors may determine the subsequent sleep response to a given event. For didactic purposes, we will consider two main strategies for the study of stress-induced sleep alterations: environmental influences, which influence the effects of stressors that may or may not represent an ethologic situation, and genetic influences, which influence how the sleep of animals with different genetic backgrounds respond to stress.

Environmental influences

In rodents, it is generally accepted that sleep is increased after an acute stressful event, and this increase is believed to function as a coping strategy and an aid for recovery. However, there seems to be a clear temporal pattern for this effect; i.e., during stress exposure, both SWS and REM sleep are inhibited and this inhibition does not seem to habituate, because it is virtually the same whether the rat is submitted to 1 or 4 hours of immobilization.[25] Sleep remains inhibited for some time after the end of the stimulus,[26] when it begins to rise, reaching the highest levels during the dark phase of the cycle.[26–29]

The length of the stimulus also influences sleep rebound. For instance, rats submitted to a 2-hour immobilization stress exhibit a 32% rebound of paradoxical sleep (PS) and no changes in SWS.[30] The effect on REM sleep is further increased when immobilization is reduced to 1 hour, when REM rebound goes up to 63% and SWS rebound increases to 16% during the dark period.[31] However, when the length of immobilization is increased to 4 hours, the sleep rebound is no longer observed and corticosterone levels are increased by 92% (against 71% observed after 1 hour of immobilization), suggesting that prolonged elevations of corticosterone may inhibit the expression of stress-induced sleep rebound.[25]

Although stress-induced sleep rebound has been reported by several authors, this is not a universal effect, since different types of stress lead to different outcomes. Acute cold stress has been shown to induce SWS, whereas acute footshock induces sustained waking during the subsequent 6 hours of recording.[32] In addition, footshock results in prolonged latency to sleep and to REM sleep; nonetheless, rebound is not expressed in the dark period, as should be expected.[33]

In mice, the association of tone with shock (conditioned fear), either in single or multiple training schedules, produces a reduction of SWS and REM sleep. For mice submitted to the multiple training schedule, sleep reduction is still evident on the day after training. Presentation of the tone to this same group up to 27 days after training elicits reduction of REM sleep, indicating that the strength of the conditioning is capable of interfering with sleep for almost 1 month after the tone–shock pairing.[34] Assessment of freezing behavior elicited by situational reminders of traumatic events may serve as a model of post-traumatic stress disorder (PTSD). With this idea in mind, Pawlyk et al[35] studied the sleep pattern of rats submitted to situational reminders from a series of five shocks. When sleeping in the same context where the shock was delivered, rats exhibit longer latencies to sleep and to REM sleep and reduced percentage of REM sleep; however, when sleeping in a neutral context, they displayed SWS and REM sleep rebound, thus being able to distinguish between neutral and aversive contexts, confirming the occurrence of aversive conditioning.

In human beings, the most powerful stressors are those involving a social context, such as social hierarchy, familiar problems, and interpersonal relationships. In rodents, one example of social manipulation is the social defeat paradigm, obtained in the laboratory via the resident–intruder paradigm. This method is based on the establishment of a territory by a male and its defense against unfamiliar male intruders. The experimental male (the 'intruder') is introduced into the home cage of an aggressive male (the 'resident'), the former being attacked and submitted by the latter.[36] Social defeat by a conspecific male induces not only strong neuroendocrine responses in plasma catecholamines, corticosterone, prolactin, and testosterone, but also acute responses in heart rate, blood pressure, and body temperature.[37] Studies of social defeat-induced sleep rebound show increased slow-wave activity (SWA), but not of the time spent in SWS, reflecting augmented intensity but not quantity of sleep. Moreover, SWA is believed to take place in order to restore the internal balance after a traumatic event.[38,39]

Genetic influences

The genetic background is a major variable for determination of behavioral expression. Therefore, the same stimulus may lead to different outcomes, depending on how the animals react to it. Animal models that attempt to represent human individual differences employ two main strategies: (1) selection of high and low responders to a given stimulus in genetically heterogeneous outbred strains; (2) comparison of inbred strains, which are genetically identical within strain but vary genetically and phenotypically across strains.

In regard to the first strategy, selection of Wistar rats, which intensely explore the open arms of the elevated plus maze (and are thus considered low anxiety-related behavior or LAB rats) or intensely avoid them (and are thus considered high anxiety-related behavior or HAB rats), has provided neuroendocrine and behavioral phenotypes that reflect different coping strategies and fearful behaviors to novel situations.[40,41] HAB rats display less baseline pre-REM sleep and greater stress-induced sleep impairment, reflected by augmented wakefulness, and reduced SWS and pre-REM sleep, than LAB animals. Interestingly, blockade of CRF1 receptors results in more SWS in HAB animals,[42] confirming, by means of a different approach, that hyperactivity of the CRF system in 'anxious' rats is most likely involved with stress-induced sleep impairment.

Using locomotor activity as the behavioral endpoint for selection of animals, Bouye et al[43] reported on the sleep pattern of high responders (HRs: high novelty-induced locomotor activity) and low responders (LRs: low novelty-induced locomotor activity) exposed to immobilization stress. Initially, there is a positive correlation between novelty-induced locomotor activity and corticosterone plasma levels. Peak corticosterone levels are similar between LRs and HRs, but the latter exhibit an impaired negative feedback. Compared with LRs, the amount of wakefulness is greater in HRs, at the expense of SWS, whereas REM sleep is similar. In response to acute immobilization, both LRs and HRs increase their time spent in REM sleep; however, for LRs, there is a reduction in the time spent in SWS, whereas for HRs, the reduction takes place in the time spent in wakefulness, which means that stress-induced sleep rebound is evident only in HRs.

The second approach consists of comparing different strains, which basically differ in their behavioral and neuroendocrine responsiveness to stress. For instance, Lewis (LEW) rats, which are deficient in CRF production, exhibit less wakefulness and more SWS than Fisher 344 (F344) and Sprague–Dawley (Sp-D) rats.[44] When compared with Sp-D or to outbred Wistar strains, F344 rats show adrenocortical and prolactin hyper-responsiveness to footshock stress and display more anxiety-related behavior in the open field and elevated plus maze. In their home cages, F344 and Wistar rats are more active during the dark period, and baseline sleep indicates that these two strains also sleep less than LEW and Sp-D rats. The smaller sleep time is due to reduction of both SWS and REM sleep, but, interestingly, the proportion of REM with regard to total sleep time is similar for all strains.[45] In response to a conditioning fear paradigm, performed in 2 days, LEW rats exhibit the greatest sleep loss during the daytime period and the least recovery during the night-time period, compared with F344 and Wistar rats. Curiously, F344 and LEW exhibit similar levels of freezing behavior, which are higher than those exhibited by Wistar rats, indicating that the reaction to an aversive stimulus does not predict the sleep alteration. Therefore, mechanisms other than activation of the HPA axis may underlie stress-induced sleep changes.[46]

In mice strains that differ in reactivity to noxious stimuli such as footshock and contextual fear conditioning, a clear and persistent loss of SWS and REM sleep is observed in the more 'anxious' BALB/cJ mice, whereas the less 'anxious' C57BL/6J mice only show a loss of REM sleep within the hour that follows shock presentation.[47,48] A similar pattern of sleep reactivity is also seen in response to non-noxious manipulations, such as exposure to an open-field[49] or restraint stress:[50] C57BL/6J mice display the characteristic stress-induced sleep rebound, whereas the BALB/cJ strain displays sleep impairment.

MECHANISMS AND MEDIATORS OF STRESS-INDUCED SLEEP CHANGES

The first hypothesis put forward to explain how stress induces sleep rebound involves the

serotoninergic system. Evidence has linked serotonin with sleep, in as much as blockade of its
synthesis or a lesion of the raphe nuclei causes insomnia.[51] Voltametry studies have shown a differential pattern of serotonin release depending on the
phase of the sleep–wake cycle: (1) from the nerve
terminal (axonal) during waking; and (2) from
the dendrites during sleep. Axonal release during
waking may be involved in the preparation for
sleep, by triggering the synthesis of hypnogenic
substances in target structures, such as the arcuate
nucleus. Therefore, according to the serotonergic
hypothesis, at the beginning of immobilization stress,
there is augmented secretion of 5-hydroxyindoles,
especially in the arcuate nucleus, with subsequent
reduction throughout the stress session induced by
corticosterone. Thus, waking is induced during
stress and sleep rebound is observed later on.[52]
Increased serotonergic transmission induces the
synthesis of pro-opiomelanocortin (POMC) mRNA
in the arcuate nucleus, which can, in turn, increase
the synthesis of POMC derivatives such as
$ACTH_{1-39}$, α-melanocyte stimulating hormone
(α-MSH) and corticotropin-like intermediate lobe
peptide (CLIP or $ACTH_{18-39}$). Although ACTH is
well known to induce waking, α-MSH and CLIP
increase sleep time.[53] The content of CLIP and its
phosphorylated form is augmented in the nucleus
raphis dorsalis immediately after the end of immobilization stress, whereas in the arcuate nucleus, the
increase is observed 4 hours after the end of the
session, when REM rebound is at its maximum[54]
(Figure 17.2). Exogenous administration of CLIP
or of its N-terminal fragments $ACTH_{20-24}$ and
$ACTH_{18-24}$ produces a significant increase of
REM sleep because of episode duration. The N-
terminus is devoid of sleep-enhancing effects.[53,55]

A second line of investigation is related to the
involvement of the noradrenergic system on stress-
induced sleep rebound. Major evidence comes from
studies reporting that lesions of the LC reduce
SWS and REM sleep rebound induced by immobilization stress.[56] Likewise, administration of
α-helical CRH, a CRF receptor antagonist, before
immobilization stress prevents the characteristic

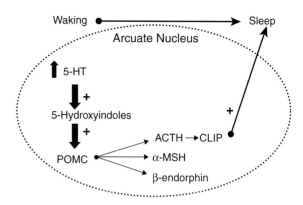

Figure 17.2   Schematic representation of the serotonergic
hypothesis of stress-induced sleep rebound, elaborated by
Cespuglio et al.[52] According to this hypothesis, serotonin
released in the arcuate nucleus would induce pro-
opiomelanocortin (POMC) cleavage, resulting in the synthesis
of ACTH derivatives, including $ACTH_{18-39}$ (CLIP)

REM sleep rebound in rats.[57] Since the effect of
immobilization stress on the LC is mediated by the
CRF system, González and Valatx[57] argued that
lesioned animals would exhibit a smaller activating
response of the LC to CRF, indicating that stress-
induced REM sleep rebound is dependent on CRF
activation. However, it is difficult to understand
how the blockade of two arousing systems would
lead to smaller sleep rebound, unless this blockade
impacts on other systems that might take part in
stress-induced sleep rebound (e.g., the POMC-
derivative peptides).

Among the many neurotransmitter/neuro-
endocrine systems that are responsive to stressful stimuli, endorphins are particularly involved, since they
are a product of POMC cleavage, being released
together with ACTH. The effects of endorphins
on sleep are somehow controversial, in so far as some
studies show that systemic or i.c.v. administration
of morphine inhibits both SWS and REM sleep,
whereas direct administration of morphine in the
LC or in the solitary tract promotes sleep. Naltrexone, a selective blocker of the μ-opioid receptors,
prevents immobilization stress-induced sleep
rebound in rats, but does not interfere with the

corticosterone response to stress, evidencing a dissociation between the endocrine and the sleep responses to stress. Curiously, naltrexone by itself affects neither hormone secretion nor sleep, indicating that it only modifies the effects of stress on these parameters.[58] This effect can be explained by the fact that stimulation of μ-opioid receptors inhibits the discharge rate of neurons in the LC.[59] If immobilization stress elicits the release of β-endorphin from neurons of the arcuate nucleus, then the stressor would inhibit LC discharge, via activation of μ-opioid receptors, leading to augmented REM sleep. An alternative explanation is that endogenous μ-agonists released in response to stress block the action of CRF on LC neurons, facilitating their inhibition and the increase of REM sleep.[58] There is a major problem, however, because the opioidergic hypothesis is difficult to reconcile with the reduced REM rebound resulting from LC lesions.

Another important peptide responsive to stressful stimuli is PRL. As mentioned already, PRL is closely related to REM sleep. In mice strains that differ in anxiety-related behavior (C57BL/6J or 'less-anxious' mice and BALB/cJ or 'anxious' mice), restraint stress was capable of eliciting sleep rebound only in the 'less-anxious' strain. Investigation of possible mediators of such distinct response led to finding that only the 'less-anxious' strain (C57BL/6J) displayed higher levels of restraint-induced prolactin when compared with handling-induced peptide secretion, whereas PRL secretion in BALB/cJ mice was as low after restraint as after handling. Interestingly, corticosterone levels were equally elevated after restraint in both strains, demonstrating a similar activation of the adrenocortical system.[60]

CONCLUDING REMARKS

In humans, stressful situations, especially those with a social character, are capable of eliciting insomnia. This, however, is not a universal outcome. Stress-induced insomnia depends on some features of the stimulus, but most of all on individual characteristics. This also seems to be the case in rodents. In general, stress induces sleep rebound, and this effect appears to be highly adaptive, since sleep is viewed as an effective strategy of recovery from either endogenous or exogenous insults. However, mouse and rat strains that are characterized by displaying high levels of anxiety-related behavior are more vulnerable to stress-induced sleep impairment.

In this regard, a likely neural substrate for insomnia related to stress is the central nucleus of the amygdala (CeA), especially because most of the evidence for the awakening properties of adverse stimuli comes from classical conditioning studies, which are known to be related to the amygdala. This structure evaluates the emotional significance of stimuli and initiates the appropriate neurobehavioral responses. In addition, the CeA exhibits reciprocal connections to each of the brainstem structures involved in sleep and waking, i.e., the dorsal raphe nucleus, the LC, and the pedunculopontino/laterodorsal tegmental nuclei (PPT/LDT).[61] Electrical stimulation of the CeA inhibits the discharge of LC neurons, ultimately resulting in augmented REM sleep. Therefore, inhibition of amygdala activity would lead to reduced REM sleep. This, in fact, is observed when muscimol (a γ-aminobutyric acid A-type receptor (GABA$_A$) agonist) is injected intra-CeA, while bicuculline (a GABA$_A$ antagonist) elicits REM sleep.[62,63] The mechanisms whereby the amygdala influences REM sleep have not yet been identified and pose an interesting line of investigation, given the close relationship between this structure, anxiety-related behavior, and sleep disturbance induced by emotionally arousing stimuli.

ACKNOWLEDGMENTS

This work was supported by Associação Fundo de Incentivo à Psicofarmacologia (AFIP) and Fundação de Amparo à Pesquisa do Estado de São Paulo (FAPESP – CEPID, Grant 98/14303-3). Paula A Tiba is a PhD student and a recipient of a fellowhip from CAPES; Sergio Tufik and Deborah Suchecki are recipients of fellowships from CNPq.

REFERENCES

1. Vgontzas AN, Bixler EO, Kales A. Sleep, sleep disorders, and stress. In: Fink G, ed. Encyclopedia of Stress. San Diego, CA: Academic Press, 2000: 449–57.
2. Cartwright RD, Wood E. Adjustment disorders of sleep: the sleep effect of a major stressful event and its resolution. Psychiatry Res 1991; 39: 199–209.
3. Vgontzas AN, Bixler EO, Lin HM, et al. Chronic insomnia is associated with nyctohemeral activation of the hypothalamic-pituitary-adrenal axis: clinical implications. J Clin Endocrinol Metab 2001; 86: 3787–94.
4. Suchecki D, Tufik S. Social stability attenuates the stress in the modified multiple platform method for paradoxical sleep deprivation in the rat. Physiol Behav 2000; 68: 309–16.
5. Suchecki D, Tiba P, Tufik S. Hormonal and behavioural responses of paradoxical sleep-deprived rats to the elevated plus maze. J Neuroendocrinol 2002; 14: 549–54.
6. Meerlo P, Koehl M, van der Borght K, Turek FW. Sleep restriction alters the hypothalamic–pituitary–adrenal response to stress. J Neuroendocrinol 2002; 14: 397–402.
7. Leproult R, Copinschi G, Buxton O, Van Cauter E. Sleep loss results in an elevation of cortisol levels the next evening. Sleep 1997; 20: 865–70.
8. Spiegel K, Leproult R, Van Cauter E. Impact of sleep debt on metabolic and endocrine function. Lancet 1999; 354: 1435–9.
9. Carrasco GA, van der Kar LD. Neuroendocrine pharmacology of stress. Eur J Pharmacol 2003; 463: 235–72.
10. Pace-Schott EF, Hobson JA. The neurobiology of sleep: genetics, cellular physiology and subcortical networks. Nat Rev Neurosci 2002; 3: 591–605.
11. Born J, Fehm HL. The neuroendocrine recovery function of sleep. Noise Health 2000; 2: 25–38.
12. Roky R, Obál F Jr, Valatx J-L, et al. Prolactin and rapid eye movement sleep regulation. Sleep 1995; 18: 536–42.
13. Roky R, Valatx JL, Jouvet M. Effect of prolactin on the sleep–wake cycle in the rat. Neurosci Lett 1993; 156: 117–20.
14. Zhang SQ, Inoue S, Kimura M. Sleep-promoting activity of prolactin-releasing peptide (PrRP) in the rat. NeuroReport 2001; 12: 3173–6.
15. Bodosi B, Obal F Jr, Gardi J, et al. An ether stressor increases REM sleep in rats: possible role of prolactin. Am J Physiol 2000; 279: R1590–8.
16. Arborelius L, Owens MJ, Plotsky PM, Nemeroff CB. The role of corticotropin-releasing factor in depression and anxiety disorders. J Endocrinol 1999; 160: 1–12.
17. Ehlers CL, Reed TK, Henriksen SJ. Effects of corticotropin-releasing factor and growth hormone-releasing factor on sleep and activity in rats. Neuroendocrinology 1986; 42: 467–74.
18. Chang F-C, Opp MR. Blockade of corticotropin-releasing hormone receptors reduces spontaneous waking in the rat. Am J Physiol 1998; 275: R793–802.
19. Chang F-C, Opp MR. IL-1 is a mediator of increases in slow-wave sleep induced by CRH receptor blockade. Am J Physiol 2000; 279: R793–802.
20. Jahn H, Kiefer F, Schick M, et al. Sleep endocrine effects of the 11-β-hydroxysteroid dehydrogenase inhibitor metyrapone. Sleep 2003; 26: 823–9.
21. Vázquez-Palacios G, Renata-Márquez S, Bonilla-Jaime H, Velásquez-Moctezuma J. Further definition of the effect of corticosterone on the sleep–wake pattern in the male rat. Pharmacol Biochem Behav 2001; 70: 305–10.
22. Bradbury MJ, Dement WC, Edgar DM. Effects of adrenalectomy and subsequent corticosterone replacement on rat sleep state and EEG power spectra. Am J Physiol 1998; 275: R555–65.
23. De Kloet ER. Brain corticosteroid receptor balance and homeostatic control. Front Endocrinol 1991; 12: 95–164.
24. Healey ES, Kales A, Monroe LJ, et al. Onset of insomnia: role of life-stress events. Psychosom Med 1981; 43: 439–51.
25. Marinesco S, Bonnet C, Cespuglio R. Influence of stress duration on the sleep rebound induced by immobilization in the rat: a possible role for corticosterone. Neuroscience 1999; 92: 921–33.
26. Tiba PA, Tufik S, Suchecki D. Effects of maternal separation on baseline sleep and cold stress-induced sleep rebound in adult Wistar rats. Sleep 2004; 27: 1146–53.
27. Dewasmes G, Loos N, Delanaud S, Dewasmes D, Ramadan W. Pattern of rapid-eye movement sleep episode occurrence after an immobilization stress in the rat. Neurosci Lett 2004; 355: 17–20.
28. Koehl M, Bouyer JJ, Darnaudéry M, Le Moal M, Mayo W. The effect of restraint stress on paradoxical sleep is influenced by the circadian cycle. Brain Res 2002; 937: 45–50.

29. Tiba PA, Palma BD, Tufik S, Suchecki D. Effects of early handling on basal and stress-induced sleep parameters in rats. Brain Res 2003; 975: 158–66.

30. Rampin C, Cespuglio R, Chastrette N, Jouvet M. Immobilization stress induces paradoxical sleep rebound in rat. Neurosci Lett 1991; 126: 113–18.

31. Cespuglio R, Marinesco S, Baubet V, Bonnet C, El Kafi B. Evidence for a sleep-promoting influence of stress. Adv Neuroimmunol 1995; 5: 145–54.

32. Palma BD, Suchecki D, Tufik S. Differential effects of acute cold and footshock on the sleep of rats. Brain Res 2000; 861: 97–104.

33. Vázquez-Palacios G, Velazquez-Moctezuma J. Effect of electric foot shocks, immobilization, and corticosterone administration on the sleep–wake pattern in the rat. Physiol Behav 2000; 71: 23–8.

34. Sanford LD, Fang J, Tang X. Sleep after differing amounts of conditioned fear training in BALB/cJ mice. Behav Brain Res 2003; 147: 193–202.

35. Pawlyk AC, Jha SK, Brennan FX, Morrison AR, Ross RJ. A rodent model of sleep disturbances in posttraumatic stress disorder: the role of context after fear conditioning. Biol Psychiatry 2005; 57: 268–77.

36. Koolhaas JM, De Boer SF, De Rutter AJ, Meerlo P, Sgoifo A. Social stress in rats and mice. Acta Physiol Scand 1997; 640(Suppl 161): 69–72.

37. Bohus B, Benus RF, Fokkema DS, et al. Neuroendocrine states and behavioural and physiological stress responses. In: De Kloet ER, Wiegant VM, De Wied D, eds. Progress in Brain Research. Amsterdam: Elsevier, 1987: 57–70.

38. Meerlo P, de Bruin EA, Strijkstra AM, Daan S. A social conflict increases EEG slow-wave activity during subsequent sleep. Physiol Behav 2001; 73: 331–5.

39. Meerlo P, Pragt BJ, Daan S. Social stress induces high intensity sleep in rats. Neurosci Lett 1997; 225: 41–4.

40. Liebsch G, Linthorst AC, Neumann ID, et al. Behavioral, physiological, and neuroendocrine stress responses and differential sensitivity to diazepam in two Wistar rat lines selectively bred for high- and low-anxiety-related behavior. Neuropsychopharmacology 1998; 19: 381–96.

41. Liebsch G, Montkowski A, Holsboer F, Landgraf R. Behavioural profiles of two Wistar rat lines selectively bred for high or low anxiety-related behaviour. Behav Brain Res 1998; 94: 301–10.

42. Lancel M, Muller-Preuss P, Wigger A, Landgraf R, Holsboer F. The CRH1 receptor antagonist R121919 attenuates stress-elicited sleep disturbances in rats, particularly in those with high innate anxiety. J Psychiatr Res 2002; 36: 197–208.

43. Bouyer JJ, Vallee M, Deminiere JM, Le Moal M, Mayo W. Reaction of sleep-wakefulness cycle to stress is related to differences in hypothalamo–pituitary–adrenal axis reactivity in rat. Brain Res 1998; 804: 114–24.

44. Opp MR, Imeri L. Rat strains that differ in corticotropin-releasing hormone production exhibit different sleep–wake responses to interleukin 1. Neuroendocrinology 2001; 73: 272–84.

45. Tang X, Liu X, Yang L, Sanford LD. Rat strain differences in sleep after acute mild stressors and short-term sleep loss. Behav Brain Res 2005; 160: 60–71.

46. Tang X, Yang L, Sanford LD. Rat strain differences in freezing and sleep alterations associated with contextual fear. Sleep 2005; 28: 1235–44.

47. Sanford LD, Yang L, Tang X. Influence of contextual fear on sleep in mice: a strain comparison. Sleep 2003; 26: 527–40.

48. Sanford LD, Tang X, Ross RJ, Morrison AR. Influence of shock training and explicit fear-conditioned cues on sleep architecture in mice: strain comparison. Behav Genet 2003; 33: 43–58.

49. Tang X, Xiao J, Liu X, Sanford LD. Strain differences in the influence of open field exposure on sleep in mice. Behav Brain Res 2004; 154: 137–47.

50. Meerlo P, Easton A, Bergmann BM, Turek FW. Restraint increases prolactin and REM sleep in C57BL/6J mice but not in BALB/cJ mice. Am J Physiol 2001; 281: R846–54.

51. Jouvet M, Renault J. Persistence of insomnia after lesions of the nuclei of the raphe in the cat. CR Seances Soc Biol Fil 1966; 160: 1461–5. [in French]

52. Cespuglio R, Houdouin F, Oulerich M, El Mansari M, Jouvet M. Axonal and somato-dendritic modalities of serotonin release: their involvement in sleep preparation, triggering and maintenance. J Sleep Res 1992; 1: 150–6.

53. Wetzel W, Balschun D, Janke S, Vogel D, Wagner T. Effects of CLIP (corticotropin-like intermediate lobe peptide) and CLIP fragments on paradoxical sleep in rats. Peptides 1994; 15: 237–41.

54. Bonnet C, Leger L, Baubet V, Debilly G, Cespuglio R. Influence of a 1 h immobilization stress on sleep states and corticotropin-like intermediate lobe peptide (CLIP or ACTH18-39, Ph-ACTH18-39) brain contents in the rat. Brain Res 1997; 751: 54–63.

55. Wetzel W, Wagner T, Vogel D, Demuth HU, Balschun D. Effects of the CLIP fragment ACTH20-24 on the duration of REM sleep episodes. Neuropeptides 1997; 31: 41–5.

56. González MM, Debilly G, Valatx JL, Jouvet M. Sleep increase after immobilization stress: role of the

noradrenergic locus coeruleus system in the rat. Neurosci Lett 1995; 202: 5–8.

57. González MMC, Valatx JL. Effect of intracerebroventricular administration of α-helical CRH (9-41) on the sleep/waking cycle in rats under normal conditions or after subjection to an acute stressful situation. J Sleep Res 1997; 6: 164–70.

58. González MMC, Valatx JL, Debilly G. Role of the locus coeruleus in the sleep rebound following two different sleep deprivation methods in the rat. Brain Res 1996; 740: 215–26.

59. Vázquez-Palacios G, Retana-Márquez S, Bonilla-Jaime H, Velázquez-Moctezuma J. Stress-induced REM sleep increase is antagonized by naltrexone in rats. Psychopharmacology 2004; 171: 186–90.

60. Yang YR, Lee EH, Chiu TH. Electrophysiological and behavioral effects of Tyr-d-Arg-Phe-Sar on locus coeruleus neurons of the rat. Eur J Pharmacol 1998; 351: 23–30.

61. Meerlo P, Easton A, Bergmann BM, Turek FW. Restraint increases prolactin and REM sleep in C57BL/6J mice but not in BALB/cJ mice. Am J Physiol 2001; 281: R846–54.

62. Morrison AR, Sanford LD, Ross RJ. The amygdala: a critical modulator of sensory influence on sleep. Biol Signals Recept 2000; 9: 283–96.

63. Sanford LD, Parris B, Tang X. GABAergic regulation of the central nucleus of the amygdala: implications for sleep control. Brain Res 2002; 956: 276–84.

18

Sleep deprivation as an antidepressant

Joseph C Wu, Blynn G Bunney, Steven G Potkin

INTRODUCTION

The identification of mechanisms associated with the rapid (within 24 hours) and often robust anti-depressant actions of sleep deprivation could potentially revolutionize the understanding, prevention, and treatment of depression. Sleep deprivation studies have been conducted for more than 45 years,[1] and despite the wide range of protocols (e.g., differing environmental settings, inpatient versus outpatient studies, diagnoses, gender, age, and medications), it is effective in an estimated 40–50% of depressed patients.[2] Further, the improvement in depressive symptoms (significant reductions on the Hamilton Depression Rating Scale, HDRS) that can occur within several hours of sleep deprivation are comparable to long-term (2–6 weeks) treatment with conventional anti-depressant medications.[3] The evidence that sleep deprivation is effective even in chronic treatment-resistant patients (albeit at lower rates than non-refractory patients)[4,5] may imply that it temporarily reverses some fundamental abnormality in depression. On the downside, recovery sleep (even short naps) precipitates relapse in approximately 80% of responders,[2,6–9] suggesting that it also affects these same networks. Analyses of recovery sleep architecture (e.g., cumulative sleep time, slow-wave sleep (SWS), and rapid eye movement (REM) sleep density) fail to account for the relapse.[2] Circadian factors are likely involved, as evidence suggests that recovery sleep in the morning

hours is more detrimental than sleep at other times of the day in some[7,9,10] but not all[11] responders. A longitudinal electroencephalographic (EEG) study conducted over a period of 60 hours showed that some patients have repeated periods of microsleep (20 seconds). It was found that an accumulation of these episodes, particularly in the morning hours, is associated with a greater number of postsleep deprivation relapses.[9] An ongoing challenge and a focus of current research is the identification of mechanisms to extend the rapid antidepressant responses of sleep deprivation by counteracting the apparent depressiogenic mechanisms associated with recovery sleep.

As a research tool, sleep deprivation provides a potentially critical experimental framework to investigate the factors associated with the switch process. It is somewhat remarkable that virtually every type of treatment that can ameliorate the symptoms of depression has the capability of switching a small percentage of patients into hypomania/mania. This holds true also for sleep deprivation. Bipolar patients have the highest risk for switches into hypomania/mania following sleep deprivation, although the risk is no greater than that for conventional antidepressants.[12,13] For example, Colombo et al[13] found switch rates in the range of 4–6% in a sample of 206 bipolar patients (10 switches into mania and 12 switches into hypomania). The exception is for a rare subgroup of rapid cyclers who switch in and out of depression and mania every 48 hours. Wehr et al[14] sleep deprived

9 drug-free rapid-cycling bipolar patients for a total of 40 hours (over 1 night) and observed that although most of them (8/9) switched out of depression, almost all (7/8) of which became hypomanic/manic.

A review of the literature reveals that there are very few, if any, clinical variables that predict sleep deprivation responses. Data from our laboratory and others report that repetitive sleep deprivation trials produce a large variation in responses from one trial to the next in the same individuals. Weigand et al[15] administered six cycles of total sleep deprivation (each cycle consisting of sleep deprivation followed by a night of recovery sleep) over a 3-week period. Prior to the beginning of subsequent trials of sleep deprivation, subjects relapsed to baseline levels, so that the presleep deprivation depression ratings were consistent throughout the protocol. Analysis of the data revealed that (i) there was no predictable pattern of response for any individual from one cycle to the next; (ii) patients who may not initially respond to sleep deprivation may still be good candidates for future sleep deprivation trials; and (iii) that repeated cycles of sleep deprivation do not produce habituation or sensitization. There is some evidence to suggest that a subgroup of patients showing diurnal worsening of depression in the morning and improvement in the late afternoon are more likely to,[2,16–18] but will not always,[5] benefit from sleep deprivation interventions. We propose that this subgroup of depressed patients may have dysregulation in functions of the core clock genes that control the master circadian clock located in the suprachiasmatic nucleus in the hypothalamus.[16,19]

FUNCTIONAL BRAIN IMAGING STUDIES

Neuroimaging data provide compelling evidence for selective regional activation of brain areas associated with sleep deprivation. There is a growing consensus from [^{18}F] fluorodeoxyglucose (FDG) position-emission tomography (PET), single photon emission computed tomography (SPECT) with technetium-99m-hexamethylpropyleneamine oxime (HMPAO), and functional magnetic resonance imaging (fMRI) data that responders to either partial (PSD) or total (1-night) (TSD) sleep deprivation have elevations in regional baseline (presleep deprivation) activity, which normalize with clinical improvement. Increased baseline activation in sleep deprivation responders is seen in regions associated with the anterior cingulate cortex, fronto-orbital cortex,[20–26] and left superior and inferior temporal cortex,[24] as well as the amygdala.[20,27] In the largest major depressive disorder (MDD) study to date, our group[24] identified 12 responders and 24 non-responders to total sleep deprivation and demonstrated that clinical improvement was linked to the activation of a region centered in the medial prefrontal cortex (BA 32). Another study using fMRI in a group of 17 unmedicated MDD patients compared with 8 controls in a partial sleep deprivation protocol reported increases in amygdala perfusion, which decreases with clinical improvement.[27] It appears that depression may be associated with hypermetabolism, a hypothesis supported by data from Nofzinger et al[28] suggesting that some depressed patients may have an overactive ventral emotional neural system, which persists during waking and sleep (non-REM: NREM) in a subgroup of depressed patients. The mechanism of action of sleep deprivation in reducing brain metabolic activity may be related to the antidepressant effects of sleep deprivation. This is supported, in part, by data in PET studies of sleep deprived healthy individuals showing that enforced wakefulness decreases global brain activity, particularly in the thalamus, prefrontal cortex, basal ganglia, posterior parietal association cortices, and cerebellum.[29,30] However, in contrast to depressed patients, data from normal subjects suggest that sleep deprivation can provoke depressive-like symptoms such as cognitive impairments (notably in working memory) and abnormalities in sleep architecture.[31–34] Although there are descriptions of depressive-like changes in mood following sleep deprivation, there are few, if any, carefully controlled studies documenting the relationship.[35]

PREVENTING RELAPSE: COMBINATION OF SLEEP DEPRIVATION WITH ANTIDEPRESSANTS, MOOD STABILIZERS, BRIGHT LIGHT, AND PHASE ADVANCE

Non-invasive circadian manipulations have been used as adjunctive therapies in an attempt to extend sleep deprivation-related antidepressant responses. Briefly, administration of bright-light therapy, sleep deprivation, and phase advance, administered individually or in combination, can produce improvement in symptoms in a subgroup of patients. It appears that the combination of these methods may exert longer-lasting antidepressant effects. A review of 20 studies reported that bright light as adjunctive therapy in non-seasonal depression is efficacious as adjunctive treatment to antidepressants, including sleep deprivation, especially when administered during the first week of treatment, in the morning, and as an adjunctive treatment to sleep deprivation responders.[36] The meta-analysis by Golden et al[37] of three studies of bright-light therapy in non-seasonal depression failed to find an effect; however, this finding may be limited by the small number of studies. Data from phase advance, in contrast, show that advancing the time of sleep can produce a rapid antidepressant response in some patients. First introduced by Wehr et al,[38] phase advance was reported to produce immediate but transient improvement in a bipolar depressed patient by advancing the time of sleep and awakening by 6 hours over 2 days. A later study by this same group[39] reported antidepressant responses in four treatment-resistant patients using phase advance. The most dramatic response was described in a patient with a severe persistent depressive episode that lasted for 30 days. Significant improvement within 48 hours followed a 5-hour phase advance.

A growing body of evidence shows that sleep deprivation in combination with circadian manipulations (e.g., bright white light or phase advance), antidepressants, and/or mood stabilizers such as lithium can maintain postsleep deprivation responses in some individuals.[4,18,40–55] Either total or partial sleep deprivation protocols were administered in each study, with the exception of the investigation by Elsenga et al,[45] where patients were treated with both (total sleep deprivation was followed by partial sleep deprivation). To summarize, there is a general consensus that (i) the combination of antidepressants and sleep deprivation has added benefit; (ii) treatment with the mood stabilizer lithium is efficacious when combined with sleep deprivation;[41,51,52,56,57] (iii) morning bright white light may modestly augment sleep-deprivation responses in some individuals; (iv) serial sleep deprivations (partial or total) are efficacious and of benefit to initial non-responders to sleep deprivation;[15,46,58] and (v) phase advances in the sleep/wake cycle may extend the antidepressant response.[6,49,50,59]

GENE RESEARCH

Advances in gene research include the combined use of gene expression data with genetic linkage analysis. Benedetti and colleagues have conducted a series of genetic studies in depressed patients treated with sleep deprivation. Results from these studies suggest a functional polymorphism located within the promoter of the serotonin transporter that may influence the antidepressant response to total sleep deprivation as well as to serotonin-related drugs. It was found that homozygotes (*l/l*) for the long variant of the serotonin transporter (5-HTTLPR) are more likely to respond to total sleep deprivation (plus bright light) compared with those who are heterozygotes and homozygotes for the short variant.[60] We have previously discussed the possible role that serotonergic system mobilization might play in the antidepressant mechanism of sleep deprivation,[61] suggesting that depressed patients who are homozygotes for 5-HTTLPR (*l/l*) have a greater capacity to mobilize the serotonergic system when sleep deprived. Other studies from Benedetti et al[62] report that the dopamine receptor variants (DRD2 and DRD3) are not associated with the antidepressant effect of sleep deprivation in bipolar depressives. This same group[63] reported possible genetic markers associated with the regulation of the biologic clock. They found that the presence of a glycogen synthase kinase 3β (GSK-3β) promoter gene single-nucleotide polymorphism (SNP) is predictive of a response to total sleep deprivation. Data from 60 bipolar inpatients showed that homozygotes for the single nucleotide polymorphism in the promoter region of the gene coding for GSK-3β had a delayed onset of the illness. GSK-3 is thought to be a target for the therapeutic actions of the mood stabilizer lithium. Work in cell cultures suggests that lithium inhibits GSK-3 via the rev-erbα component of the circadian clock.[64] Benedetti et al[65] have proposed that the chronobiologic genotype for GSK-3β could play a protective role in bipolar illness in terms of delayed onset and increased antidepressant responsiveness to sleep deprivation. However, the interpretation is limited due to the small number of bipolar patients carrying the GSK-3 (C/C) genotype. If the replication of these findings prevails, it can offer a totally new perspective on the treatment of depression.

COMMENTS AND FUTURE DIRECTIONS

Since 80% of MDD patients complain of insomnia,[66] it is somewhat counterintuitive that depriving depressed patients of sleep can produce rapid antidepressant responses. Moreover, normals suffering from primary insomnia (a sleep disturbance that is unrelated to any other medical conditions) for a 2-week period have a significantly increased risk for developing depression over the subsequent 1–3 years.[67] The interplay between depressive illness and sleep loss needs further investigation. Data suggest that the neurobiologic substrates underlying depression vary over the course of a depressive episode. In rapidly cycling bipolar patients, it was reported that increased responses to sleep deprivation

occurred later rather than earlier in the course of an episode.[68] Pflug,[69] in contrast, found that the sleep deprivation applied earlier within an episode in MDD patients had a greater effect.

Sleep deprivation research provides intriguing clues to the pathophysiologic mechanisms underlying depression. In view of recent technological advances, it seems that studies of sleep deprivation can be sequentially studied (pre- and postsleep deprivation) to help determine genetic variables that may contribute to antidepressant responses. The major research question is how sleep deprivation differentially affects the brain of depressed patients to produce an antidepressant response. Is there a common neuronal pathway underlying the many diverse interventions that can alleviate depression such as electroconvulsive therapy (ECT), transcranial magnetic stimulation, at least 30 antidepressant medications, mood stabilizers, phase advance, bright light, vagal stimulation, and various forms of psychotherapy in addition to sleep deprivation? Basic studies in sleep deprived mammals are beginning to provide potentially exciting clues to candidate genes and relevant pathways.[70–72]

REFERENCES

1. Schulte W. Sequelae of sleep deprivation. Med Klin (Munich) 1959; 54: 969–73. [in German]
2. Wu JC, Bunney WE. The biological basis of an antidepressant response to sleep deprivation and relapse: review and hypothesis. Am J Psychiatry 1990; 147: 14–21.
3. Gillin JC, Buchsbaum M, Wu J, Clark C, Bunney W Jr. Sleep deprivation as a model experimental antidepressant treatment: findings from functional brain imaging. Depress Anxiety 2001; 14: 37–49.
4. Benedetti F, Barbini B, Fulgosi MC, et al. Combined total sleep deprivation and light therapy in the treatment of drug-resistant bipolar depression: acute response and long-term remission rates. J Clin Psychiatry 2005; 66: 1535–40.
5. Leibenluft E, Moul DE, Schwartz PJ, Madden PA, Wehr TA. A clinical trial of sleep deprivation in combination with antidepressant medication. Psychiatry Res 1993; 46: 213–27.

6. Berger M, Hohagen F, Konig A, et al. Chronotherapeutic approaches in depressive disorders. Wien Med Wochenschr 1995; 145: 418–22. [in German]

7. Wiegand M, Riemann D, Schreiber W, Lauer CJ, Berger M. Effect of morning and afternoon naps on mood after total sleep deprivation in patients with major depression. Biol Psychiatry 1993; 33: 467–76.

8. Reist C, Chen CC, Choeu A, Berry RB, Bunney WE Jr. Effects of sleep on the antidepressant response to sleep deprivation. Biol Psychiatry 1994; 35: 794–7.

9. Hemmeter U, Bischof R, Hatzinger M, Seifritz E, Holsboer-Trachsler E. Microsleep during partial sleep deprivation in depression. Biol Psychiatry 1998; 43: 829–39.

10. Riemann D, Wiegand M, Lauer CJ, Berger M. Naps after total sleep deprivation in depressed patients: Are they depressiogenic? Psychiatry Res 1993; 49: 109–20.

11. Gillin JC, Kripke DF, Janowsky DS, Risch SC. Effects of brief naps on mood and sleep in sleep-deprived depressed patients. Psychiatry Res 1989; 27: 253–65.

12. Riemann D, Voderholzer U, Berger M. Sleep and sleep–wake manipulations in bipolar depression. Neuropsychobiology 2002; 45 (Suppl 1): 7–12.

13. Colombo C, Benedetti F, Barbini B, Campori E, Smeraldi E. Rate of switch from depression into mania after therapeutic sleep deprivation in bipolar depression. Psychiatry Res 1999; 86: 267–70.

14. Wehr TA, Goodwin FK, Wirz-Justice A, Breitmaier J, Craig C. 48-hour sleep–wake cycles in manic-depressive illness: naturalistic observations and sleep deprivation experiments. Arch Gen Psychiatry 1982; 39: 559–65.

15. Wiegand MH, Lauer CJ, Schreiber W. Patterns of response to repeated total sleep deprivations in depression. J Affect Disord 2001; 64: 257–60.

16. Bunney WE, Bunney BG. Molecular clock genes in man and lower animals: possible implications for circadian abnormalities in depression. Neuropsychopharmacology 2000; 22: 335–45.

17. Reinink E, Bouhuys N, Wirz-Justice A, van den Hoofdakker R. Prediction of the antidepressant response to total sleep deprivation by diurnal variation of mood. Psychiatry Res 1990; 32: 113–24.

18. Elsenga S, Van den Hoofdakker RH. Response to total sleep deprivation and clomipramine in endogenous depression. J Psychiatr Res 1987; 21: 151–61.

19. Bunney BG, Potkin SG, Bunney WE. Dysregulation of circadian rhythms in mood disorders: molecular mechanisms. In: Lucinio J, ed. Biology of Depression. Weinheim: Wiley VCH, 2005: 467–92.

20. Ebert D, Feistel H, Barocka A. Effects of sleep deprivation on the limbic system and the frontal lobes in affective disorders: a study with Tc-99m-HMPAO SPECT. Psychiatry Res 1991; 40: 247–51.

21. Wu JC, Gillin JC, Buchsbaum MS, et al. Effect of sleep deprivation on brain metabolism of depressed patients. Am J Psychiatry 1992; 149: 538–43.

22. Volk SA, Kaendler SH, Hertel A, et al. Can response to partial sleep deprivation in depressed patients be predicted by regional changes of cerebral blood flow? Psychiatry Res 1997; 75: 67–74.

23. Holthoff VA, Beuthien-Baumann B, Pietrzyk U, et al. Changes in regional cerebral perfusion in depression. SPECT monitoring of response to treatment. Nervenarzt 1999; 70: 620–6. [in German]

24. Wu J, Buchsbaum MS, Gillin JC, et al. Prediction of antidepressant effects of sleep deprivation by metabolic rates in the ventral anterior cingulate and medial prefrontal cortex. Am J Psychiatry 1999; 156: 1149–58.

25. Smith GS, Reynolds CF 3rd, Houck PR, et al. Glucose metabolic response to total sleep deprivation, recovery sleep, and acute antidepressant treatment as functional neuroanatomic correlates of treatment outcome in geriatric depression. Am J Geriatr Psychiatry 2002; 10: 561–7.

26. Ebert D, Feistel H, Barocka A, Kaschka W. Increased limbic blood flow and total sleep deprivation in major depression with melancholia. Psychiatry Res 1994; 55: 101–9.

27. Clark CP, Brown GG, Archibald SL, et al. Does amygdalar perfusion correlate with antidepressant response to partial sleep deprivation in major depression? Psychiatry Res 2005; 146: 43–51.

28. Nofzinger EA, Buysse DJ, Germain A, et al. Alterations in regional cerebral glucose metabolism across waking and non-rapid eye movement sleep in depression. Arch Gen Psychiatry 2005; 62: 387–96.

29. Wu JC, Gillin JC, Buchsbaum MS, et al. The effect of sleep deprivation on cerebral glucose metabolic rate in normal humans assessed with positron emission tomography. Sleep 1991; 14: 155–62.

30. Thomas M, Sing H, Belenky G, et al. Neural basis of alertness and cognitive performance impairments during sleepiness. I. Effects of 24 h of sleep deprivation on waking human regional brain activity. J Sleep Res 2000; 9: 335–52.

31. Chee MW, Choo WC. Functional imaging of working memory after 24 hr of total sleep deprivation. J Neurosci 2004; 24: 4560–7.

32. Mu Q, Nahas Z, Johnson KA, et al. Decreased cortical response to verbal working memory following sleep deprivation. Sleep 2005; 28: 55–67.

33. Habeck C, Rakitin BC, Moeller J, et al. An event-related fMRI study of the neurobehavioral impact of sleep deprivation on performance of a delayed-match-to-sample task. Brain Res Cogn Brain Res 2004; 18: 306–21.

34. Chee MW, Chuah LY, Venkatraman V, et al. Functional imaging of working memory following normal sleep and after 24 and 35 h of sleep deprivation: correlations of fronto-parietal activation with performance. Neuroimage 2006; 31: 419–28.

35. Durmer JS, Dinges DF. Neurocognitive consequences of sleep deprivation. Semin Neurol 2005; 25: 117–29.

36. Tuunainen A, Kripke DF, Endo T. Light therapy for non-seasonal depression. Cochrane Database Syst Rev 2004; (2): CD004050.

37. Golden RN, Gaynes BN, Ekstrom RD, et al. The efficacy of light therapy in the treatment of mood disorders: a review and meta-analysis of the evidence. Am J Psychiatry 2005; 162: 656–62.

38. Wehr TA, Wirz-Justice A, Goodwin FK, Duncan W, Gillin JC. Phase advance of the circadian sleep–wake cycle as an antidepressant. Science 1979; 206: 710–13.

39. Sack DA, Nurnberger J, Rosenthal NE, Ashburn E, Wehr TA. Potentiation of antidepressant medications by phase advance of the sleep–wake cycle. Am J Psychiatry 1985; 142: 606–8.

40. Caliyurt O, Guducu F. Partial sleep deprivation therapy combined with sertraline affects subjective sleep quality in major depressive disorder. Sleep Med 2005; 6: 555–9.

41. Benedetti F, Colombo C, Barbini B, Campori E, Smeraldi E. Ongoing lithium treatment prevents relapse after total sleep deprivation. J Clin Psychopharmacol 1999; 19: 240–5.

42. Loving RT, Kripke DF, Shuchter SR. Bright light augments antidepressant effects of medication and wake therapy. Depress Anxiety 2002; 16: 1–3.

43. Fritzsche M, Heller R, Hill H, Kick H. Sleep deprivation as a predictor of response to light therapy in major depression. J Affect Disord 2001; 62: 207–15.

44. Neumeister A, Goessler R, Lucht M, et al. Bright light therapy stabilizes the antidepressant effect of partial sleep deprivation. Biol Psychiatry 1996; 39: 16–21.

45. Elsenga S, Beersma D, Van den Hoofdakker RH. Total and partial sleep deprivation in clomipramine-treated endogenous depressives. J Psychiatr Res 1990; 24: 111–19.

46. Kuhs H, Farber D, Borgstadt S, Mrosek S, Tolle R. Amitriptyline in combination with repeated late sleep deprivation versus amitriptyline alone in major depression. A randomised study. J Affect Disord 1996; 37: 31–41.

47. Kuhs H, Kemper B, Lippe-Neubauer U, Meyer-Dunker J, Tolle R. Repeated sleep deprivation once versus twice a week in combination with amitriptyline. J Affect Disord 1998; 47: 97–103.

48. Bump GM, Reynolds CF 3rd, Smith G, et al. Accelerating response in geriatric depression: a pilot study combining sleep deprivation and paroxetine. Depress Anxiety 1997; 6: 113–18.

49. Riemann D, Hohagen F, Konig A, et al. Advanced vs. normal sleep timing: effects on depressed mood after response to sleep deprivation in patients with a major depressive disorder. J Affect Disord 1996; 37: 121–8.

50. Voderholzer U, Valerius G, Schaerer L, et al. Is the antidepressive effect of sleep deprivation stabilized by a three day phase advance of the sleep period? A pilot study. Eur Arch Psychiatry Clin Neurosci 2003; 253: 68–72.

51. Baxter LR Jr. Can lithium carbonate prolong the antidepressant effect of sleep deprivation? Arch Gen Psychiatry 1985; 42: 635.

52. Baxter LR Jr, Liston EH, Schwartz JM, et al. Prolongation of the antidepressant response to partial sleep deprivation by lithium. Psychiatry Res 1986; 19: 17–23.

53. Colombo C, Lucca A, Benedetti F, et al. Total sleep deprivation combined with lithium and light therapy in the treatment of bipolar depression: replication of main effects and interaction. Psychiatry Res 2000; 95: 43–53.

54. Holsboer-Trachsler E, Hemmeter U, Hatzinger M, et al. Sleep deprivation and bright light as potential augmenters of antidepressant drug treatment – neurobiological and psychometric assessment of course. J Psychiatr Res 1994; 28: 381–99.

55. Souetre E, Salvati E, Pringuey D, et al. Antidepressant effects of the sleep/wake cycle phase advance. Preliminary report. J Affect Disord 1987; 12: 41–6.

56. Grube M, Hartwich P. Maintenance of antidepressant effect of sleep deprivation with the help of lithium. Eur Arch Psychiatry Clin Neurosci 1990; 240: 60–1.

57. Szuba MP, Baxter LR Jr, Altshuler LL, et al. Lithium sustains the acute antidepressant effects of sleep deprivation: preliminary findings from a controlled study. Psychiatry Res 1994; 51: 283–95.

58. Telger K, Tolle R, Fischer H. Repeating antidepressive sleep deprivation therapy (partial sleep deprivation). Psychiatry Prax 1990; 17: 121–5. [in German]

59. Riemann D, Konig A, Hohagen F, et al. How to preserve the antidepressive effect of sleep deprivation: a comparison of sleep phase advance and sleep phase delay. Eur Arch Psychiatry Clin Neurosci 1999; 249: 231–7.

60. Benedetti F, Colombo C, Serretti A, et al. Antidepressant effects of light therapy combined with sleep deprivation are influenced by a functional polymorphism within the promoter of the serotonin transporter gene. Biol Psychiatry 2003; 54: 687–92.

61. Wu JC, Buchsbaum M, Bunney WE Jr. Clinical neurochemical implications of sleep deprivation's effects on the anterior cingulate of depressed responders. Neuropsychopharmacology 2001; 25(5 Suppl): S74–8.

62. Benedetti F, Serretti A, Colombo C, et al. Dopamine receptor D2 and D3 gene variants are not associated with the antidepressant effect of total sleep deprivation in bipolar depression. Psychiatry Res 2003; 118: 241–7.

63. Benedetti F, Serretti A, Colombo C, et al. A glycogen synthase kinase 3-β promoter gene single nucleotide polymorphism is associated with age at onset and response to total sleep deprivation in bipolar depression. Neurosci Lett 2004; 368: 123–6.

64. Yin L, Wang J, Klein PS, Lazar MA. Nuclear receptor Rev-erbα is a critical lithium-sensitive component of the circadian clock. Science 2006; 311: 1002–5.

65. Benedetti F, Serretti A, Pontiggia A, et al. Long-term response to lithium salts in bipolar illness is influenced by the glycogen synthase kinase 3-β -50 T/C SNP. Neurosci Lett 2005; 376: 51–5.

66. Ohayon MM. Epidemiology of insomnia: what we know and what we still need to learn. Sleep Med Rev 2002; 6: 97–111.

67. Riemann D, Voderholzer U. Primary insomnia: a risk factor to develop depression? J Affect Disord 2003; 76: 255–9.

68. Gill DS, Ketter TA, Post RM. Antidepressant response to sleep deprivation as a function of time into depressive episode in rapidly cycling bipolar patients. Acta Psychiatr Scand 1993; 87: 102–9.

69. Pflug B. The influence of sleep deprivation on the duration of endogenous depressive episodes. Arch Psychiatr Nervenkr 1978; 225: 173–7.

70. Cirelli C. How sleep deprivation affects gene expression in the brain: a review of recent findings. J Appl Physiol 2002; 92: 394–400.

71. Naidoo N, Giang W, Galante RJ, Pack AI. Sleep deprivation induces the unfolded protein response in mouse cerebral cortex. J Neurochem 2005; 92: 1150–7.

72. Tononi G, Cirelli C. Sleep function and synaptic homeostasis. Sleep Med Rev 2006; 10: 49–62.

19

Fibromyalgia and the neurobiology of sleep

Daniel J Wallace

INTRODUCTION

Fibromyalgia (FM) is not a disease, but a syndrome, characterized by centralized sensitization of afferent inputs into the spinal cord from tactile, chemical, thermal, and nociceptive stimuli that leads to amplified pain. Sleep pathology is a unifying feature of the syndrome, and improvement in sleep architecture is the principal treatment goal.

CLINICAL ASPECTS OF FIBROMYALGIA

Evolution of the concept

References to the symptoms of FM date back to biblical times and can be found in the books of Job and Jeremiah among individuals whose insomnia was associated with musculoskeletal discomfort.[1] Modern understanding stems from observations in 1904 by Sir William Gowers, who coined the term 'fibrositis' for tender points in patients with lumbago (back pain). Serious investigation into tender points first took place in the early 1800s, but the connection with fatigue and systemic symptoms is credited to Hugh Smythe and Harvey Moldofsky at the University of Toronto in the 1970s, who described alpha-wave intrusion into delta-wave sleep on polysomnograms and correlated it with the presence of tender points.[2] Work by Muhammad Yunus and colleagues in 1981 statistically correlated tender points with fatigue, functional bowel disease, sleep pathology, tension headache, and other systemic symptoms.[3] The American College of Rheumatology published statistically validated working criteria for the syndrome in 1990, and this was followed by epidemiologic surveys to define what constituted FM[4] (Table 19.1 and Figure 19.1).

Clinical overview[5,6]

From an operational standpoint, FM requires 3 months of discomfort in individuals with 11 of 18 specified tender points in all four quadrants of the body. The presence of fewer FM-like tender points in one to three quadrants is termed *myofascial pain syndrome* or *regional myofascial pain*. Approximately 6 million people in the USA have FM (2% of the adult population), and another 6 million have FM-related complaints but never seek medical attention for it (termed *community fibromyalgia*). This is the third most common reason for referral to a rheumatologist. Eighty-five percent of patients are female, and most develop the syndrome during their reproductive years. *Primary fibromyalgia* is of unknown cause, but patients with *secondary fibromyalgia* can trace the onset of their symptoms to an inciting event or cumulative emotional or physical trauma. The most common of these events include inception after a motor vehicle accident, a viral process, untreated inflammatory arthritis, or lifting heavy loads with poor body mechanics.

Table 19.1   1990 American College of Rheumatology criteria for the classification of fibromyalgia

1. **History of widespread pain**

Definition: Pain is considered widespread when all of the following are present: pain in the left side of the body; pain in the right side of the body; pain above the waist; pain below the waist. In addition, axial skeletal pain (cervical spine or anterior chest or thoracic spine or low back) must be present. In this definition, shoulder and buttock pain is considered as pain for each involved side. 'Low-back' pain is considered lower-segment pain.

2. **Pain in 11 of 18 tender point sites on digital palpation**

Definition: Pain, on digital palpation, must be present in at least 11 of the following 18 tender point sites:

- Occiput: bilateral, at the suboccipital muscle insertions
- Low cervical: bilateral, at the anterior aspects of the intertransverse spaces at C5–C7
- Trapezius: bilateral, at the midpoint of the upper border
- Supraspinatus: bilateral, at origins, above the scapula spine near the medial border
- 2nd rib: bilateral, at the 2nd costochondral junctions, just lateral to the junctions on upper surfaces
- Lateral epicondyle: bilateral 2 cm distal to the epicondyles
- Gluteal: bilateral, in upper outer quadrants of buttocks in anterior fold of muscle
- Greater trochanter: bilateral, posterior to the trochanteric prominence
- Knees: bilateral, at the medial fat pad proximal to the joint line
- For a tender point to be considered 'positive', the subject must state that the palpation was painful. 'Tender' is not to be considered painful

Note: For classification purposes, patients will be said to have fibromyalgia if both criteria are satisfied. Widespread pain must have been present for at least 3 months. The presence of a second clinical disorder does not exclude the diagnosis of fibromyalgia

Reproduced from Wolfe F et al. Arthritis Rheum 1990; 33: 160–72.[4]

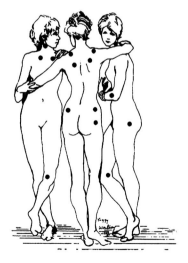

Figure 19.1   Fibromyalgia tender points – based on 'The Three Graces' (Louvre, Paris) (reproduced from Wallace DJ, Wallace JB. All About Fibromyalgia. New York: Oxford University Press, 2003 with permission)

Most of these individuals have preexisting risk factors such as psychosocial stressors, poor sleep habits, or myofascial pain syndrome.

The principal symptoms and signs of FM are listed in order of prevalence in Table 19.2. Fatigue is a nearly universal complaint. Although some patients complain of fevers, the 'feverish' sensation reflects autonomic or hormonal imbalance, and true FM patients are always afebrile unless infected. Tender lymph glands without lymphadenopathy are a frequent complaint. FM patients have tenderness in their muscle regions without inflammation, weakness, or myositis. The most tender areas are in the neck, upper back, anserine bursa, proximal hip, and shoulder girdle region. Similarly, joint discomfort or stiffness is common, always without synovitis. Stiffness or aching is worse in the late afternoons, and tends to spare the hands or feet, which are the opposite of what is reported in rheumatoid arthritis or systemic lupus. Tension headaches are common, and cervical osteoarthritis, sinusitis, and migraine need to be ruled out. Migraine is more frequent in FM patients due to vasomotor instability. Alterations in blood flow patterns to the brain, documented by single photon emission computed tomography (SPECT) imaging, account for some of the headache-related complaints as well as intermittent symptoms of cognitive impairment (also termed 'fibro fog'). The sympathetic nervous system is dysfunctional in FM, which leads to vasomotor hyperreactivity and is manifested by a resting decrease in oncotic pressure, higher prevalence of Raynaud's phenomenon, mitral valve prolapse, livedo reticularis, self-reported edema, as well as complaints of numbness, burning and tingling. Dysautonomia can also be associated with 'hypervigilance syndromes' where sensitivity to loud noises and bright lights and the sensation of dizziness are common along with anxiety disorders. One percent of patients with FM evolve dramatic sympathetic pathology associated with frank swelling, burning, and tenderness, which is termed *reflex sympathetic dystrophy*, or *regional complex pain syndrome, type 1*.

Association with other central sensitization syndromes[7-9]

Patients with FM-like complaints often have symptoms that are more bothersome than musculoskeletal ones and consult physicians who diagnose them with conditions also associated with central sensitization. A listing of these and their prevalence is given in Table 19.3. Chronic fatigue syndrome has its own statistically validated criteria, but differs from FM in that fatigue is more prominent than myofascial discomfort, and many more chronic fatigue patients have documented evidence that an infectious process induced their symptoms. Postinfectious fatigue syndrome patients (e.g., Epstein–Barr or Lyme) often manifest myofascial symptomatology. There is considerable overlap between FM and conditions associated with visceral hyperalgesia, such as irritable bowel syndrome, non-cardiac chest pain, non-ulcer dyspepsia, and esophageal spasm. Pathophysiologically, there is greater emphasis on parasympathetic dysfunction and smooth muscles, as opposed to

Table 19.2 Prevalence of frequently observed symptoms and signs in fibromyalgia

Symptom or sign	Percentage
Widespread pain with tender points	100
Muscle and joint aches	80
Non-restorative sleep	80
Fatigue	60
Tension headache	53
Dysmenorrhea	40
Irritable colon	40
Subjective numbness, tingling	35
Livedo reticularis	30
Complaints of fever	20
Complaints of swollen glands	20
Significant cognitive impairment	20
Restless legs syndrome	15
Irritable bladder	12
Chronic pelvic pain	5

Table 19.3 Fibromyalgia (FM)-associated conditions

Condition	Percentage with FM	Percentage with FM-associated conditions
Chronic fatigue syndrome	50	50
Functional bowel spectrum	20	40
Autoimmune disease	10	2
Lyme disease	30	2
Reflex sympathetic dystrophy	100	1
Irritable bladder	10	12
Chronic pelvic pain	50	5
Tension headache	20	53
US population	2	—

sympathetic dysfunction and striated muscle involvement in FM. Dysmenorrhea, chronic pelvic pain, vulvodynia, vaginismus, interstitial cystitis, and irritable bladder are found in a minority with FM, but once mechanical problems or hormonal imbalances have been taken into account, there is an increased prevalence of sexual abuse, rape experiences, pelvic trauma, or guilt surrounding sexual feelings. Other regional (not necessarily four-quadrant) associated syndromes include repetitive strain, temporomandibular joint dysfunction, and scoliosis.

Clinical evaluation and differential diagnosis

FM patients have normal blood chemistry panels, complete blood counts, immune profiles, imaging studies, and electrodiagnostic testing. It is often a diagnosis of exclusion. Many individuals diagnosed with FM turn out not to have the syndrome. Other disorders and conditions are associated with myofascial symptoms and need to be differentiated from FM. These include multiple sclerosis, hypothyroidism, rheumatoid arthritis, bipolar illness, early pregnancy, allergies, nutritional deficiencies, anorexia, cancer, substance (e.g., steroids, alcohol, heroin, and cocaine) withdrawal, and opportunistic infections.

Psychologic profiles[10,11]

The majority of FM patients have a history of depression, but only 18% are depressed at any given visit. Individuals with FM tend to have more anxiety, poorer coping skills, and psychosocial stressors than control populations. In 20–30% of patients with FM, there are no psychologic problems (e.g., those with scoliosis) influencing the syndrome, but two personality profiles predominate. Post-traumatic stress disorder (PTSD) is found in 20% of patients with FM, and another 20% are females of above average intelligence with perfectionistic tendencies, chronic anxiety, and hypervigilance symptoms who find it difficult to relax and often have no hobbies.

THE ETIOPATHOGENESIS OF FIBROMYALGIA

Pain pathways in healthy and FM patients[12-15]

What causes the 'pain without purpose' of FM? FM affects chronic but not acute pain. Chronic pain states consist of psychogenic or organic pain. Within the realm of organic pain, the discomfort can be localized (which plays a minor role in FM) or central. The sources of central pain are either neuropathic (not part of FM), nociceptive, or non-nociceptive. In FM, nociceptive pain, or pain associated with discomfort, when amplified by repetitive inputs leads to hyperalgesia, neuroplasticity, hyperpathia, and/or (rarely) causalgia. Non-nociceptive inputs (e.g., gentle stroking) that should not be uncomfortable become painful – a phenomenon known as allodynia.

In FM and healthy individuals, thin non-myelinated C-fibers in the skin are easily activated by chemical, mechanical, or thermal stimuli. Even without noxious stimuli, signals can arise spontaneously that are converted into neural impulses. Once sensitized by this stimulus, the C-fiber nerves convey this afferently to the dorsal root ganglion of the spinal cord. The constant bombardment of noxious inputs by C-fibers produces a 'wind-up' phenomenon that leads to central sensitization and ultimately FM. Large, myelinated Aδ-fibers, which normally transmit very noxious signals, start carrying some of the signals usually carried by the C-fibers. Even autonomic B-fibers start carrying nociceptive stimuli to handle the overload. Non-nociceptive fibers begin to carry nociceptive signals. In the dorsal root ganglion, increased discharges of second- and third-rung neurons takes place via the secretion of nerve growth factor (NGF) and substance P. Numerous studies have documented that cerebrospinal levels of substance P are increased in FM. Excitatory amino acids (e.g., glutamate) result in *N*-methyl-D-aspartate (NMDA) receptors in the spinal column, normally dormant, enhancing electrical depolarization and thus calcium influx into nerve cells, which makes them more excitable. These impulses ascend via the spinothalamic tract to the thalamus (and autonomic fibers via the spino-reticular tract to the limbic system). The brain now responds with inhibitory actions via neurotransmit-ters (e.g., dopamine, norepinephrine (noradrena-line), epinephrine (adrenaline), serotonin, and opioids) in the descending system. However, in FM, the responses are diminished (e.g., serotonin prod-ucts are decreased in cerebrospinal fluid). Recently, it has been shown that glial cells make cytokines,

substance P, and other chemicals that may perpetu-ate the process. These factors are influenced by hormones, emotional stress, cytokines, and sleep disorders. The end result is amplified pain. Figures 19.2 and 19.3 summarize these interactions.

Role of sleep in the etiopathogenesis of fibromyalgia

Between 2% and 15% of any given population and between 60% and 90% of FM patients have

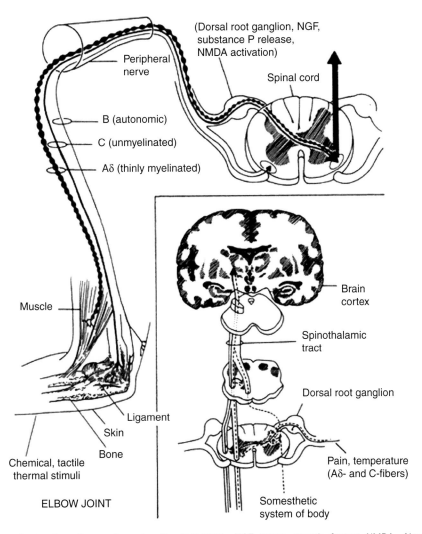

Figure 19.2 Ascending pair pathways in a healthy individual. NGF, nerve growth factor; NMDA, *N*-methyl-D-aspartate (reproduced with revisions from Wallace DJ, Wallace JB. All About Fibromyalgia. New York: Oxford University Press, 2003 with permission)

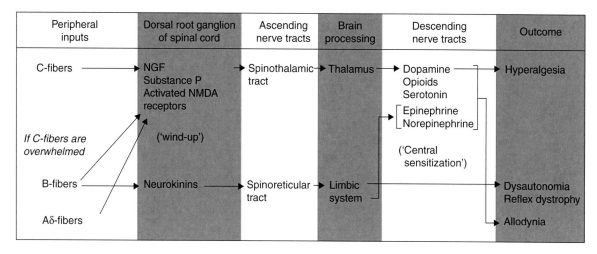

Figure 19.3 Ascending and descending pathways in fibromyalgia. NGF, nerve growth factor; NMDA, N-methyl-D-aspartate (reproduced with revisions from Wallace DJ, Wallace JB. All About Fibromyalgia. New York: Oxford University Press, 2003 with permission)

non-restorative sleep.[16] First reported with FM in the 1970s by Moldofsky's group in Toronto, alpha-wave intrusion into delta-wave sleep is noted on polysomnograms during stages 2–4 of non-rapid eye movement (NREM) sleep.[2] Other findings noted include an increase in stage 1 sleep, a reduction in delta sleep, and an increase in the number of arousals.[17,18] This leads to one being in bed for 8 hours or so, but waking up not feeling rested. Moldofsky's group has identified three distinct patterns of alpha sleep activity in FM: phasic alpha–delta activity (50%), tonic alpha continuous throughout NREM sleep (20%), and low alpha in the remaining 30%.[19] The phasic group had the greatest number of symptoms and lowest sleep time. Increased fragmented sleep has been documented additionally by greater numbers of arousals and alpha–K complexes (which promotes arousal, fatigue, and muscular symptoms) in the syndrome. Electrocardiograms demonstrate increased sympathetic nervous system activity overnight, while healthy individuals report a decline with sleep. FM and pain have been associated with a higher proportion of stage 1 NREM sleep, fewer sleep spindles and less sleep spindle frequency activity (usually seen in stage 2 sleep), suggesting that the mechanism relates to thalamocortical mechanisms of spindle generation. Cyclic altering

patterns during sleep, which express instability of the level of vigilance that manifests the brain's fatigue in preserving and regulating the macrostructure of sleep, are more often present in FM.[20]

Non-restorative sleep is felt to derive from decreases in growth hormone secretion as measured by insulin-like growth factor I (IGF-I). We have 640 muscles in our body which undergo microtrauma during our daytime activities. During sleep, there are increases in growth hormone and melatonin secretion, which heal the microtrauma experienced by our muscles.[21,22] In other words, abnormal electrical activity interferes with a sound sleep. These changes are more pronounced with menstruation, stress, pain, trauma, infection, nocturia, and barometric changes.

From 10% to 30% of FM patients exhibit another pattern of sleep pathology, which can be documented via a sleep study: restless legs syndrome, also known as sleep myoclonus or periodic limb movement syndrome.[23,24] These patients experience an alpha-wave burst followed by limb movement, and may have excess sympathetic tone, more movement arousals, and less stage 3 and 4 sleep. They do not respond to usual sleep aids, and report that their legs shoot out, lift, jerk, or go into spasm. Bed partners are often the first to alert

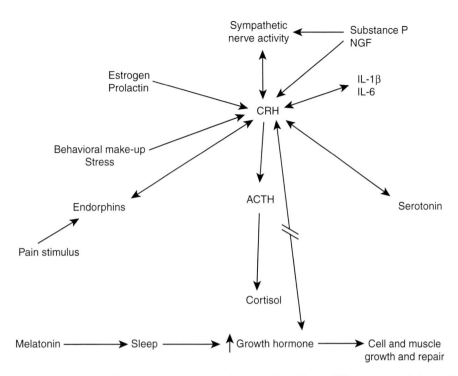

Figure 19.4 Influence upon sleep of hormones, neurotransmitters, and cytokines. NGF, nerve growth factor; IL, interleukin; CRH, corticotropin-releasing hormone; ACTH, adrenocorticotropic hormone (reproduced with revisions from Wallace DJ, Wallace JB. All About Fibromyalgia. New York: Oxford University Press, 2003 with permission)

patients that this is present. Respiratory flow dynamics during sleep in FM are just beginning to be surveyed. While initial reports suggested that it may correlate with an increased number with sleep apnea (especially in men), its true prevalence is only 5%, Gold's group has associated upper-airway resistance syndrome (UARS) rather than sleep apnea or hypopnea in the overwhelming majority of FM patients.[25–27]

Hormones and cytokines play an important role in the disturbances reported in FM.[28–30] Behavioral make-up, stress, estrogen release and sympathetic nerve activity, and interleukin-1β (IL-1β) all lead to the release of corticotropin-releasing hormone (CRH), which indirectly blocks growth hormone secretion. IL-1 independently promotes fatigue, sleep, and muscle aches, and blocks the release of substance P. Chronic insomnia is associated with a shift of IL-6 and tumor necrosis factor (TNF) secretion from night-time to daytime, as well as hypersecretion of cortisol. This leads to

daytime fatigue and difficulty sleeping. See Figure 19.4.

MANAGEMENT OF SLEEP DISORDERS IN FIBROMYALGIA

Before treating sleep problems in a FM patient, a medical work-up should classify the nature of the problem. Does the patient have classic fibromyalgia? Is periodic limb movement syndrome part of the picture? Is sleep apnea, hypopnea, UARS, or bruxism present? Are there psychiatric considerations? Are medical comorbidities such as hypothyroidism or inflammatory arthritis present? Is the patient taking medications (especially for fatigue) that keep them up during the day or make it more difficult to sleep? Is the patient taking analgesic agents that interfere with sleep? These aspects may influence the medications or treatment regimens advocated.

Ascertainment methodologies

Improved quality of sleep in FM has been correlated with decreased musculoskeletal pain, better quality of life, and less fatigue. A review of studies examining sleep in FM found that multiple methodologies, most validated for non-FM conditions, were used as methods of ascertainment.[31] These included interviewing patients, keeping a sleep–wake diary, self-rating scales (Beck Depression Inventory, Multidimensional Fatigue Inventory, and Fatigue Severity Scale), sleepiness scales (e.g., Stanford Sleepiness Scale and Epworth Sleepiness Scale), qualitative and quantitative self-rating scales of sleep (e.g., Pittsburgh Sleep Quality Index, Sleep Assessment Questionnaire, and Karolinska Sleep Diary), and looking at performance tasks. These metrics and inventories are complemented by polysomnography.

Sleep hygiene

The rules of sleep hygiene are reviewed in Chapter 8. Briefly, they include making sure that the room is dark, the mattress firm, bed partners do not snore, children and/or pets are not in the bedroom, taking a hot shower before sleeping, not napping during the day, creating a restful environment during the hour before going to sleep, eliminating alcohol or caffeine after 6 PM, not exercising in the evenings, and going to sleep and waking up at the same times, among other actions. If one is up in the middle of the night and unable to sleep, it is desirable to do an activity or read for less than an hour and then return to bed and wake up at the same time as usual. In FM, any actions that reduce anxiety or improve body mechanics are appropriate additional considerations.

Medication

Since few studies have evaluated sleep therapies for FM, textbooks and experience from rheumatic disease practices have evolved the following set of general concepts:

1. Medication should only be used in patients who have failed implementation of sleep hygiene regimens.

2. Is the diagnosis correct, and are there other medical or psychiatric considerations that apply? (See the first paragraph of this section.)

3. If medication is to be used, a tricyclic antidepressant (TCA) that promotes sleep with or without muscle relaxation can be prescribed. These include cyclobenzaprine, trazodone, amitriptyline, or doxepin in low doses given 1–2 hours before going to bed.

4. Selective serotonin reuptake inhibitors (SSRIs) may make sleep more problematic, but can be used with TCAs. Non-steroidal anti-inflammatory agents have no effect on sleep. Diphenhydramine and other sedating antihistamines do not adequately address the problem.

5. Failure to respond or a partial response to the above regimens is followed by the introduction or addition of a benzodiazepine. These agents are effective, and may ameliorate anxiety, but can tolerize (e.g., diazepam) and sometimes lead to depression (e.g., clonazepam). The most commonly prescribed drugs in FM patients include tenazepam and zolpidem.

6. Severe anxiety may warrant innovative interventions such as atypical antipsychotics (e.g., quetiapine), and concomitant burning and tingling agents such as gabapentin.

7. Failure to respond to the usual measures warrants a psychiatric evaluation and polysomnogram, with a sleep center consultation.

Evidence-based review of sleep interventions in fibromyalgia[32–48]

A Pub Med search of sleep interventions for fibromyalgia using agents available in the USA that met criteria for Evidence Based Levels A, B, or

C was conducted in March 2006. Eighteen studies met the criteria for inclusion. Five involved non-medication interventions: hypnotherapy, cognitive-behavioral therapy, electroacupuncture, and a stress reduction program were helpful, but a cardiovascular fitness program was not. Thirteen publications explored specific medication regimens. Over-the-counter preparations studied included melatonin and 5-hydroxytryptophan and were slightly beneficial. Of the remaining 11 papers, four examined amitriptyline (efficacious in two and not in two – in one of these, sleep architecture did not change), three cyclopenzaprine (definitely useful), one prednisone (a disaster), one pregabalin (helpful), and one zolpidem (improved sleep but had no effect upon fibromyalgia) and sodium oxybate (helpful for both sleep and fibromyalgia).

SUMMARY

Fibromyalgia is a pain amplification syndrome produced by persistent afferent sensory stimulation and manifested as a central sensitization syndrome. It is not a disease, but is present in a variety of medical and behavioral conditions. FM is modified by hormonal, cytokine, neurotransmitter, and autonomic influences. The overwhelming majority with FM have sleep disorders, with the alpha–delta abnormality being the principal pathology. Managing sleep pathology in FM appropriately ameliorates the symptoms and signs of the syndrome more than almost any other intervention.

REFERENCES

1. Wallace DJ, The history of fibromyalgia. In: Wallace DJ, Clauw DJ, eds. Fibromyalgia and Other Central Pain Syndromes. Philadelphia, PA: Lippincott, Williams & Wilkins, 2005; 1–8.
2. Smythe HA, Moldofsky H. Two contributions to understanding of the fibrositis syndrome. Bull Rheum Dis 1977/78; 28: 928–31.
3. Yunus M, Masi AT, Calabro JJ, et al. Primary fibromyalgia (fibrositis): clinical study of 50 patients with matched normal controls. Semin Arthritis Rheum 1981; 11: 151–70.
4. Wolfe F, Smythe HA, Yunus MB, et al. The American College of Rheumatology 1990 criteria for the classification of fibromyalgia. Report of the Multicenter Criteria Committee. Arthritis Rheum 1990; 33: 160–72.
5. Wallace DJ, Wallace JB. Fibromyalgia: An Essential Guide for Patients and Their Families. New York: Oxford University Press, 2003.
6. Wallace DJ. The fibromyalgia syndrome. Ann Med 1997; 29: 9–21.
7. Yunus MB. The concept of central sensitivity syndromes. In: Wallace DJ, Clauw DJ, eds. Fibromyalgia and Other Central Pain Syndromes. Philadelphia, PA: Lippincott, Williams & Wilkins, 2005: 29–44.
8. Wallace DJ, Clauw DJ, eds. Fibromyalgia and Other Central Pain Syndromes. Philadelphia, PA: Lippincott, Williams & Wilkins, 2005.
9. Clauw DJ, Crofford LJ. Chronic widespread pain: what we know and what we need to know. Best Pract Res Clin Rheumatol 2003; 17: 685–701.
10. Hallegua DS, Wallace DJ. Managing fibromyalgia: a comprehensive approach. J Musculoskeletal Med 2005; 22: 382–90.
11. Wallace DJ, Clauw DJ, Hallegua DS. Adressing behavioral problems in fibromyalgia. J Musculoskeletal Med 2005; 22: 562–79.
12. Russell IJ. Neurotransmitters, cytokines, hormones and the immune system in chronic non-neuropathic pain. In: Wallace DJ, Clauw DJ, eds. Fibromyalgia and Other Central Pain Syndromes, Philadelphia, PA: Lippincott, Williams & Wilkins, 2005: 63–80.
13. Staud R. The neurobiology of chronic musculoskeletal pain. In: Wallace DJ, Clauw DJ, eds. Fibromyalgia and Other Central Pain Syndromes. Philadelphia, PA: Lippincott, Williams & Wilkins, 2005: 45–62.
14. Russell IG, Orr MD, Littman B, et al. Elevated cerebrospinal fluid levels of substance P in patients with fibromyalgia syndrome. Arthritis Rheum 1994; 37: 1593–601.
15. Staud R, Vierck CJ, Cannon RL, et al. Abnormal sensitization and temporal summation of second pain (wind up) in patients with fibromyalgia syndrome. Pain 2001; 91: 165–75.
16. Ohayon MM. Prevalence and correlates of non-restorative sleep complaints. Arch Intern Med 2005; 165: 35–41.
17. Landis CA, Lentz MJ, Rothermel J, Buchwald D, Shaver JL. Decreased sleep spindles and spindle activity in midlife women with fibromyalgia and pain. Sleep 2004; 27: 741–50.

18. Moldofsky H. Sleep, neuroimmune and neuro-endocrine functions in fibromyalgia and chronic fatigue syndrome. Adv Neuroimmunol 1995; 5: 39–56.

19. Roizenblatt S, Moldofsky H, Benedito-Silva AA, Tufik S. Alpha sleep characteristics in fibromyalgia. Arthritis Rheum 2001; 44: 222–30.

20. Rizzi M, Sarzi-Puttini P, Atenzi F, et al. Cyclic alternating pattern: a new marker of sleep alteration in patients with fibromyalgia. J Rheumatol 2004; 31: 1193–9.

21. Ruhr UD, Herold J. Melotonin deficiencies in women. Mauritas 2002; 41 (Suppl 1): S85–104.

22. Bagge E, Bengstsson BA, Carlsson L, Carlsson J. Low growth hormone secretion in patients with fibromyalgia – a preliminary report on 10 patients and 10 controls. J Rheumatol 1998; 25: 145–8.

23. Moldofsky H, Tullis C, Lue FA. Sleep related myoclonus in rheumatic pain modulation disorder (fibrositis syndrome). J Rheumatol 1986; 13: 614–17.

24. Bara-Jimenez W, Aksu M, Graham B, et al. Periodic limb movements in sleep: state-dependent excitability of the spinal flexor reflex. Neurology 2000; 54: 1609–16.

25. Gold A, Dipalo F, Gold MS, Broderick J. Respiratory airflow dynamics during sleep in women with fibromyalgia. Sleep 2004; 27: 459–66.

26. Vgontzas AN, Zoumakis M, Papanicolaou DA, et al. Chronic insomnia is associated with a shift of interleukin-6 and tumor necrosis factor secretion from nighttime to daytime. Metabolism 2002; 51: 887–92.

27. Chen LX, Baqir M, Schumacher HR, et al. Increased incidence of sleep apnea in fibromyalgia patients. Arthritis Rheum 2004; 50: S494 (abst).

28. Bennett RM, Clark SR, Campbell SM, Burkhardt CS. Low levels of somatomedin C in patients with the fibromyalgia syndrome. A possible link between sleep and muscle pain. Arthritis Rheum 1992; 35: 1113–16.

29. Landis CA, Lentz MJ, Rothermel J, et al. Decreased nocturnal levels of prolactin and growth hormone in women with fibromyalgia. J Clin Endocrinol Metab 2001; 86: 1672–8.

30. Wikner J, Hirsch Y, Wetterberg L, Rojdmark S. Fibromyalgia – a syndrome associated with decreased nocturnal melatonin secretion. Clin Endocrinol 1998; 49: 179–83.

31. Moldofsky H, MacFarlane JG. Sleep and its potential role in chronic pain and fatigue. In: Wallace DJ, Clauw DJ, eds. Fibromyalgia and Other Central Pain Syndromes. Philadelphia, PA: Lippincott, Williams & Wilkins, 2005: 115–24.

32. Citera G, Arias MA, Maldonado-Cocco JA, et al. The effect of melatonin in patients with fibromyalgia: a pilot study. Clin Rheumatol 2000; 19: 9–13.

33. Clark S, Tindall E, Bennett RM. A double blind crossover trial of prednisone versus placebo in the treatment of fibrositis. J Rheumatol 1985; 12: 908–83.

34. Goldenberg DL, Felson DT, Dinerman H. A randomized controlled trial of amitryptyline and naproxen in the treatment of patients with fibromyalgia. Arthritis Rheum 1986; 29: 1371–7.

35. McCain GA, Bell DA, Mai FM, Halliday PD. A controlled study of the effects of a supervised cardiovascular fitness training program on the manifestations of primary fibromyalgia. Arthritis Rheum 1988; 31: 1135–41.

36. Caruso I, Sarzi Puttini P, Cazzola M, et al. Double blind study of 5-hydroxytryptophan versus placebo in the treatment of primary fibromyalgia syndrome. J Int Med Res 1990; 18: 201–9.

37. Haanen HC, Hoenderdos HT, van Rommunde RK, et al. Controlled trial of hypnotherapy in the treatment of refractory fibromyalgia. J Rheumatol 1991; 18: 72–5.

38. Reynolds WJ, Moldofsky H, Saskin P, Lue FA. The effects of cyclobenzaprine on sleep physiology and symptoms in patients with fibromyalgia. J Rheumatol 1991; 18: 452–4.

39. Fossaluzza V, de Vita S. Combined therapy with cyclobenzaprine and ibuprofen in primary fibromyalgia syndrome. Int J Clin Pharmacol Res 1992; 12: 99–102.

40. Deluze C, Bosia L, Zirbs A, et al. Electroacupuncture in fibromyalgia: results of a controlled trial. BMJ 1992; 305: 1249–52.

41. Santandrea S, Montrone F, Sarzi-Puttini P, et al. A double-blind crossover study of two cyclobenzaprine regimens in primary fibromyalgia syndrome. J Int Med Res 1993; 21: 74–80.

42. Carette S, Oakson G, Guimont C, Steriade M. Sleep electroencephalography and the clinical response to amitriptyline in patients with fibromyalgia. Arthritis Rheum 1995; 38: 1211–17.

43. Kaplan KH, Goldenberg DL, Galvin-Nadeau M. The impact of a mediation-based stress reduction program on fibromyalgia. Gen Hosp Psychiatry 1993; 15: 284–9.

44. Moldofsky H, Lue FA, Mously C, et al. The effect of zolpidem in patients with fibromyalgia: a dose ranging, double blind, placebo controlled, modified crossover study. J Rheumatol 1996; 23: 529–33.

45. Goldenberg D, Mayiskiy M, Mossey C, et al. A randomized, double-blind crossover trial of fluoxetine and amitriptyline in the treatment of fibromyalgia. Arthritis Rheum 1996; 39: 1852–9.

46. Scharf MB, Baumann M, Berkowitz DV. The effects of sodium oxybate on clinical symptoms and sleep patterns in patients with fibromyalgia. J Rheumatol 2003; 30: 1070–4.

47. Crofford LJ, Rowbotham MC, Mease PJ, et al. Pregabalin for the treatment of fibromyalgia syndrome: results of a randomized, double-blind, placebo-controlled trial. Arthritis Rheum 2005; 52: 1264–73.

48. Edinger JD, Wohlgemuth WK, Krystal AD, et al. Behavioral insomnia therapy for fibromyalgia patients: a randomized clinical trial. Arch Intern Med 2005; 165: 2527–35.

Index

Printed and bound by CPI Group (UK) Ltd, Croydon, CR0 4YY

01/11/2024

01782639-0002